FIRST EXPOSURE TO

GENERAL SURGERY

Danny O. Jacobs, MD, MPH
Professor and Chairman
Department of Surgery
Duke University School of Medicine
Durham, North Carolina

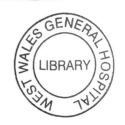

McGRAW-HILL
MEDICAL PUBLISHING DIVISION

New York / Chicago / San Francisco / Lisbon / London / Madrid / Mexico City
Milan / New Delhi / San Juan / Seoul / Singapore / Sydney / Toronto

First Exposure to General Surgery

Copyright © 2007 by The McGraw-Hill Companies, Inc. All rights reserved. Printed in the United States of America. Except as permitted under the United States Copyright Act of 1976, no part of this publication may be reproduced or distributed in any form or by any means, or stored in a data base or retrieval system, without the prior written permission of the publisher.

1 2 3 4 5 6 7 8 9 0   DOC/DOC   0 9 8 7 6

ISBN-13: 978-0-07-144140-7
ISBN-10: 0-07-144140-9

This book was set in Palatino by International Typesetting and Composition.
The editors were Jason Malley, Christie Naglieri, and Regina Y. Brown.
The production supervisor was Sherri Souffrance.
The cover designer was Janice Bielawa.
The indexer was Susan Hunter.
RR Donnelley was printer and binder.

This book is printed on acid-free paper.

Notice

Medicine is an ever-changing science. As new research and clinical experience broaden our knowledge, changes in treatment and drug therapy are required. The authors and the publisher of this work have checked with sources believed to be reliable in their efforts to provide information that is complete and generally in accord with the standards accepted at the time of publication. However, in view of the possibility of human error or changes in medical sciences, neither the editors nor the publisher nor any other party who has been involved in the preparation or publication of this work warrants that the information contained herein is in every respect accurate or complete, and they disclaim all responsibility for any errors or omissions or for the results obtained from use of the information contained in this work. Readers are encouraged to confirm the information contained herein with other sources. For example and in particular, readers are advised to check the product information sheet included in the package of each drug they plan to administer to be certain that the information contained in this work is accurate and that changes have not been made in the recommended dose or in the contraindications for administration. This recommendation is of particular importance in connection with new or infrequently used drugs.

Library of Congress Cataloging-in-Publication Data

First exposure to general surgery/ [edited by] Danny O. Jacobs.–1st ed.
  p. ; cm.–(First exposure series)
Includes bibliographical references and index.
ISBN 0-07-144140-9 (softcover)
  1. Surgery–Problems, exercises, etc. I. Jacobs, Danny O. II. Series.
  [DNLM: 1. Surgical Procedures, Operative–methods. WO 500 F527 2006]
RD37.2.F7 2006
617.0076–dc22   2006042002

International Edition ISBN-13: 978-0-07-110551-4; ISBN-10: 0-07-1105514 copyright © 2007. Exclusive rights by the McGraw-Hill Companies, Inc., for manufacture and export. This book cannot be re-exported from the country to which it is consigned by McGraw-Hill. The International edition is not available in North America.

To all students of surgery and we honor those
who have taught us.

CONTENTS

SECTION III   FUNDAMENTAL PROCEDURES   369

CONTRIBUTORS

Jennifer H. Aldrink, MD
General Surgery Resident
Department of Surgery
Duke University Medical Center
Durham, North Carolina
Chapter 15

Steffen Baumeister, MD
Research Fellow
Division of Plastic, Reconstructive,
    Maxillofacial and Oral Surgery
Department of Surgery
Duke University Medical Center
Durham, North Carolina
Chapter 17

C. Denise Ching, MD
General Surgery Resident
Department of Surgery
Duke University Medical Center
Durham, North Carolina
Chapter 4

Bradley H. Collins, MD, FACS
Assistant Professor of Surgery
Division of General Surgery,
    Transplantation
Department of Surgery
Duke University Medical Center
Durham, North Carolina
Chapter 12

Wendy R. Cornett, MD
Assistant Professor of Surgery
Department of Surgery
Medical University of South Carolina
Charleston, South Carolina
Chapter 3

Dev M. Desai, MD, PhD
Assistant Professor of Surgery
Division of General Surgery
Department of Surgery
Duke University Medical Center
Durham, North Carolina
Chapter 13

Detlev Erdmann, MD, PhD
Assistant Professor of Surgery
Division of Plastic, Reconstructive,
    Maxillofacial and Oral Surgery
Department of Surgery
Duke University Medical Center
Durham, North Carolina
Chapter 7

Matthew G. Hartwig, MD
General Surgery Resident
Department of Surgery
Duke University Medical Center
Durham, North Carolina
Chapter 18

Danny O. Jacobs, MD, MPH
Professor and Chairman
Department of Surgery
Duke University School
    of Medicine
Durham, North Carolina

Paul C. Kuo, MD, MBA
Professor and Chief
Division of General Surgery
Department of Surgery
Duke University Medical Center
Durham, North Carolina
Chapter 6

Sandhya Lagoo-Deenadayalan, MD, PhD
Assistant Professor of Surgery
Department of Surgery
Duke University Medical Center
Durham, North Carolina
Chapter 1

Anthony Lemaire, MD
General Surgery Resident
Department of Surgery
Duke University Medical Center
Durham, North Carolina
Chapter 18

L. Scott Levin MD, FACS
Professor and Chief
Division of Plastic/Reconstructive/
    Oral Surgery
Professor of Orthopaedic Surgery
Duke University Medical Center
Durham, North Carolina
Chapter 5, 17

Brian Lima, MD
General Surgery Resident
Department of Surgery
Duke University Medical Center
Durham, North Carolina
Chapter 18

Shu S. Lin, MD, PhD
Assistant Professor of Surgery
Division of Thoracic and
    Cardiovascular Surgery
Department of Surgery
Duke University Medical Center
Durham, North Carolina
Chapter 8

Carlos E. Marroquin, MD
Assistant Professor of Surgery
Department of Surgery
Duke University Medical Center
Durham, North Carolina
Chapter 9

John A. Olson, Jr., MD, PhD
Associate Professor of Surgery
Division of General Surgery
Department of Surgery
Duke University Medical Center
Durham, North Carolina
Chapter 15

Kumash R. Patel, MD
Assistant Professor of Surgery
Department of Surgery
Tulane University Hospital
New Orleans, LA
Chapter 2

Mayur B. Patel, MD
General Surgery Resident
Department of Surgery
Duke University Medical Center
Durham, North Carolina
Chapter 18

Rebecca P. Petersen, MD, MSc
General Surgery Resident
Department of Surgery
Duke University Medical Center
Durham, North Carolina
Chapter 18

Aurora D. Pryor, MD
Assistant Professor of Surgery
Division of General Surgery
Department of Surgery
Duke University Health System
Durham, North Carolina
Chapter 4

Keshava Rajagopal, MD, PhD
General Surgery Resident
Department of Surgery
Duke University Medical Center
Durham, North Carolina
Chapter 16

Jacob N. Schroder, MD
General Surgery Resident
Department of Surgery
Duke University Medical Center
Durham, North Carolina
Chapter 18

Rebecca A. Schroeder, MD
Associate Professor
Department of Anesthesiology
Durham Veterans Affairs
   Medical Center
Chapter 6

David Sindram, MD, PhD
General Surgery Resident
Department of Surgery
Duke University Medical Center
Durham, North Carolina
Chapter 11

Tracey H. Stokes, MD
Chief Resident in Plastic Surgery
Division of Plastic, Reconstructive,
   Maxillofacial and Oral Surgery
Department of Surgery
Duke University Medical Center
Durham, North Carolina
Chapter 7

Jose L. Trani, Jr., MD
General Surgery Resident
Department of Surgery
Duke University Medical Center
Durham, North Carolina
Chapter 18

Janet E. Tuttle-Newhall, MD
Assistant Professor of Surgery
Division of General Surgery/
   Transplant Surgery/Critical Care
Department of Surgery
Duke University Medical Center
Durham, North Carolina
Chapter 11

Steven N. Vaslef, MD, PhD
Associate Professor of Surgery
Director, Trauma Services and
   Chief, Section of Trauma and
   Critical Care
Division of General Surgery
Department of Surgery
Duke University Medical Center
Durham, North Carolina
Chapter 2

Philip Y. Wai, MD
General Surgery Resident
Yale School of Medicine
New Haven, Connecticut
Chapter 6

Tamarah J. Westmoreland, MD
General Surgery Resident
Department of Surgery
Duke University Medical Center
Durham, North Carolina
Chapter 18

Rebekah R. White, MD
Surgical Oncology Fellow
Memorial Sloan-Kettering
   Cancer Center
New York, New York
Chapter 10

Jin S. Yoo, MD
General Surgery Resident
Department of Surgery
Duke University Medical Center
Durham, North Carolina
Chapter 18

Michael R. Zenn, MD, FACS
Associate Professor
Division of Plastic/Reconstructive
   Oral Surgery
Department of Surgery
Duke University Medical Center
Durham, North Carolina
Chapter 14

PREFACE

We have endeavored to prepare a concise "mini-textbook" that would be most useful for medical students as they begin their first clinical rotations on general surgery services. Our goal was to present the material as succinctly as possible while emphasizing the fundamental principles relevant to each topic area. We asked ourselves, what do we wish had been written in the texts we read as medical students and used the answers to these questions to guide our efforts.

Danny O. Jacobs, MD, MPH

ACKNOWLEDGMENTS

We'd like to thank Michelle Fisher for her many contributions that helped to make "First Exposure to Surgery" possible.

FUNDAMENTAL PRINCIPLES

PREOPERATIVE ASSESSMENT AND PREPARATION

Sandhya Lagoo-Deenadayalan, MD, PhD

INTRODUCTION

The aim of a *preoperative evaluation* of a patient is to assess the fitness of the individual for anesthesia and surgery. Given a choice of any one test for pre-operative assessment of a patient, a thorough history and physical examination will be the test of choice. This time—honored and inexpensive test can account for more than two-thirds of all diagnoses made and should direct all preoperative testing.

A well-conducted history and physical examination answer several important questions:

- Is this a healthy patient?
- What is the indication for surgery?
- Is the surgical procedure low risk, intermediate risk, or high risk?
- What is the functional status of the patient?
- What is the effect of the present condition on the patient?
- What improvement is expected after surgery?

Answers to these questions should then direct preoperative testing and management.[1] Preoperative tests rarely detect unsuspected medical conditions. The tests selected should therefore evaluate existing illness, screen for conditions that could affect outcomes in the perioperative period, and help to determine perioperative risks. Existing illnesses that need evaluation and possible treatment prior to surgery include hypertension, diabetes mellitus, cardiac, vascular, pulmonary, renal, and hepatic diseases. The pregnant patient, the geriatric patient, the patient with oncologic disease, malnutrition, or coagulation disorders also needs directed evaluations.

THE HEALTHY PATIENT

The initial preoperative evaluation of a patient should be supplemented by a complete assessment of the patient's general health. This involves a thorough history and physical examination. Complete blood counts should be obtained in all adult women, men over 60 years of age, and patients with hematologic disorders. Blood urea and electrolytes should be tested in all patients over 60 years of age, and in patients with known cardiovascular and renal disease, diabetes, and in patients on steroids, diuretics, and angiotensin-converting enzyme (ACE) inhibitors. An electrocardiogram (ECG) is indicated in men over 40 years, women over 50 years, and in patients with cardiovascular diseases and diabetes. Posteroanterior and lateral chest x-rays are indicated in patients with cardiovascular and respiratory diseases, in patients with malignancy, and those undergoing major thoracic or abdominal surgery.[2]

A history of the current diagnosis and the planned procedure should be obtained. The history should include information regarding any known medical problems and ongoing treatment, previous surgical procedures, and problems if any during previous anesthesia. These can include difficult intubation, bleeding tendencies, and anesthetic jaundice. Family history of problems during anesthesia or surgery should be obtained. These can make the anesthesiologist aware of potential problems such as malignant hyperthermia, bleeding tendencies, or thrombophilia. In addition to routine information about family history, a strong family history of allergies should alert the surgeon to the possibility of hypersensitivity to drugs.

An exhaustive history of drug allergies, sensitivities, and current or recently taken medications should be obtained. Medications such as digitalis, insulin, and corticosteroids should be maintained and their doses carefully regulated in the perioperative period. If the patient is on corticosteroids or if it has been discontinued within a month of surgery, he or she may have a hypofunctioning adrenal cortex resulting in impaired physiologic response to surgical stress. This may necessitate administration of steroids in the perioperative period. Long-term use of barbiturates, opiates, and alcohol may be associated with increased tolerance to anesthetic drugs. History of smoking and alcohol use should be obtained. A review of constitutional symptoms—fever, weight loss, heartburn, and regurgitation—is critical.

PHYSICAL EXAMINATION

A thorough physical examination should be conducted. Assessment of general appearance, vital signs, body mass index, jugular venous pressure and pulsation, evaluation of the head and neck to gauge airway problems and lack of supple neck movements, auscultation of the lung, precordial palpation and auscultation, abdominal inspection for scars from previous surgery and abdominal palpation, examination of peripheral arterial pulses (carotid, radial, femoral, popliteal, posterior tibial, and dorsalis pedis) and of the extremities for edema are critical. Cyanosis, pallor, jaundice, dyspnea, nutritional status, skeletal deformity, and anxiety should be recognized. An assessment of mental status and a brief neurologic examination should be conducted. A rectal and pelvic examination should be performed unless contraindicated. Surgery-specific risk can be determined based on several criteria (Table 1-1).

Briefly, high-risk cases in which the incidence of morbidity and mortality may be greater than 5 percent include aortic and major vascular procedures, intra-abdominal resections, surgery with major fluid shifts, and gynecologic and oncology procedures. Intermediate-risk cases have a morbidity of 1–5 percent and include head and neck resections, carotid endarterectomy, major orthopedic procedures, laparoscopic intra-abdominal procedures, and hysterectomy or radical prostatectomy. Low-risk cases include most endoscopic procedures, breast surgery, ophthalmologic procedures, and hernia repair.

Table 1-1 **Surgery-specific Risk**

High Risk >5%

Emergencies
Aortic and major vascular procedures
Major intra-abdominal resections
Surgery with major fluid shifts
Gynecologic and oncology procedures

Intermediate Risk 1–5%

Head and neck resections
Carotid endarterectomy
Major orthopedic procedures
Laparoscopic intra-abdominal procedure
Hysterectomy or radical prostatectomy

Low Risk

Endoscopic procedures
Breast surgery
Ophthalmologic procedures
Hernia repair

Table 1-2 **ASA Classification**

ASA Class	Description
1	No gross organic disease, healthy patient
2	Mild or moderate systemic disease without functional impairment
3	Organic disease with definite functional impairment
4	Severe disease that is life threatening
5	Moribund patient, not expected to survive

Identification of functional status is a critical part of a preoperative evaluation and is accomplished during a physical examination. The American Society of Anesthesiologists (ASA) Physical Status Classification is a commonly used grading system that accurately correlates functional status with morbidity and mortality following surgery (Table 1-2). *ASA Class 1* indicates a healthy patient with no gross organic disease. *ASA Class 2* indicates a patient with mild or moderate systemic disease without functional impairment, while *ASA Class 3* indicates a patient with organic disease with definite functional impairment. A *Class 4* patient is one with a severe disease that is life threatening and a *Class 5* patient is one who is moribund and has a low likelihood of survival. Mortality is expected to be 0.05 percent in ASA Class 1 patients, 0.4 percent in ASA Class 2 patients, 4.5 percent in ASA Class 3 patients, 25 percent in Class 4 patients, and 50 percent in ASA Class 5 patients.

HYPERTENSION

Hypertension is a minor clinical predictor of increased preoperative cardiovascular risk. Hypertension is classified as *primary* (essential or idiopathic) in 95 percent of cases. *Secondary* hypertension is found in 5 percent of patients. The five most common causes of secondary hypertension include renal artery stenosis, primary hyperaldosteronism, Cushing syndrome, pheochromocytoma, and aortic stenosis. Several studies have suggested that intraoperative blood pressure changes may be greater in untreated hypertensive patients. Patients are therefore advised to take their antihypertensive medications on the day of surgery, with the exception of diuretics. These are withheld to avoid hypovolemia or hypokalemia.

Application of ASA grading to hypertensive disease classifies those patients with well-controlled hypertension on a single agent as ASA Class 2 patients and those patients with poorly controlled hypertension and on multiple drugs as ASA Class 3 patients. Elegant studies by Goldman[3] revealed that elective surgery in patients with inadequately controlled hypertension was not associated with increased risk of perioperative cardiac morbidity provided the diastolic blood pressure was less than 110 mmHg and perioperative blood pressure was closely monitored. Discontinuation of antihypertensive therapy can be dangerous. Examples include rebound hypertension after discontinuation of a centrally acting α_2-adrenergic agonist such as clonidine or congestive heart failure (CHF) in the perioperative period after withholding ACE inhibitors. β-Adrenergic blockade should be continued throughout the preoperative period. Myocardial ischemia is associated with tachycardia but not with acute changes in blood pressure. Beta-blockers such as atenolol are found to be cardio protective. A study by Mangano and Goldman[4] has shown that beta-blockers given pre- and postoperatively can reduce the risk of death in patients with known coronary artery disease (CAD) or at risk for CAD. Contraindications to the use of beta-blockers include a heart rate of less than 55, systolic blood pressure of less than 100, bronchospasm, CHF, and patients with second- or third-degree heart block. A recent myocardial infarction (MI) is the single most important factor that can predict perioperative infarction. The risk is greatest within the first 3 months after an infarction. In a patient with a recent MI, elective surgery should be postponed to after 6 months, when the risk of reinfarction drops to 4.5 percent as opposed to 30 percent within 3 months. Urgent surgery should be preceded by coronary artery bypass or stenting.

In cases of emergency surgery, uncontrolled hypertension should not be a deterrent to proceeding with surgery. Short-acting beta-blockers can be used to control hypertension in the perioperative period. Ketamine should be avoided, as tachycardia, hypertension, and increased intracranial pressure are all associated with its use. Most importantly, perioperative treatment of hypertension with the parenterally administered drugs mentioned earlier should be undertaken only after optimization of ventilation, oxygenation, and circulation in the patient.

CARDIAC DISEASE

A careful history and physical examination can shed light on risk factors for coronary disease such as smoking, hypertension, diabetes, hypercholesterolemia, and a family history of CAD, valvular disease, CHF, arrhythmias, cerebrovascular disease, and peripheral vascular disease. Clinical predictors, cardiac risk for the procedure (Table 1-3), and functional status of the patient should determine the need for preoperative cardiac workup.[5]

Perioperative cardiac and long-term risks are increased in patients unable to meet a 4-MET demand. MET is a *metabolic equivalent*. Greater than

Table 1-3 **Clinical Predictors of Increased Perioperative Cardiovascular Risk**

Major Risk

Unstable coronary syndromes—recent MI, unstable angina
Decompensated CHF
Significant arrhythmias
Severe valvular disease

Intermediate Risk

Mild angina
Prior MI
Compensated CHF
Diabetes mellitus

Minor Risk

Advanced age
Abnormal ECG
Uncontrolled systemic hypertension

10 METs indicate an individual with excellent functional status, a patient involved in competitive sports, aerobics, jogging, and so on. Between 4 and 10 METs indicates a patient who can climb one flight of steps, walk up a hill, or walk a mile in 15 min. Less than 4 METs indicates a patient unable to meet the above criteria. Stable angina with occasional use of nitroglycerin classifies a patient as an ASA Class 2 patient, whereas unstable angina or regular use of nitroglycerin classifies a patient as ASA Class 3. Major clinical risk factors should be stabilized before surgery. This may require intervention such as coronary angiography, angioplasty or stenting, or cardiac surgery. Patients with intermediate clinical risk and poor functional capacity should undergo noninvasive testing. Those with good functional capacity need invasive testing only for high-risk procedures. Patients with minor or no clinical risk and poor functional capacity need invasive testing only in case of high-risk procedures. Those with good functional capacity can undergo surgery without further testing.

New invasive studies are designed to determine the presence and severity of reversible ischemia induced by stress. The stress can be induced by exercise or with drugs such as dobutamine or dipyridamole in patients who cannot exercise. Test tools include ECG, echocardiography, and radionuclide studies using thallium and/or sestamibi. Patients with low- or intermediate-risk noninvasive testing can proceed with surgery, while those with high-risk noninvasive testing should undergo coronary angiography and a revascularization procedure prior to noncardiac surgery. In high-risk cardiac patients, perioperative hemodynamic monitoring is essential. This may involve arterial lines and central venous lines or pulmonary artery catheters that can help assess hemodynamic status. Such monitoring can help optimize perioperative volume resuscitation or restriction, diuretics, afterload reduction, and the use of inotropic drugs.

PULMONARY DISEASE

An accurate preoperative prediction of pulmonary risk associated with abdominal surgery is not well-defined. Clinical factors that have been shown to be useful in the prediction of postoperative pulmonary complications include a history of smoking, chronic bronchitis, airflow obstructions, obesity, and prolonged preoperative hospital stay. The presence of colonizing bacteria in the stomach and the use of nasogastric intubation increase the specific risk of postoperative pneumonia. Smaller incisions and the use of laparoscopic techniques reduce the incidence of pulmonary complications due to decreased postoperative pain and early ambulation. The most important predictive factors appear to be the overall condition of the patient (based on the ASA classification) and patient age. Patients with controlled cough or wheeze and asthma well controlled on inhalers belong to ASA Class 2, and those with breathlessness on minor exertion, and poorly controlled asthma that limits lifestyle are considered ASA Class 3.

Early and late postoperative pulmonary complications were leading causes of morbidity and mortality in surgery. A detailed history should be obtained to evaluate the history of asthma, bronchospasm, duration of prior asthma therapy, previous hospitalization, steroid use, and prior need for mechanical ventilation. Elective surgery should be postponed in cases of acute upper respiratory tract infections. Additional information regarding smoking history (pack-years), nutritional status, concomitant heart disease, and current therapy including home oxygen use should be sought. Physical findings that suggest right ventricular failure include peripheral edema, a prominent right ventricular impulse, or neck vein distention.

A preoperative chest radiograph helps to evaluate lung disease and serves as a basis for comparison in the perioperative period. Significant airflow obstructions can be associated with a normal x-ray. Findings such as depression of the right hemidiaphragm at or below the seventh rib in an anteroposterior view, a cardiac silhouette with a transverse diameter of less than 11.5 cm, and a retrosternal air space of greater than 4.4 cm on a lateral view should raise concern for chronic lung disease. Laboratory studies such as elevated serum bicarbonate suggest respiratory acidosis and polycythemia may suggest chronic anemia.

Patients at high risk for pulmonary complications include those with documented pulmonary disease (chronic obstructive pulmonary disease [COPD] or chronic bronchitis), those with history of heavy smoking and cough, poor perioperative nutrition, and those undergoing thoracic surgery or upper abdominal surgery. Arterial blood gases on room air and pulmonary function testing should be performed in these patients. An arterial oxygen tension (PaO_2) of less than 60 mmHg correlates with pulmonary hypertension and a partial arterial pressure ($PaCO_2$) of greater than 45 mmHg is associated with increased perioperative morbidity. Pulmonary function criteria that indicate increased risk include a forced vital capacity (FVC) less than 50 percent of predicted, forced expiratory volume (FEV_1) less than 50 percent of predicted or less than 2.0 L, or an FEV_1/FVC ratio of less than 0.65. If spirometric parameters improve with bronchodilator therapy, the therapy should be continued during the perioperative period. This improves airflow obstruction, lung mechanism, and gas exchange. Patients undergoing pulmonary resection should have split function studies with either bronchospirometry or radionuclide imaging. An FEV_1 of 800 mL in the contralateral lung is required to proceed with a pneumonectomy.

Cessation of cigarette smoking is helpful in patients smoking more than 10 cigarettes per day. Smoking doubles the risk of pulmonary complications and the risk persists for 3–4 months after the cessation of smoking. However, patients should be informed that even 48 h of cessation could decrease carboxyhemoglobin levels to that of a nonsmoker, abolish the effect of nicotine on the cardiovascular system, and improve mucosal ciliary function. Patients should be educated about the merits of deep breathing, coughing, incentive spirometry, and early ambulation in the postoperative periods. Various preoperative risk reduction strategies suggested by Smetana[6] include advice regarding cessation of cigarette smoking, treatment of airflow obstruction in patients with COPD or asthma, administering antibiotics and delaying surgery when respiratory infection is present, and educating patients regarding lung-expansion maneuvers (Table 1-4).

Table 1-4 **Preoperative Pulmonary Risk Reduction Strategies**

- Encourage cessation of cigarette smoking for at least 8 weeks
- Treat airflow obstruction in patients with COPD or asthma
- Administer antibiotics and delay surgery if respiratory infection is present
- Begin patient education regarding lung-expansion maneuvers

RENAL DISEASE

Preexisting renal insufficiency (RI) is an independent risk factor for cardiovascular death after elective surgery due to the presence of multiple risk factors such as hypertension, hyperlipidemia, and abnormal carbohydrate metabolism. Renal function is classified into three categories based on serum creatinine: normal function with creatinine less than 1.5 mg/dL, mild RI with serum creatinine of 1.5–3 mg/dL, and severe chronic RI with serum creatinine greater than 3.0 mg/dL.

Patients with mild RI have a high incidence of coexisting cardiovascular disease. In patients with mildly elevated creatinine that has not been previously evaluated, urinalysis, 24-h urine for creatinine clearance, and consultation with an internist are indicated before an elective operation. Serum creatinine is a good estimate of renal function; however, it may be inaccurate in patients with ascites, pregnancy, obesity, and edema. Glomerular filtration, which can be calculated from the 24-h creatinine clearance, is the gold standard for renal function. In patients with severe chronic RI, elective surgery should be coordinated with their nephrologist for optimal timing of dialysis; preferably within 24 h of surgery. Perioperative fluid management is critical in these patients and even more so in patients who are not dialysis dependent. Laboratory values to be monitored include hematocrit, prothrombin time (PT), activated partial thromboplastin time (aPTT), and platelets and electrolytes before and after surgery (serum potassium, calcium phosphate, and magnesium). Stable normochromic-normocytic anemia (hematocrit of 25–30) is well tolerated in these patients. Nephrotoxic agents such as contrast dyes and aminoglycosides should be avoided. Enflurane should be avoided due to the potential for fluorane nephrotoxicity.

The acutely ischemic kidney is more vulnerable to subsequent ischemic insults than the normal kidney. Any acute deterioration in renal function preoperatively should therefore be investigated before proceeding with anesthesia and surgery.

HEPATIC DISEASE

Mortality from anesthesia and surgery can be high in patients with liver disease even with simple procedures. This is especially true in the case of unrecognized liver disease or in the case of acute deterioration of liver function. Common causes of jaundice include nonhepatic, obstructive, and acute parenchymal jaundice and jaundice associated with chronic liver disease.

Evaluation of a patient with hepatic disease should include a history of jaundice, hepatotoxic drugs, history of alcoholism, and symptoms of liver disease. Signs of chronic liver disease and scleral icterus should be recognized. Liver function tests, albumin, and PT should be measured. The most

Table 1-5 **Child's Classification**

	Bilirubin	Albumin	Nutrition	Encephalopathy	Ascites
A	<2	<3.5	Excellent	None	None
B	2–3	3–3.5	Good	Minimal	Easily
C	>3	<3	Poor	Severe	Poorly controlled

useful classification regarding the risk of surgery in patients with liver disease is *Child's Classification*. Factors taken into account include bilirubin, albumin, nutrition, encephalopathy, and ascites (Table 1-5).

Modifiable risk factors that should be addressed in these patients prior to surgery include correction of ascites, preservation of renal function, control of glucose and electrolyte abnormalities, improved nutrition, and treatment of encephalopathy. Cirrhotic patients present a significant challenge in the perioperative period. Factors that demand specific attention include intravascular volume, optimization of medical management of ascites, avoidance of hyponatremia, prevention of gastrointestinal bleeding, and providing nutrition supplemented with thiamine. Stress ulcer prophylaxis should be implemented with parenteral H_2-blocker or antacids. Risk of encephalopathy in patients with advanced disease can be decreased by gut decontamination and/or lactulose administration.

VASCULAR DISEASE

Many of the risk factors contributing to peripheral vascular disease (e.g., diabetes mellitus, tobacco use, and hyperlipidemia) are also risk factors for CAD. Peripheral vascular disease is invariably an indicator of cardiac disease. Morbidity and mortality in the perioperative period are generally related to cardiac causes. The usual symptomatic presentation for CAD in these patients may be obscured by exercise limitations imposed by advanced age or intermittent claudication, or both. Major arterial operations often are time consuming and may be associated with substantial fluctuations in intravascular fluid volumes, cardiac filling pressure, systemic blood pressure, heart rate, and thrombogenicity. Marked improvement in management of hemodynamics and myocardial oxygen supply and demand in the operating room have resulted in improved outcomes due to the reduced incidence of major hypoxic episodes. Preoperative cardiac evaluation in patients with vascular disease is crucial in order to optimize perioperative care. It is generally felt that preoperative coronary artery revascularization should be reserved only for patients with unstable cardiac symptoms. A study conducted by McFalls et al.[7] illustrates this point. Patients scheduled to undergo vascular surgery and found to be at increased risk for perioperative cardiac complications and clinically significant CAD were randomized to two treatment arms. These were revascularization or no vascularization before elective vascular surgery. They concluded that coronary revascularization before elective surgery does not significantly affect long-term outcome. Therefore, patients with stable cardiac symptoms cannot be recommended to undergo coronary revascularization. If a carotid bruit is found during a routine preoperative physical evaluation in a patient undergoing nonvascular surgery, further studies may be needed to determine the need and timing for carotid surgery. In patients undergoing cardiopulmonary bypass, carotid atherosclerosis is a risk factor for hemispheric stroke.[8]

ANEMIA AND COAGULATION DISORDERS

Patients with hemoglobin of less than 9 g/dL can have significant surgical morbidity. A peripheral blood smear may indicate the etiology of the anemia. Macrocytosis or microcytosis suggests significant anemia, target cells are seen in splenic hypofunction, and spherocytes and schistocytes are seen in hemolytic anemias. The usual initial screening coagulation tests include a PT, aPTT, and a platelet count.

Platelet Disorders

Qualitative and quantitative defects are seen in platelets in the presence of uremia and liver disease. Platelet aggregation studies and a bleeding time test can identify qualitative defects in platelets. In idiopathic thrombocytopenic purpura, intravenous immune globulin 2 g/kg over 2–4 days can be given to increase platelet counts. If the thrombocytopenia is drug induced, the drug should be stopped and the patient allowed to recover prior to operation. If the surgery cannot be delayed, platelet transfusion should be undertaken.

Sickle Cell Anemia

In patients with sickle cell anemia or trait, deoxygenated hemoglobin undergoes polymerization and forms characteristic sickle cells. These can block small vessels resulting in vasoocclusion. Diagnosis is confirmed by the sickle solubility test and high-performance liquid chromatography. Patients will need to be transfused with hemoglobin of 9–10 g/dL prior to surgery. Dehydration, hypoxia, and pain should be avoided with intravenous hydration, oxygen, and adequate pain control to decrease the risk of a sickle cell crisis.

Von Willebrand Disease

Desmopressin 0.3 µg/kg IV is administered every 12–24 h for 5–7 days. The Factor VIII: vWF ratio should be 60 percent for minor surgery and 80 percent for major surgery. If no effect is seen, cryoprecipitate can be administered (cryoprecipitate contains 80–100 units of vWF/10 U).

Hemophilia A

Mild hemophilia A can be treated with desmopressin; severe hemophilia A may require Factor VIII concentrate.

Hemophilia B

Mild hemophilia B can be treated with desmopressin; severe hemophilia A may require Factor IX concentrate.

Liver Disease

Fresh frozen plasma can be given to keep PT/aPTT less than 1.3 times the control. Vitamin K should be administered if vitamin K deficiency is suspected. Cryoprecipitate can be administered if fibrinogen and Factor VIII levels are low.

Uremia

Patients with uremia may require aggressive dialysis, maintenance of a hematocrit of 30, and a trial of desmopressin and cryoprecipitate.[9]

DIABETES AND ENDOCRINE DISORDERS

Diabetes Mellitus

Diabetes mellitus is one of the most common metabolic diseases encountered. The prevalence of diabetes mellitus in both adults and children has been steadily rising in the past 20–30 years. Improved glycemic control has a beneficial effect on microvascular and neuropathic complications in type 2 diabetes, but has no effect on the incidence of macrovascular disease. However, light control of blood pressure (with an ACE inhibitor or a beta-blocker) in patients with type 2 diabetes and hypertension reduces the risk of diabetes-related death, including that secondary to macrovascular complications, as well as the risk of other diabetes-related complications and eye disease.[10] Good control of diabetes also decreases the potential for postoperative infection. Diabetic patients need careful treatment with adjusted doses or infusions of short-acting insulin based on frequent blood sugar determinations.

The main concern for the anesthetist in the perioperative management of diabetic patients is the avoidance of harmful hypoglycemia; mild hyperglycemia is more acceptable. This has been attributed to the difficulties of measuring blood glucose when the reduced level of consciousness preoperatively masks signs and symptoms of hypoglycemia. The immediate perioperative problems facing the diabetic patient are (1) surgical induction of the stress response with catabolic hormone secretion; (2) interruption of food intake, which may be prolonged following gastrointestinal procedure; (3) altered consciousness, which masks the symptoms of hypoglycemia and necessitates frequent blood glucose estimations; and (4) circulatory disturbances associated with anesthesia and surgery, which may alter the absorption of subcutaneous insulin.

In patients who are dehydrated, vomiting, have severe abdominal pain, and are on the verge of obtundation, there should be a high index of suspicion for diabetic ketoacidosis (DKA). Diagnostic criteria for DKA include blood glucose greater than 700 mg/dL, serum osmolarity greater than 340 mOsmol/L, and acidosis. Treatment includes obtaining an ECG to rule out a silent infarct, fluid replacement with hypotonic saline, administering 5 percent dextrose after the blood glucose falls below 250 mg/dL, and monitoring and supplementing potassium.

Carcinoid Tumors

Adequate hydration is extremely important in patients who present with carcinoid syndrome resulting from vasoactive substances released by the tumor. Increased levels of serotonin cause diarrhea, abdominal cramping, respiratory distress due to bronchospasm, and hypertension. In patients with long-standing carcinoid, an echocardiogram should be obtained to test for right heart failure. Antihistaminics can be used to counteract the effect of histamines and octreotide can be used to block the release of hormonal substances.

Pheochromocytoma

A patient with pheochromocytoma needs preoperative pharmacologic manipulation with alpha-blockade first, followed by possible beta-blockade. This is best accomplished by coordinated treatment of the patient by the surgeon, the anesthesiologist, and the referring physician. Alpha-blockade is suggested for 7–10 days preoperatively using phenoxybenzamine 10–40 mg orally twice daily (titrated to onset of nasal congestion and orthostatic hypotension). Beta-blockade is used only after adequate alpha-blockade. Beta-blockade is attained over the last three preoperative days with propranolol 10 mg orally twice daily. Beta-blockade is indicated in patients with tachycardia or tachyarrhythmia, and is not necessary in all patients.[11]

THE GERIATRIC PATIENT

The risks of a major procedure in patients over 60 years of age are increased only slightly in the absence of cardiovascular, renal, and other systemic diseases. Changes associated with generalized arteriosclerosis are to be expected, as are limitations of cardiac and renal reserve. The incidence of silent MI increases with age. A thorough comprehensive preoperative evaluation is therefore very critical. Occult cancer is also frequently seen in this age group, and therefore minor gastrointestinal and other complaints should be investigated. Older patients show less heart rate response to hypotension, and therefore are at increased risk for orthostatic hypotension. In addition, the ventilatory responses to hypoxia and hypercapnia are both reduced.

In an elderly patient, it is particularly important to establish the indication for surgery, the likelihood of progression of the disease, the quality of life with and without surgery, and the risk of a negative outcome. Negative outcomes are influenced by the nature of the disease process and the type of intervention planned. In addition to morbidity and mortality, attention should be paid to the quality of life and the return to preoperative functional status. The presence of a comorbid disease increases with age. Major perioperative complications increase with the number of comorbid conditions in all age groups but the effects are most pronounced in the youngest[12] and in the oldest groups (over 75 years of age). In a study of patients with colon cancer, by age 75, 50 percent of male and female patients had at least five other disorders in addition to the cancer.[13] While only a minimal increase in mortality and morbidity is seen in older patients who lack coexisting disease, there is a threefold increase associated with as few as two additional comorbidities.

A thorough history and evaluation should direct further workup and laboratory testing. In addition to the routine workup, special attention should be paid to nutritional assessment and mental status evaluation. Deficits in nutritional and mental status have been found to be largely unrecognized prior to admission in the hospital.[14] Baseline cognitive function in the elderly can be evaluated using the Holstein Mini Mental Status test. This tests the ability for orientation, registration, attention, and the use of language.

The prevalence and predictive value of abnormal preoperative laboratory tests in elderly patients (abnormal preoperative electrolyte values and thrombocytopenia) is small and has low predictive values. Although more prevalent, abnormal hemoglobin, creatinine, and glucose values were also not predictive of postoperative adverse outcomes. Routine preoperative testing for hemoglobin, creatinine, glucose, and electrolytes on the basis of age only may not be indicated in geriatric patients. Rather, selective laboratory testing is indicated as suggested by history and physical examination, which will determine patient's comorbidities and surgical risk.[15]

THE PREGNANT PATIENT

Surgery in a pregnant patient involves the care of two patients: the mother and the fetus. One to two percent of pregnant women require surgery for indications not related to the pregnancy. A thorough understanding of changes in the cardiovascular and respiratory physiology during pregnancy is critical. Anesthesia does not increase the risk of fetal anomalies; however, it could lead to preterm labor. Therefore, elective surgery should be avoided during the first trimester. Attention should be paid in the preoperative period to the maintenance of uterine blood flow and fetal oxygenation, avoidance of teratogenic drugs, and the prevention of preterm labor. When possible, fetal monitoring should be performed preoperatively and continued in the perioperative period. α-Adrenergic agonists cause uterine vasoconstriction and should be avoided. Hypotension in pregnant patients can be treated with ephedrine, a mixed α and β agonist that protects uterine blood flow.

The pregnant patient is at increased risk for aspiration of gastric contents. She should not have any oral intake for 6 h before surgery. Magnesium sulfate should be readily available for the treatment of preterm labor. Hydralazine is the drug of choice for hypertensive crisis in preeclamptic patients. Labetalol is an alternative drug that can be used. When possible, regional anesthesia should be administered instead of general anesthesia (spinal or epidural).

PATIENTS WITH A HISTORY OF VENOUS THROMBOEMBOLISM

Elective surgery should be avoided in the first month after an acute episode of venous thromboembolism. If this is not possible, intravenous heparin should be given before and after the procedure while the international normalized ratio (INR) is below 2.0. If the aPTT is in the therapeutic range, stopping continuous intravenous heparin therapy 6 h before operation is usually sufficient for heparin to be cleared.

Heparin therapy should not be restarted until 12 h after major surgical procedure and should be delayed even longer if there is any evidence of bleeding from the surgical site. Heparin should be restarted without a bolus, at no more than the expected maintenance infusion rate. The aPTT should be checked 12 h after restarting therapy to allow time for a stable anticoagulant response.

If the patient has been receiving anticoagulant therapy for less than 2 weeks after a pulmonary embolism or a proximal deep vein thrombosis or if the risk of bleeding during intravenous heparin therapy is considered unacceptable, a vena caval filter should be inserted.

THE ONCOLOGY PATIENT

Airway management in patients with head and neck tumors can be challenging because of the potential for airway distortions. Since maintenance of an airway is a major concern in the perioperative period, the anatomic effects of a larger tumor must be assessed preoperatively to minimize adverse effects. Large tumors with extrinsic compression of the trachea often require awake intubation using fiber-optic guidance. Preoperative review of the CT scan of the neck is important because some large tumors may be relatively asymptomatic prior to attempts at intubation, but may make intubation extremely difficult. Another important management tool is the use of tracheotomy in patients with large tumors. Patients in whom a difficult fiber-optic intubation is anticipated should undergo tracheotomy prior to the planned procedure.[11]

A careful history is important to identify episodes of dyspnea, stridor, wheezing, or orthopnea. A history of these problems and/or findings, from a physical examination consistent with possible mediastinal compression should warn the surgeon to avoid general anesthesia, and obtain necessary biopsy specimens using local anesthesia. Preoperative workup of the asymptomatic patient with an anterior or middle mediastinal mass should include CT scan of the chest, inspiratory and expiratory flow volume loops with pulmonary function tests, and echocardiography to rule out tracheobronchial, pulmonary artery, or cardiac compression.

NUTRITIONAL STATUS

Patients should undergo a preoperative nutritional assessment in advance of surgery. Signs and symptoms of malnutrition should be actively sought. Malnutrition leads to a significant increase in the operative death rate. Weight loss of more than 20 percent caused by illnesses such as cancer or gastrointestinal disease results in a higher death rate and a threefold increase in postoperative infection rate. The dietary history should be obtained as well as information that can indicate basic nutritional deficiencies associated with disease states, especially vitamin deficiencies.

In addition to a thorough history and physical examination, nutritional assessment may include measuring serum transferrin, albumin and prealbumin, and total urinary nitrogen (TUN). Values that suggest severe impairment in the visceral protein mass include serum albumin of less than 2.5 g/dL, serum transferrin of less than 150 mg/dL, serum prealbumin of less than 10 mg/dL, and TUN of greater than 12 g/24 h.

Well-nourished patients undergoing surgical procedures may benefit from early postoperative feeding within 48 h. If the patient is able to meet greater than two-thirds of nutritional needs by mouth, nutritional support can be provided by the oral route. Every effort should be made to replete the severely malnourished patient preoperatively. Supportive measures should be instituted in cases of weight loss greater than 10 percent of body weight, and of an anticipated prolonged postoperative recovery period during which the patient cannot be fed (>5–10 days for patients with preexisting severe malnutrition). These include perioperative hyperalimentation either through the enteral or parenteral routes. Enteral feeding can be provided either through nasogastric or nasoduodenal tubes or gastrostomy tubes. The purported advantages of enteral feeding are better substrate utilization, maintenance of gut mucosal integrity, and immunocompetence. Patients in whom the gastrointestinal tract is nonfunctional, parenteral nutrition is provided via a central rein. Central parenteral formulas are highly concentrated and tailored to meet the need for proteins, carbohydrates, fat, electrolytes, multivitamins, and minerals.

PREOPERATIVE MANAGEMENT OF SPECIFIC PROBLEMS

Prophylaxis for Deep Venous Thrombosis and Pulmonary Embolism

The morbidity and mortality of deep vein thrombosis and pulmonary embolism make it mandatory to provide prophylaxis against these catastrophes. Patients at high risk include older individuals, those with previous abdominal surgery, varicose veins, increased antithrombin III levels, history of cigarette smoking, and high platelet counts. The risk is increased in patients older than 40 years who undergo general anesthesia for more than 30 min.

The routine use of sequential compression devices on both lower extremities began in the operating room even prior to induction of anesthesia is advised. This can be continued until the patient is ambulating. These devices stimulate endothelial cell fibrinolytic activity and as such can be used on one leg alone or on the upper extremity if lower extremity application is contraindicated.

Low-dose heparin, 5000 units administered 2 h prior to induction and continued twice a day on a daily basis is effective prophylaxis. However, it is not advisable for patients with major fractures, recent head injury, or gastrointestinal bleeding. In such patients, prophylactic percutaneous placement of an inferior vena cava filter is appropriate.

Therapeutic Anticoagulation

There are several recommendations for the perioperative management of anticoagulation in patients who cannot tolerate oral anticoagulants. If a patient's INR is between 2.0 and 3.0, four scheduled doses of warfarin should be withheld to allow the INR to fall spontaneously to 1.5 or less before surgery. Warfarin should be withheld for a longer period if the INR is normally maintained above 3.0 or if it is necessary to keep it at a lower value (i.e., less than 1.3). The INR should be measured a day before surgery to ensure adequate progress in the reversal of anticoagulation; the physician then has the option of administering a small dose (1 mg subcutaneously) of vitamin K, if required (i.e., if the INR is 1.8 or higher). Alternative preoperative or postoperative prophylaxis, or both, against thromboembolism should be considered[16] for the period during which the INR is less than 2.0.

Antimicrobial Prophylaxis

Prophylactic antibodies are indicated for clean contaminated or contaminated cases. Even for clean cases, prophylactic antibodies may decrease the rate of infection. This includes cases where prosthetic mesh is to be used. A prophylactic antibiotic covering typical skin organisms is adequate in these cases. In cases where an infection is already established, the choice of the antibiotic should be based on culture and sensitivity results and continued for the appropriate length of time. Antibiotics should be administered in a timely fashion so that therapeutic blood levels of the antibiotic are present at the start of the procedure.

In patients with open wounds or ongoing infections, culture and antibiotic sensitivities should be obtained. Surface cultures do not yield adequate information. Instead quantitative cultures of punch biopsies from the wounds are more precise indicators. Greater than 10^5 organisms per gram of tissue correspond to greater than 50 percent graft failure, whereas below 10^5 organisms per gram of tissue correspond to greater than 80 percent graft take.

Duration of the procedure correlates with higher rate of wound infection, and therefore in procedures lasting more than 4 h a second dose of the antibiotic should be administered intraoperatively. Recent work suggests that better glycemic control with insulin infusions may reduce the incidence of deep sternal wound infections in diabetic patients who have undergone cardiac surgery. This observation is supported by a study demonstrating better preservations of neutrophil function with aggressive glycemic control using an insulin infusion compared with intermittent therapy, in diabetic cardiac patients.

Preoperative Orders Regarding Diet

Patients should avoid solid foods for 12 h and liquids for 8 h prior to surgery. They are generally advised to remain nil by mouth after midnight on the night before operation. Patients undergoing esophageal surgery for achalasia are requested to begin clear liquids 2 days prior to surgery and continue this until midnight, the night before surgery. Similarly, patients undergoing surgery on the small intestine, colon, and rectum are advised to start clear liquids 2–3 days prior to surgery.

Bowel Preparation

In addition to limiting intake of clear liquids, starting 3 days prior to surgery, patients undergoing small intestine, colon, and rectal surgery are advised to undergo a bowel preparation. Various preparations can be used. The polyethylene glycol electrolyte preparation consists of 4 L of solution that should be consumed over a 2–3 h period the day before surgery, before administration of the oral antibiotics. Alternatively, two doses of a $1^1/2$ fl oz bottle of Fleet's Phospho-Soda (hypertonic sodium phosphate solution) diluted with half a glass of water can be consumed the day before surgery; one in the early afternoon and the other in the early evening. A bottle of magnesium citrate taken 3 days prior to surgery and then again the morning before surgery can also provide an adequate bowel preparation. As part of the bowel preparation, patients are advised to take neomycin and erythromycin base, 1 g each orally at 1, 2, and 11 p.m. the day before surgery. Metronidazole can be substituted for erythromycin.

Preoperative Orders Regarding Medications

Long-acting sulfonylureas should be stopped 48 h prior to surgery; short-acting agents should be omitted on the morning of surgery. These medications should be restarted when the patient resumes adequate oral intake. Patients are advised to take their antihypertensive medications on the day of surgery, with the exception of diuretics. These are withheld to avoid hypovolemia or hypokalemia. The route of administration of certain drugs may need to be changed to parenteral in the preoperative period. This may be necessary for drugs such as digitalis, other cardiac drugs, and immunosuppressive drugs in transplant patients.

Information Regarding Postoperative Hospital Stay, Diet, Exercise, and Return to Work

Patients should be advised about what to expect in the perioperative period. Information regarding duration of the procedure, ambulatory or in-patient status following surgery, and duration of hospital stay should be given. Advice regarding diet, exercise, and possible return to work allays some of the traditional fears about surgery. Intraoperative risks of bleeding, infection, injury to adjacent structures, and need for conversion to open procedures for laparoscopic cases should be discussed, as also the perioperative risks of developing an MI, pulmonary embolism, or loss of life. The technical details of the procedure should be explained and informed consent obtained.

REFERENCES

1. Rosenthal RA, Zenilman ME, Katlic MR. *Principles and Practice of Geriatric Surgery.* New York: Springer, 2001.

2. Rogers MC, Tinker JH, Covino BG, et al. *Principles and Practice of Anesthesiology.* New York: Mosby, 1993.

3. Goldman L. Cardiac risk in noncardiac surgery: an update. *Anesth Analg* 80:810–820, 1995.

4. Mangano D, Goldman L. Preoperative assessment of patients with known or suspected coronary disease. *N Engl J Med* 333:1749–1756, 1995.

5. Norton LW, Stiegmann GV, Eiseman B. *Surgical Decision Making.* Philadelphia, PA: W.B. Saunders, 2000.

6. Smetana G. Preoperative pulmonary evaluation. *N Engl J Med* 340(12):937–944, 1999.

7. McFalls EO, Ward HB, Moritz TE. Coronary-artery revascularization before elective major vascular surgery. *N Engl J Med* 351:2795–804, 2004.

8. Schwartz LB, Bridgman AH, Keiffer RW. Asymptomatic carotid artery stenosis and stroke in patients undergoing cardiopulmonary bypass. *J Vasc Surg* 21:146–153, 1995.

9. Nyhus LM, Baker RJ, Fischer JE. *Mastery of Surgery.* New York: Little, Brown and Company, 1997.

10. McAnulty GR, Robertshaw HJ, Hall GM. Anesthetic management of patients with diabetes mellitus. *Br J Anaesth* 85:80–90, 2000.

11. Lefor AT. Perioperative management of the patient with cancer. *Chest* 115:165S–171S, 1999.

12. Tiret L, Desmonts JM, Hatton F, et al. Complications associated with anesthesia: a prospective survey in France. *Can Anaesth Soc J* 33:336–344, 1986.

13. Yancick R,Wesley MN, Ries LA, et al. Comorbidity and age as predictors of risk for early mortality of male and female colon carcinoma patients based study. *Cancer* 82:2123–2134, 1998.

14. Pinholt EM, Kroenke K, Hanley JF, et al. Functional assessment of the elderly: a comparison of standard instruments with clinical judgment. *Arch Intern Med* 147:484, 1987.

15. Dzankic S, Pastor D, Gonzalez C, et al. The prevalence and predictive value of abnormal preoperative laboratory test in elderly patients. *Anesth Analg* 93:301–308, 2001.

16. Kearon C, Hirsh J. Management of anticoagulation before and after elective surgery. *N Engl J Med* 336:1506–1511, 1997.

TRAUMATIC INJURY

Kumash R. Patel, MD
Steven N. Vaslef, MD, PhD

HISTORIC PERSPECTIVE

Trauma has been a part of humanity since before the dawn of civilization and is not isolated to only the human race. Traumatic events occur in all species on earth and the known universe. Despite this obvious logic, the first recording of a traumatic event being treated is traced back to the ancient Egyptians. At the great pyramid at Giza, mummies were found with splints on partially healed fractures of the radius and ulna and healed ends of amputations. These mummies were dated back to 2465 B.C. Formal treatment of injuries was evidenced in the Edwin Smith Papyrus,[1] dating to 1600 B.C. (Fig. 2-1). These papers describe 48 surgical cases of treated wounds to the head, neck, shoulders, chest, and breasts. Avicenna's Canon of Medicine written in 1012 is the next major text on treatment of injuries, in which he describes, "There are three principles to follow when treating loss of continuity in fleshy tissues. (1) Stabilize the part which is insufficiently firm, arrest the bleeding, and if there be a discharge strive to reduce its amount. (2) Make the immobilized part consolidated by administering appropriate medicines and suitable articles of food. (3) Prevent sepsis as much as possible. If all three cannot be achieved, concentrate on the two that can. You know how the arrest of bleeding is achieved. Consolidation of the part is secured by opposing the edges of the wound and by applying desiccant remedies and by taking agglutinative food."[1] These tenets established the basic guidelines for treating not only traumatic wounds, but also most pathologic diseases. This knowledge continued to accumulate over the years until the first successful trauma resuscitation occurred in London on July 16, 1774. A 3-year-old child had fallen on the flagstones and had been pronounced dead until an apothecary arrived on the scene 20 min later and proceeded to deliver electric shocks via a portable electrostatic generator. The child regained a pulse and respiration and eventually recovered fully.[1]

Despite these advances that have been recorded through history, modern trauma care originated with Dominique Jean Larrey. He was the physician to

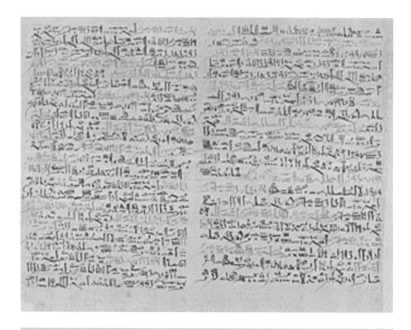

Figure 2-1 **The Edwin Smith Papyrus, ca. 1600 B.C., is the oldest known text describing treatments of injuries.**

the French army who in 1797 designed the *ambulance volante*. These flying ambulances were horse drawn wagons that carried the wounded from the battlefield to a base hospital, the first mobile army surgical hospital (MASH), a self-contained United States Army military unit. This improved treatment and survival, being able to treat the wounded immediately rather than waiting for the end of the battle. He also developed the concept of triage during this time. "The best plan that can be adopted in such emergencies, to prevent the evil consequences of leaving soldiers who are severely wounded without assistance, is to place the ambulance as near as possible to the line of the battle, and to establish headquarters to which the wounded, who require delicate operations, shall be collected to be operated on by the surgeon general. Those who are dangerously wounded should receive the first attention, without regard to rank or distinction. Those who are injured to a less degree may wait until their brethren-in-arms, who are badly mutilated, have been operated and dressed, otherwise the latter would not survive many hours, rarely until the succeeding day."[1]

With these foundations, trauma care evolved over the next two centuries into an intricate system of care that is universally adopted. As medical knowledge improved and research revealed the hidden truths of human physiology, so did trauma care. Collectively, the knowledge became advanced trauma life support.

MECHANISMS OF INJURY

With the discussion of trauma and its associated injuries, consideration and understanding to the mechanism must be achieved to properly care for the patient and the injuries that are present. These injuries result from energy transfer based on the laws of motion and energy. Since energy cannot be created or destroyed and objects have both stationary and mobile energy, it can be deduced that the force generated in a traumatic event is transferred to the patient resulting in various soft tissue and osseous injuries. This transfer of energies leaves two types of cavities. On initial impact, the force *pushing* the tissue and the cellular particles create a *temporary cavity*. Once the forces have dissipated, the tissues will recoil back to their previous position depending on the amount of elasticity and compliance they possess. This process occurs in a fraction of a second. A *permanent cavity* is noticed when the tissue has the inability to recoil due to destruction or crushing. Both these cavities occur due to two main types of mechanisms: *blunt* and *penetrating*.[2]

Blunt Trauma

Blunt trauma leads to compression, shear, and overpressure injuries. *Compression injuries* occur due to the force crushing the cells that it comes into contact with. *Shear injuries* appear from an organ accelerating or decelerating at a different velocity than the surrounding tissues or cavity. The stretching and rupturing of surrounding tissues when excessive pressure is placed on the tissue cause *overpressure injuries*.[2]

Causes of blunt trauma are categorized into motor vehicle crashes, pedestrian injuries, falls, and assaults. *Motor vehicle crashes* are associated with frontal, lateral, rear, off-center, rotational, and ejectional collisions.[2] *Pedestrians* struck by a motorized vehicle sustain injuries that are associated with multiple mechanisms and multiple points of force. The initial impact is followed by a *fall* on another impact point. These types of mechanisms potentially lead to many occult injuries; therefore, a high index of suspicion should be maintained. Falls occur from various heights, leading to various amounts of force on impact and variable injury patterns. Once again, a high index of suspicion needs to be maintained for occult injuries. *Assaults* come in a myriad of types and sizes, but are generally more localized than the other mechanisms mentioned. Injuries are isolated to the area of impact, for the most part. It must be kept in mind that any of these mechanisms can overlap into penetrating trauma (Fig. 2-2), depending on if an object violated the exterior barrier to enter the soft tissue in the process of the blunt trauma.

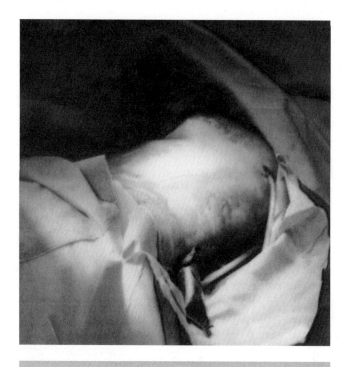

Figure 2-2 **Combined blunt and penetrating mechanisms of injury in a patient who was impaled by a metal fence post. The post is seen entering the upper abdomen and exiting the left flank.**

Penetrating Trauma

Penetrating trauma encompasses those of bullet/missile injuries and stab injuries from various objects (Fig. 2-3). These injuries lead to direct tissue destruction, various sizes of temporary cavities, and a more permanent cavity. The amount of tissue destruction is dependent on the type of object, its size, and the velocity at which the object was traveling. The density of the tissue the object interacts with will also affect cavity formation. As the object moves through the tissue, energy is transferred to the tissue. The tissue in contact with the object is crushed and destroyed while the surrounding tissue is stretched all along the path of the object until the force is dissipated and the tissue recoils.[2]

Stab injuries will have very small temporary cavities created as the object is entering the tissue, but will have a permanent cavity dependent on the size of the object and the velocity it was traveling when entering the tissue planes. Bullets and projectile missiles, on the other hand, will create larger

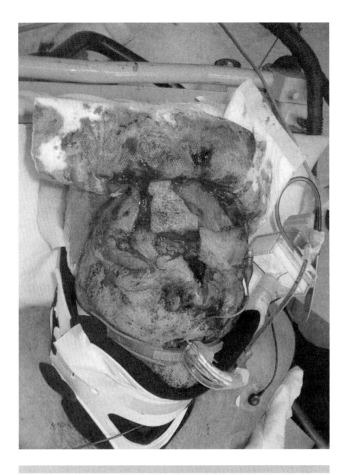

Figure 2-3 **Penetrating trauma to the head resulting in multiple wounds from a machete attack.**

temporary cavities and obvious permanent cavities with greater secondary trauma. The size of the frontal area of the projectile is a major factor in the size of the cavity it creates. The larger the area in contact with tissue, the larger the cavity formed, both permanent and temporary. The projectile can create a temporary cavity of 20–25 times that of its frontal area. Therefore, as a projectile encounters a tissue and becomes deformed, a larger frontal area will be created which will lead to larger cavities. Other factors that will increase the projectile's frontal area are its ability to tumble through the tissue due to changes in momentum between the front and the back of the projectile; its ability to fragment on encountering tissue; and its ability to explode on tissue contact.

Generally, penetrating injuries are classified as low-velocity or high-velocity injuries. Most stab injuries and handguns are *low-velocity injuries* due to the projectiles traveling at speeds less than 450 m/s. Projectiles with speeds greater than 450 m/s are considered to cause *high-velocity injuries*. Kinetic energy is proportional to the square of the projectile's velocity. Thus, higher-velocity projectiles cause much greater injuries, mostly due to temporary cavitation and secondary tissue destruction.[2]

TRAUMA RESUSCITATION

Personnel

Preparing for a trauma is just as daunting as the trauma itself. Designation of personnel to specific duties and responsibilities is of the utmost importance. Without knowledge of each team member's responsibilities, a simple trauma can turn into a chaotic event and lead to a patient's demise. The most important person in the team is the team leader, who should be the most senior surgeon. The team leader should always be standing at the foot of the bed, able to visualize all the proceedings clearly and to be heard effectively. Not only is the team leader responsible for directing patient care, but he or she must also be able to keep tranquility amongst the team during the resuscitation. If the level of noise and discordance rises too high, errors will occur.

The next most important member is at the head of the bed, responsible for managing the airway and cervical spine. Various members may play this role, including the anesthesiologist, certified nurse anesthetist, respiratory technician, or ER physician. Regardless, this should be the most experienced person in airway management. Included in this role is the protection of the cervical spine at all times.

On either side of the patient should be a physician and a nurse. The physician proceeds with the primary survey while the nurse obtains peripheral venous access. Also aiding the physician or the nurse is any trauma team member, either by removing articles of clothing, assisting with the primary survey, or obtaining peripheral venous access. Besides these members of the trauma team, no one else should be near the bedside during the resuscitation phase. Other members that are present should be aiding by obtaining necessary equipment that is required by the bedside team.

The other important aspect of the trauma resuscitation is the documentation. There should be a nurse documenting all the proceedings that are going on. The nurse should have a clear field of vision to observe the process and be able to clearly hear the team leader to document history and physical examination findings as well as any procedures that are being done.

Besides the team members at the bedside, ancillary aid should be available. This includes radiology for immediate plain radiographs, computed tomography (CT), or emergent angiography. The blood bank should be ready to type and cross-match the patient's blood and other appropriate blood products.

In accordance with being prepared, prior to the arrival of the patient, all possible equipments necessary for the resuscitation should be readily available. Mandatory items include large bore peripheral IVs, large bore central venous catheter, rapid fluid infuser, Foley catheter kit, nasogastric tube, warm IV fluids, warm blankets, various-sized endotracheal tubes, and an ultrasound machine. Other items that should be nearby and ready for use include emergency cricothyroidotomy set, chest tube insertion set, and thoracotomy set.

Primary Survey

The evaluation of a trauma patient begins with the primary survey. The purpose of the primary survey is to identify and treat immediately life-threatening injuries. While all the aspects of the primary survey are discussed as individual components, they are in actuality addressed altogether, along with the resuscitation of the patient. While the primary survey—the *ABCDEF*—is undertaken, an *AMPLE* history (Table 2-1) is also obtained to aid in the resuscitation.[3]

The first component of the ABCDEF mnemonic is *A*irway management with cervical spine immobilization. Evaluation of the airway starts with asking the patient questions. If the patient can answer, then the airway is patent. If the response is absent, garbled, or hoarse, the airway may be compromised. Other signs that the airway may be compromised are agitation or combativeness, cyanosis, noisy breathing, or use of accessory muscles. Compromised airways need to be secured with intubation and mechanical ventilation. Intubation may also be required for those patients who may not be able to protect their airway due to concomitant injuries. Injuries that require intubation include severe facial trauma, significant burns or inhalation injury, laryngeal injury, neck trauma, and depressed mental status due to significant head injuries or consciousness altering medications.

Table 2-1 **Components of the AMPLE History**

Allergies
Medications currently being taken
Past medical-surgical history
Last time a meal was eaten
Events and **E**nvironment related to the trauma

Source: Adapted from American College of Surgeons Committee on Trauma: Initial Assessment and Management. In *Advanced Trauma Life Support Program for Doctors*, 7th ed. Chicago, IL: American College of Surgeons, 2004: 11–29.

Once the decision has been made to secure the airway, various methods are available, depending on the urgency and ability to secure the airway. Chemical agents may be used in aiding this process. The most common method of intubation is insertion of an endotracheal tube via the oral route. This should be done by the most experienced member of the team, who should be cognizant at all times of the possibility of a cervical spine injury, and keep the spine immobilized during the intubation. Cervical spine immobilization is generally performed at this time by a second member of the team. Special problems may arise during oral intubation attempts, such as the inability to intubate the patient via this method. Other options must be employed in a rapid fashion to maintain adequate oxygenation. Fiber-optic intubation may be employed, in which the endotracheal tube is placed over a fiber-optic bronchoscope and under direct visualization is inserted into the trachea. Nasotracheal intubation may be performed as well, either blindly or with the aid of the bronchoscope. Intubation over a laryngeal mask airway can also be accomplished. If these nonsurgical methods fail to secure an airway or the urgency is great, then a surgical airway must be performed. A cricothyroidotomy (Table 2-2) is the quickest method of securing a surgical airway. This method is performed for patients older than 12 years of age. For those patients less than 12 years of age, a needle cricothyroidotomy is performed and jet ventilation instituted. Definitive airway control can then be achieved under more controlled circumstances.

After the airway has been intubated, it must be confirmed that the endotracheal tube is adequately placed in the trachea and can be used for ventilation. Breathing and ventilation should then be assessed. Inspecting the chest wall for equal rise with insufflation of air into the endotracheal tube accomplishes this quickly. Next, auscultation of the chest for appropriate breath sounds is undertaken. An end-tidal CO_2 monitor may be placed on the endotracheal tube to confirm placement. Pulse oximetry should also be used for verification of adequate oxygenation during ventilation.

Table 2-2 **Steps in Performing a Cricothyroidotomy**

1. A vertical incision is made in the midline of the neck over the cricothyroid and thyroid cartilage.
2. Dissection is carried down with a scalpel or hemostat to the cricothyroid membrane.
3. A transverse incision is made into the cricothyroid membrane with the scalpel.
4. The incision is enlarged and dilated with the hemostat.
5. A no. 6–7 French endotracheal tube is inserted into the trachea.
6. Placement is assured by auscultation and end-tidal CO_2 monitor.
7. The endotracheal tube is then secured to the skin using 0 silk or nylon suture.

Depressed levels of oxygen or ventilation need to be addressed immediately, for injuries related to these signs are life threatening. Pathologies to evaluate for include tension pneumothorax, flail chest, pulmonary contusion, pericardial tamponade, tracheobronchial injuries, and massive hemothorax. These entities will be discussed under the section Thoracic Injury.

The next vital component in the primary survey is Circulation. There must be a sufficient amount of blood volume circulating to and from the heart to maintain adequate perfusion and prevent the shock state. To ensure this, a quick estimation of the patient's blood loss must be made by summating the blood loss from the potential injuries (Table 2-3) and by checking the patient's heart rate and blood pressure. Volume replacement must be immediate with either isotonic saline solution or packed red cells, depending on the patient's condition. This replacement should be given via two 16-gauge or larger peripheral IVs, which should be placed immediately on the patient's arrival into the trauma bay. Fluid infusion via the 16-gauge peripheral IVs occurs at the fastest rate because of the lower resistance to flow that exists. If peripheral IVs are unable to be obtained, then a large bore central venous catheter should be inserted. Ideally, this should be a no. 9 French cordis catheter in either the femoral vein or subclavian vein. The femoral vein carries less risk and may be easier to obtain than the subclavian vein. Once venous access is obtained, warm fluid should be infused rapidly into the patient with the rapid infuser. Two liters of saline solution should be infused prior to reassessing the need for more crystalloid fluid or blood product requirements. If the patient remains hemodynamically unstable or does not respond to the 2 L of saline solution, consideration for blood product infusion should be given along with continued crystalloid infusion.

A key component to the assessment of circulation is to cease any obvious source of external hemorrhage. Any superficial source of bleeding should be controlled immediately by either direct pressure or ligation. Obvious fractures should be noted and care should be taken when these injuries are moved so

Table 2-3 **Potential Blood Loss**

Skin	Infinite
Cranium	100 mL
Chest	>2 L
Abdomen	>2 L
Forearm	250 mL
Arm	500 mL
Thigh	1 L
Leg	500 mL

as to not cause further bleeding by disrupting any clot that has already been formed.

An aspect of assessing adequate circulation is the distal extremity examination. Distal extremities should be checked for pulses as well as warmth. The patient's hemodynamic status can be easily assessed with this examination. Palpation of a carotid, femoral, radial, and dorsalis pedis pulse will correlate to rough estimations of systolic blood pressures: 60, 70, 80, and 90 mmHg, respectively. The warmth or coolness of the distal extremity can also give a good estimation of the patient's shock state.

The *D* in our mnemonic stands for Disability. That is, what kind of neurologic deficit does the patient have? Obviously, until the patient is stable, a complete neurologic examination is difficult to perform. Instead, a brief examination is performed for trauma patients during the initial evaluation. The Glasgow Coma Scale (GCS) (Table 2-4) is a measurement of the patient's level of consciousness in relation to the severity of head injuries. The best response in each of three categories (*eye opening, verbal,* and *motor*) is scored

Table 2-4 **Glasgow Coma Scale**

Best Motor Response	
Obeys commands	6
Localizes to pain	5
Withdraws to pain	4
Decorticate (abnormal flexion)	3
Decerebrate (abnormal extension)	2
None	1

Best Verbal Response	
Oriented	5
Confused	4
Inappropriate words	3
Incomprehensible sounds	2
None	1

Eye Opening	
Spontaneous	4
To command	3
To pain	2
None	1

and recorded, and the three values are totaled, yielding a value that correlates with the severity of the patient's injury. A score of 13–15 reflects a mild injury, 9–12 a moderate injury, and less than or equal to 8 a severe injury. Any patient with a score of less than or equal to 8 requires airway protection and mechanical ventilation, as well as urgent evaluation for intracranial trauma. This examination is repeated during the secondary survey with the full neurologic examination. During this part of the examination, care should be taken in noting the voluntary and involuntary movement of all extremities. This will reveal if any spinal cord injury (SCI) exists.

To fully assess the patient, complete *Exposure* of the body must be undertaken. All clothing must be removed in an expedient fashion, particularly if the articles of clothing are adding to any potential injury or future complications. All jewelry must be removed because during the resuscitation digits and extremities may become edematous. Obvious wounds and injuries should be noted and addressed as needed. Thereafter, the patient should be covered in warm blankets to prevent heat loss and hypothermia.

The *Focused* abdominal sonography for trauma (FAST) examination, if available, should be performed as soon as possible for all blunt trauma and select penetrating trauma. This is an ultrasound examination of the abdominal compartment and pericardial space. It is a safe, rapid, easily performed examination that can be easily repeated if necessary. The specificity of the examination ranges from 90 to 100 percent, whereas the sensitivity ranges from 60 to 100 percent. A 3.5-Hz convex probe is placed in four positions with the goal of detecting free fluid in areas that should be free of fluid. The first area to examination is the pericardial space. The probe is placed in the midline subxiphoid region, directed toward the left shoulder, to detect fluid in the pericardial space. As little as 200 mL of fluid can lead to tamponade, so any fluid seen should be taken into consideration in the content of the clinical scenario. Next, the probe is placed inferior to the right ribs in the anterior axillary line to visualize the hepatorenal space. Fluid here would be indicative of a hepatic injury. Position three is at the left tenth rib in the posterior axillary line to visualize the splenorenal space, looking for a splenic injury. Lastly, the probe is placed in the suprapubic position to look for pelvic fluid. Depending on the patient's overall condition, decisions regarding further care can be made based on the findings on a FAST examination. In performing this diagnostic examination, the limitations should be remembered. The FAST does not identify retroperitoneal or bowel injuries, nor does it identify injuries to the diaphragm, adrenal, pancreas, spine, pelvis, mesentery, or the vascular system.[4]

Secondary Survey

After the stabilization of the patient has occurred and any life-threatening injuries have been addressed, the secondary survey is undertaken. In essence, this is the formal history and physical examination that would be done for any patient who seeks medical care. Pertinent history must be obtained, including the events leading to the trauma, the trauma itself, and any medical-surgical history. This should be followed by a thorough physical examination, seeking any occult injury. Discovered injuries should be addressed at this time as well. That is, fractures should be stabilized; lacerations and open wounds should be irrigated and dressed.

Laboratory data should be used as an adjunct to elucidating injuries not obvious on physical examination. In the hemodynamically unstable patient, the only mandatory laboratory test is the cross-match for any transfusions that may be required. In the more stable patient, data should be obtained to aid in identifying occult injures and physiologic status. These include, but are not limited to, arterial blood gas, complete blood count, coagulation studies, blood chemistries, urinalysis, and toxicology screen.

Radiologic studies have become key components in the triage of the trauma patient. The studies that are obtained should be selected based on clinical evidence and suspicion of possible injuries since the armamentarium is quite wide and varied. Besides the FAST examination already discussed, other modalities include plain radiographs, CT, angiography, and magnetic resonance imaging (MRI).

A chest radiograph, lateral cervical spine radiograph, and pelvic radiograph constitute the trauma triple for blunt trauma. Based on the appearance of the chest radiograph, either further workup or definitive treatment can be made. Further workup generally consists of a computer tomography or angiogram looking for great vessel injury. Pneumothorax and hemothorax are easily identified on the radiograph, as are parenchymal disease and osseous injury. A lateral cervical spine film is used for screening purposes, but is limited and cannot be used solely to rule out spine injury. Pelvic radiograph is also used to discover any osseous fractures. Other plain radiographs are obtained for suspicion of injury from the clinical examination. Their greatest benefit is for extremity injuries and for serial follow-up after osseous injury repair.[5]

CT is becoming the major diagnostic test for traumatic injuries. It allows easy visualization of solid tissue and osseous tissue; it easily differentiates blood from ascites, as well as air from tissue or fluid; it allows visualization of the retroperitoneal space and other potential spaces; it has the ability to quantify or grade injuries; it provides for specific recognition of injuries; and it can visualize joint spaces. And now with the newer helical scanners, vascular injuries can be easily identified. Despite the wide usage of CT, its limitations should also be remembered. Evaluation for diaphragmatic, mesenteric, and bowel injuries remains limited by this modality, although new scanners, as well as two- and three-dimensional reconstructions of scanned images, have curtailed its shortcomings.[5,6]

MRI is a useful test to determine soft tissue injuries, particularly neural tissue. Not only is this test time consuming, it also requires the patient to be able to tolerate confined spaces and not have any ferromagnetic alloys in the body.

Angiography is helpful in diagnosing and possibly treating vascular injuries. Indication is once again based on clinical suspicion. Unusual findings on CT may also require further investigation with angiography. Care must be taken when performing this test, since it is more invasive than the other tests already mentioned. Significant complications can occur, including formation of a dissection, pseudoaneurysm, hematoma, or laceration. Contrast-induced nephropathy can also occur due to the contrast load that may be required, particularly if contrast was given for a previous CT.[5]

Trauma care has evolved into more nonoperative management strategies. The majority of the blunt trauma that occurs can be managed nonoperatively in the hospital, either on a regular ward floor or in the intensive care unit (ICU). This has led to more concise indications for operative management. In general, an operation is indicated for those patients with life-threatening injuries or those who fail nonoperative treatment. Both operative and nonoperative management are discussed later in the chapter.

SHOCK

Shock is one of the most formidable challenges the trauma surgeon faces. It is defined as a lack of oxygenation to cells due to inadequate perfusion, leading to loss of high-energy phosphates and electrochemical gradients and terminating in cellular death. It is a self-sustaining syndrome that has already begun and manifested its potential before the trauma patient has even arrived at the hospital. The basic tenet of shock treatment is based on early recognition and intervention. Not only does resuscitation need to occur, but also the cause must be elucidated and treated. In general, shock occurs due to a problem with the perfusate, the pump, or the pipes. That is, the intravascular volume is not adequate, a problem with the heart exists, or there is a problem with the vasculature.

Hypovolemic or hemorrhagic shock occurs due to the lack of adequate intravascular volume. This generally occurs due to exsanguination from the traumatic injury. Early recognition and treatment of the shock state, including stopping any ongoing blood loss, are of paramount importance. The degree of hemorrhagic shock can be grouped into four classes (Table 2-5).[7] Various clinical signs can aid in determining the shock class, which will also guide resuscitation to replace the intravascular volume, restore hemodynamic stability, and provide adequate oxygen.

Distributive shock occurs when sepsis, systemic inflammatory response syndrome, adrenal insufficiency, or anaphylaxis causes a profound vasodilation. Cytokines and other inflammatory mediators produce a redundant cascade of events that produce loss of vasomotor tone. Besides the supported resuscitation that ensues, the inciting event must be eliminated.[8]

Table 2-5 **Classes of Hemorrhagic Shock** [a]

	I	II	III	IV
Blood loss (mL)	<750	750–1500	1500–2000	>2000
Blood loss (%)	<15	15–30	30–40	>40
Pulse	<100	>100	>120	>140
Systolic blood pressure	Normal	Normal	90–110	<90
Pulse pressure	Normal or increased	Narrowed	Narrowed	Narrowed
Urine output (mL/h)	>30	15–30	5–15	<5
Mental status	Anxious	Agitated	Confused	Lethargic

[a]Based on 70 kg man's body weight.

Source: Adapted from American College of Surgeons Committee on Trauma: Shock. In *Advanced Trauma Life Support Program for Doctors*, 7th ed. Chicago, IL: American College of Surgeons, 2004: 69–97.

Shock due to loss of sympathetic tone is classified as neurogenic in nature. This may occur due to spinal cord trauma or compression, either from hematoma or tumor. Injuries above T4 usually have cardiac compromise along with the vascular system compromise, whereas injuries below T4 are usually not associated with cardiac compromise.[9]

Cardiogenic shock occurs when the pump fails. This may be due to myocardial failure, valvular disease, cardiac tamponade, or lack of venous return. Treatment will vary, depending on the etiology.

Each state will have different clinical parameters and measured values to aid in diagnosing the type of shock (Table 2-6). Parameters that are observed include heart rate, right heart filling pressure, cardiac output, left

Table 2-6 **Parameters in Shock States**

	Heart Rate	CVP	WP	CO	SVR	SVO$_2$
Hemorrhagic	↑	↓	↓	↓	↑	↓
Distributive	↑	↓	↓	↑	↓	↑
Cardiogenic	↓	↑	↑	↓	↑	↓
Neurogenic	N	↓	↓	N	↓	↓

heart filling pressure, systemic vascular resistance, and oxygen consumption. Treatment is aimed at optimizing filling pressures, cardiac output, and oxygen delivery.

COMMON ORGAN INJURIES

Head Injury

Traumatic brain injuries are a significant cause of morbidity and mortality among patients sustaining trauma, particularly from motor vehicle crashes and falls. According to the Brain Injury Association of America, 1.5 million Americans sustain a traumatic brain injury (TBI) each year, ranging from mild concussions to fatal brain injuries.[10] From 1995 to 2001 there were over 1.1 million emergency department visits, 235,000 hospitalizations, and 50,000 deaths attributed to TBI.[11,12] Falls are the leading cause of TBI in children from 0 to 4 years and in adults 75 years or older, but motor vehicle—traffic causes still result in the greatest number of TBI-related hospitalizations and deaths. Assaults account for about 11 percent of annual TBI-related emergency department visits, hospitalizations, and deaths. It is estimated that 80,000–90,000 people annually experience the onset of long-term disability as the result of TBI. The cost of TBI is estimated to be $48.3 billion each year in the United States.[13]

The primary mechanisms of head injury include concussion, compression, deceleration, and rotational acceleration. These mechanisms can account for a number of different pathologic conditions associated with head injury, including skull fracture, concussion, brain contusion, extradural hematoma, subarachnoid hemorrhage, and diffuse axonal injury (DAI). Skull fractures may be linear or stellate, depressed or nondepressed, and may involve the cranial vault or the skull base. Basilar skull fractures may be associated with cerebrospinal fluid (CSF) leak and a higher risk for subsequent meningeal infection.

Concussion is a transient loss of consciousness that may not be associated with apparent tissue injury or neurologic deficit, although retrograde and/or antegrade amnesia is not an uncommon finding.

Cerebral contusion, or intracerebral hematoma, typically occurs in the frontal or temporal lobe and is characterized by localized tissue injury and hemorrhage. It may lead to further bleeding, elevated intracranial pressure (ICP), or posttraumatic seizure disorder.

In addition to intracerebral hematoma, intracranial hematomas may be subdural (beneath the dura) or epidural (between the skull and dura) (Fig. 2-4). *Acute subdural hematomas* generally are due to rupture of bridging veins between the brain and dura, whereas *epidural hematomas* are typically due to arterial laceration, most notably the middle meningeal artery where it crosses underneath the temporal bone. Subdural hematomas are more common, are frequently associated with underlying cerebral contusion, and the prognosis

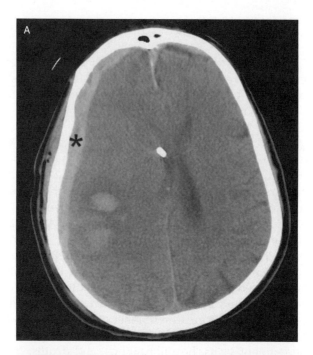

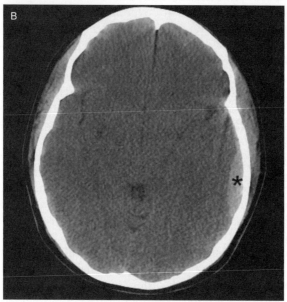

Figure 2-4 *(A) CT scan images of an acute sub-dural hematoma and (B) a lens-shaped epidural hematoma (asterisks). The subdural hematoma is also associated with an intraparenchymal brain contusion in the right parietal area.*

is worse than for epidural hematomas because of the associated brain injury. Epidural hematomas have been classically described as producing a *lucid interval* in which the patient initially loses consciousness (concussion), then recovers, and finally develops progressive neurologic deterioration as the lesion expands.

DAI is a generalized shear-type injury involving axons in the brain white matter. Damaged axons are typically interspersed among normal axons and may show up on CT scan as petechial hemorrhage. MRI scanning, however, is more sensitive than CT for detecting DAI. A wide spectrum of clinical presentations—and neurologic outcomes—may result from DAI.

It is important to conduct a thorough neurologic evaluation when assessing a patient for TBI. The GCS score, as previously described, provides an objective clinical measure of the extent of the brain injury based on the patient's best eye opening, verbal, and motor responses (Table 2-4). Frequent reevaluation of a patient's neurologic status is imperative to ascertain neurologic deterioration that may require neurosurgical intervention.

Diagnosis of TBI is best accomplished by noncontrasted CT scan. This will identify any areas of hemorrhage, as well as skull fractures, retained missile fragments, and evidence of generalized brain edema or midline shift.

Prevention of secondary brain injury due to decreased perfusion and hypoxemia of the brain is of paramount importance during the initial management of TBI. *Cerebral perfusion pressure* (CPP), defined as the difference in mean arterial pressure (MAP) and ICP, should be kept at least at 70 mmHg. Thus, the management strategy necessarily involves controlling systemic blood pressure as well as ICP. Systolic hypotension to less than 90 mmHg has been shown to be associated with a worse neurologic outcome in patients with TBI. Such patients should be resuscitated, as any trauma patient, with crystalloid solutions and perhaps even hypertonic saline solution to maintain MAP and decrease cerebral edema. Once hypovolemia is corrected, the judicious use of vasopressors may be required to maintain the MAP in the desired range. ICP monitoring, as well as mechanical ventilation, is generally indicated for severe TBI, and may be accomplished with an intraparenchymal ICP monitor or with a ventriculostomy catheter. The latter method also allows for drainage of CSF. ICP should be kept below 20 mmHg. First-line treatments to lower the ICP include elevation of head to 30°, hyperventilation to PCO_2 of 30–35 mmHg to decrease intracerebral vascular volume, and administration of mannitol, an osmotic diuretic, to reduce brain edema.[14] Additionally, patients with moderate to severe TBI should receive prophylactic anticonvulsant medication. There is no role for corticosteroids in the management of TBI.[15]

Indications for operative intervention include increasing neurologic impairment or a mass effect causing more than 5 mm midline shift. Additionally, depressed skull fractures may need to be elevated or debrided.

If the ICP is controllable with the methods outlined above and the clinical status is stable, continued close observation is indicated.

Spine and Spinal Cord Injury

Spinal cord injury has an incidence of about 11,000 new cases each year in the United States. The average age at the time of injury is 38 years, and 78 percent of SCI occur in males. Motor vehicle crashes account for about half of the injuries, while falls are responsible for 24 percent, acts of violence cause 11 percent, and recreational sporting activities comprise about 9 percent of SCI.[16]

SCI can be categorized as complete or incomplete. An *incomplete* injury is one in which there is any degree of sensory or motor function below the level of the injury. Incomplete quadriplegia is the most common lesion, occurring about 35 percent of the time, followed by complete paraplegia (25 percent), complete quadriplegia (22 percent), and incomplete paraplegia (18 percent).[16] A diagnosis of a *complete* SCI cannot be made with certainty during the first few days following injury because of possible confounding spinal shock. Spinal shock is a reversible condition that refers to muscle flaccidity and areflexia seen not infrequently after SCI. It is differentiated from neurogenic shock, which is due to interruption of descending sympathetic pathways, producing vasodilatation, bradycardia, and hypotension.

Incomplete SCI may also be associated with several syndromes, including the central cord syndrome, Brown-Séquard syndrome, and anterior spinal cord syndrome. The *central cord syndrome*, the most common of these syndromes, is characterized by greater motor loss in the upper extremities than in the lower extremities; sensory loss is variable. It commonly occurs as a hyperextension injury (e.g., a fall forward) in a patient who has cervical spondylosis and spinal canal narrowing. The *Brown-Séquard syndrome* is uncommon following trauma, usually with penetrating injuries to the spine. This syndrome clinically manifests as motor loss on the side ipsilateral to the lesion and pain and temperature loss on the contralateral side. The *anterior spinal cord syndrome* is due to trauma or ischemia in the territory of the anterior spinal artery. Motor, pain, and temperature sensation are lost, but posterior column functions of vibration, position, and deep pressure sense are preserved. It has the worst prognosis for recovery of the incomplete syndromes discussed.

Patients, sustaining significant trauma, who have neck or spine tenderness, distracting injuries, or altered mental status due to injury or substance abuse, must be evaluated further for spine or SCI. They must remain immobilized in a cervical collar and logrolling precautions should be undertaken. A complete physical examination should be carried out, paying particular attention to any spine tenderness, deformities, and sensorimotor examination. Sacral sparing, or preservation of some perianal sensation, and the presence or absence of a bulbocavernosus reflex should be documented.

The presence of either of these findings indicates an incomplete SCI, hence a better prognosis.

Radiographic evaluation of spine and SCIs is evolving. In the past, multiple plain radiographs were used to identify fractures or subluxation. More recently, CT scanning of the cervical, thoracic, and lumbar spine with coronal and sagittal reformats have become popular due to greater sensitivity compared to plain films.[17–19] MRI is usually reserved to detect soft tissue lesions, such as a herniated disk, a spinal epidural hematoma, or spinal cord contusion, that are less likely to be diagnosed with CT scan in patients with neurologic deficits. The stability or instability of spine fractures must be determined before removing spinal or logrolling precautions. This may entail further radiologic imaging, such as flexion and extension films of the cervical spine, to determine if ligamentous injury, in addition to skeletal injury, has occurred.

Airway management principles should be followed, as is the case with any trauma patient. Inline stabilization of the cervical spine must be done in preparation for orotracheal intubation. Patients with high- or midlevel cervical SCI may have respiratory insufficiency due to loss of diaphragm and/or accessory muscle function. These patients may become ventilator-dependent and are at high risk for infectious pulmonary complications.

The use of corticosteroids for SCI is somewhat controversial, but should be considered for patients who have sustained a blunt, nonpenetrating, mechanism of injury. Data from the National Spinal Cord Injury studies indicate that neurologic outcome is improved (though slightly) if steroids are given intravenously within the first 8 h of injury. Methylprednisolone is given as a bolus dose of 30 mg/kg, followed by an infusion of 5.4 mg/kg/h. If given within 3 h of injury, the infusion should last for 24 h. If given between 3 and 8 h after injury, the infusion should be continued for 48 h. The immunosuppressive effect of high-dose steroids must be weighed against the potential benefit, particularly if the steroids are to be continued for 48 h.[20–22]

Surgical management of spine and SCIs may be indicated to decompress the spinal cord and to stabilize an unstable axial skeleton. Once subluxation is reduced, the involved vertebrae may be operatively fused using a number of techniques incorporating bone graft, plates, and screws. External braces, such as the halo vest, may also be used to immobilize the spine without surgical intervention.

Neck Injury

The high concentration of vital structures in the neck makes the evaluation of neck injuries somewhat problematic. Consideration must be given to injuries of the aerodigestive tract, cervical vascular structures, nerves, and the cervical spine. Unfortunately, symptoms and signs may be absent or poorly predictive of injury, for example, to the esophagus, carotid, or vertebral arteries. Thus, a high index of suspicion must be maintained and multiple diagnostic modalities may be required to exclude occult injuries.

Blunt injuries to the neck are usually due to direct blows, deceleration and stretch-type mechanisms, or strangulation. Cervical spine injuries must be ruled out by careful examination, radiographic study, or both. The neck should be kept immobilized in a cervical collar until evaluation of the cervical spine is complete. Airway injury to the larynx or trachea may present with subcutaneous emphysema, shortness of breath, hemoptysis, hoarseness, or complete airway obstruction. Immediate or early control of the airway by cricothyroidotomy or tracheostomy may be required. Fiber-optic evaluation of the upper airway and the tracheobronchial tree is a useful adjunct to determine the presence or absence of an airway injury.

Blunt esophageal injuries are extremely rare, but the morbidity associated with missed pharyngoesophageal injuries mandates that patients with possible neck injuries should undergo thorough evaluation. Barium or Gastrografin swallow examination should be performed for suspected pharyngoesophageal injury; esophagoscopy should also be considered to further increase diagnostic accuracy.

Blunt cervical vascular injuries to the carotid and vertebral arteries may be completely asymptomatic or may present with a neurologic deficit either immediately or in a delayed fashion. There is likely an under appreciation of the mechanism of injury, usually a sudden deceleration, hyperextension/neck rotation, or direct compression by automobile safety belts.[23] Most blunt injuries to the carotid or vertebral arteries consist of intimal dissection, intramural hematoma, thrombotic occlusion, or pseudoaneurysm formation. Conventional angiography is considered the gold standard method of diagnosis, but the role of CT angiography is evolving.[24] The majority of these patients are treated nonoperatively. Systemic anticoagulation is the therapy of choice to prevent thrombus formation, although prospective, randomized data are lacking.[25] Endovascular stenting of carotid artery injuries and angioembolization of pseudoaneurysms have also added to the nonoperative management of these injuries.

Penetrating neck injuries from stab wounds or gunshot wounds have historically been classified based on the anatomic zone of injury (Fig. 2-5). *Zone I* injuries are those near the thoracic inlet, below the level of the cricoid cartilage. From a practical standpoint, such injuries cannot be accessed surgically by a cervical incision and require sternotomy or thoracotomy. *Zone II* injuries are those from the level of the cricoid cartilage to the angle of the mandible. *Zone III* injuries are those that occur above the angle of the mandible.

Zone I injuries are associated with injuries to the tracheobronchial tree, esophagus, and the great vessels. Evaluation of these structures by bronchoscopy, barium swallow/esophagoscopy, and angiography or CT angiography is indicated.

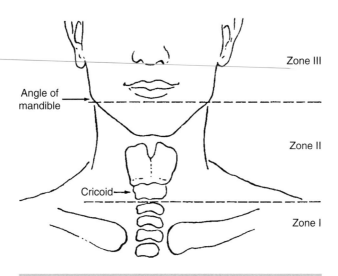

Figure 2-5 **Zones of the neck used to classify penetrating neck wounds.** (*Source:* Adapted from Wilson RF, Diebel L. Injuries to the neck. In Wilson RF, Walt AJ, eds., *Management of Trauma: Pitfalls and Practice*, 2nd ed. Baltimore, MD: Williams & Wilkins, 1996: 270–287.)

The diagnosis and management of Zone II injuries are controversial.[26] In the past, mandatory exploration of Zone II penetrating injuries was advocated for all wounds that disrupted the platysma. However, the negative exploration rate was as high as 67 percent, and the morbidity of a negative neck exploration was not insignificant.[27,28] The advantage of mandatory neck exploration is close to 0 percent missed injury rate and possibly a reduction in hospital costs associated with obtaining multiple diagnostic studies. Presently, a selective surgical approach is generally indicated, reserving operative neck exploration for injuries found on examination or by diagnostic study and, perhaps, for high caliber or bilateral Zone II gunshot wounds to the neck. If a policy of selective surgical management is followed, it is imperative that diagnostic studies are promptly available to rule out aerodigestive tract and vascular injuries. The expanded use of CT scanning, including CT angiography, as a screening modality to evaluate the carotid and vertebral arteries, as well as the aerodigestive tract, may limit the need for other, conventional, diagnostic studies.

Finally, Zone III injuries are high in the neck, usually precluding operative intervention. Injuries to consider in Zone III are to the carotid and vertebral arteries, thus, either CT angiography or conventional arteriography is indicated.

Thoracic Injury

Thoracic injuries, whether from penetrating or blunt mechanisms, account for significant morbidity and mortality following trauma. It is likely that thoracic injuries, such as traumatic aortic injury, tension pneumothorax, and cardiac tamponade, are a major cause of mortality in patients who die at the scene of injury or prior to arrival at the hospital.[29]

Evaluation of a patient following chest injury must be expeditious. Cardiogenic or hemorrhagic shock and respiratory failure may ensue quickly after sustaining traumatic chest injuries. Injuries that must be immediately considered in an unstable patient after arrival to the emergency department include tension pneumothorax, cardiac tamponade, massive hemothorax, traumatic aortic injury, and diaphragmatic rupture.

Tension pneumothorax should be a clinical, not a radiographic, diagnosis in the majority of cases. Tension pneumothorax occurs when lung or open chest wall injury results in an accumulation of air in the pleural space under pressure as the result of a *one-way valve* phenomenon. The lung on that side totally collapses, and the pressure in the hemithorax causes the mediastinum to shift to the opposite side. Cardiac diastolic filling is impaired, resulting in cardiogenic shock. Diagnosis of tension pneumothorax is made by the observation of respiratory distress, tachycardia, hypotension, distended neck veins, and unilateral absence of breath sounds. Immediate treatment is needle decompression of the affected hemithorax by a large bore needle in the second intercostal space in the midclavicular line. This maneuver decompresses the *tension* component of the pneumothorax and allows for the placement of a thoracostomy tube as the definitive treatment of the pneumothorax.

Cardiac tamponade is another entity to consider in an unstable patient following chest trauma. Beck's triad, consisting of hypotension, distended neck veins, and muffled heart sounds, is the classic description of cardiac tamponade, but it is not uncommon for the complete triad to be absent.[30] Hypovolemia due to blood loss, for example, may result in flat neck veins, even in the presence of tamponade. The finding of pulsus paradoxus, whereby the systolic pressure falls by more than 10 mmHg with inspiration, is another sign of cardiac tamponade, but may be difficult to ascertain in the emergency setting. Ultrasound may be a very useful diagnostic adjunct to evaluate for fluid in the pericardial sac, but it should not delay resuscitation or intervention. Pericardiocentesis using a subxiphoid approach may be lifesaving in instances of cardiac tamponade. Thoracotomy or median sternotomy are best performed in the operating room for definitive diagnosis and treatment.

Massive hemothorax may occur following penetrating or blunt trauma. Signs and symptoms of unilateral chest injury, such as multiple rib fractures, dullness to percussion, and decreased ipsilateral breath sounds are suggestive of hemothorax, which can be confirmed by a portable chest radiograph.

It is important to keep in mind that several hundred milliliters or more of fluid in the chest cavity are needed to appreciate a significant hemothorax on a supine radiograph. The initial treatment of a hemothorax is a large bore (at least no. 32 or 36 French catheter) chest tube. Most hemothoraces, approximately 90 percent, are treated only with a chest tube and do not require operative intervention. Indications for surgery are (1) greater than 1500 mL out of the chest tube on insertion, or (2) continued chest tube output of greater than 200–300 mL/h for several hours.

Traumatic aortic injury may occur following a deceleration-type injury such as a motor vehicle crash or a fall from a significant height. It is estimated that 16 percent of deaths, due to immediately fatal automobile crashes, are due to rupture of the aorta; it is estimated that approximately 8000 deaths a year in the United States are attributable to great vessel injury.[31,32] The most common site of aortic injury following blunt trauma is at the ligamentum arteriosum just past the takeoff of the left subclavian artery. This location of injury, corresponding with the area of maximal fixation of the aorta, is subject to high shear stress and torsion with deceleration-type mechanisms of injury. A high index of suspicion for aortic injury must be maintained in patients sustaining a significant mechanism of injury. Due to the potential for multiple injuries in patients who present with possible aortic injury, the initial workup consists of an anteroposterior (AP) chest radiograph. Although limited, particularly in obese patients, the chest radiograph may provide important findings that are associated with traumatic aortic rupture (Table 2-7). Helical contrast-enhanced CT scanning of the chest has emerged as a highly sensitive and specific screening test for blunt aortic rupture.[33,34] If the CT scan shows no periaortic hematoma or irregularity of the contour of the aorta, aortic injury can be ruled out. Aortography, however, is still considered the gold standard for diagnosis at this time. Figure 2-6 depicts some of the radiographic findings associated with traumatic aortic injury. Patients diagnosed with aortic injury should have their blood

Table 2-7 **Findings Associated with Traumatic Aortic Injury on Plain Chest Radiograph**

- Widened mediastinum
- Obliteration of the aortic knob and aortopulmonary window
- Apical cap
- Deviation of trachea, esophagus, or nasogastric tube to the right
- Depression of left mainstem bronchus
- Fractures of sternum, scapula, first or second ribs
- Widened paratracheal stripe

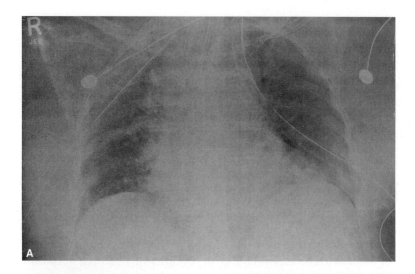

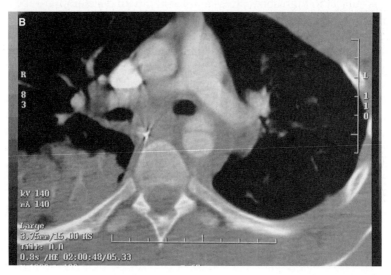

Figure 2-6 **Radiographic findings in traumatic aortic injury. (A) Plain chest radiograph showing a widened mediastinum. (B) CT scan showing intimal flap in the descending thoracic aorta, which is surrounded by hematoma. (C) Aortogram demonstrating aortic disruption distal to the left subclavian takeoff, the usual site for blunt aortic injury.**

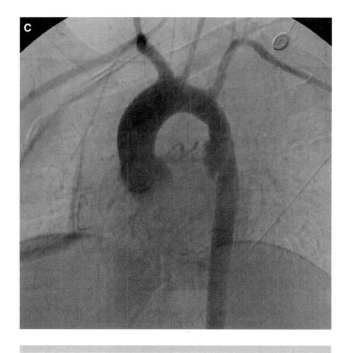

Figure 2-6 (**Continued**)

pressure tightly controlled to below a systolic pressure of 110 or 120 mmHg to diminish the chance of in-hospital free rupture and exsanguination. Repair of the aorta is indicated with an interposition graft or, if feasible from a technical standpoint, the more recent method of endovascular stenting.[35]

Traumatic diaphragmatic rupture with herniation of abdominal viscera into the chest (Fig. 2-7) can also be life threatening. Hemorrhage, torsion of the herniated abdominal contents leading to ischemia, and mediastinal shift from mass effect leading to cardiac failure all must be considered in the acute setting. These injuries should be treated via an abdominal approach to fully assess the extent of abdominal visceral injury.

In addition to the immediately life-threatening thoracic injuries described above, several other specific entities related to blunt or penetrating chest trauma deserve mention. Among these are rib fractures/flail chest, pulmonary contusion, blunt cardiac injury, and transmediastinal gunshot wounds.

Flail chest is defined as an unstable chest wall resulting from fractures to three or more adjacent ribs, with each rib fractured in more than one location. Paradoxical motion of the chest wall occurs during respiration. There is frequently an underlying pulmonary contusion that contributes to respiratory insufficiency and increased work of breathing, necessitating mechanical

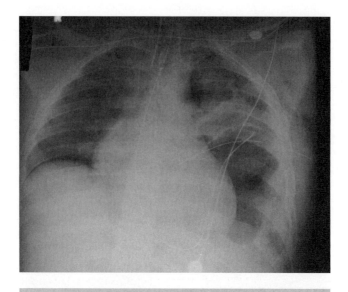

Figure 2-7 **Plain chest radiograph depicting traumatic diaphragmatic herniation. Note the indistinct left hemidiaphragm and the nasogastric tube extending into the left chest.**

ventilation. Treatment involves careful fluid management to prevent fluid overload, vigorous pulmonary toilet to prevent atelectasis and pneumonia, and adequate analgesia, including consideration of a thoracic epidural catheter.

Blunt cardiac injury can rarely result in chamber rupture, valvular disruption, or pericardial tamponade, but more commonly, myocardial contusion occurs. Definitive diagnosis of myocardial contusion can be established only by pathology, but the clinical diagnosis is inferred by ECG changes, including conduction abnormalities and arrhythmias, and echocardiography, which may be indicated to look for wall motion abnormality. Most arrhythmias will manifest in the first 24 h following injury, so patients should be placed in a monitored setting during this time period.[36]

With regard to penetrating trauma, transmediastinal gunshot wounds may be associated with injuries to multiple structures, including the heart and great vessels, lung parenchyma, tracheobronchial tree, esophagus, bones, and spinal cord. Helical CT scanning is a useful test to help define the missile tract and specific injuries, but it may not obviate the need for further diagnostic tests such as esophagography/esophagoscopy and bronchoscopy.[37] Indications for surgery depend on the findings of the diagnostic workup.

Abdominal and Pelvic Injury

The evaluation and management of abdominal trauma must be done in the context of the mechanism of injury. Abdominal injuries resulting from blunt forces must be specifically sought out with diagnostic testing, whereas those resulting from gunshot wounds, for example, may not require any diagnostic tests prior to operative intervention.

The evaluation of blunt abdominal trauma due to motor vehicle crashes, direct blows, or falls has evolved in the past decade. Diagnostic peritoneal lavage (DPL) used to be the standard, rapid method to detect intraperitoneal blood. This has been largely replaced by the FAST examination in most trauma centers. The FAST examination is a quick, noninvasive bedside examination that uses ultrasound to detect peritoneal or pericardial fluid. It has a reported sensitivity rate of up to 88 percent, a specificity rate of about 99 percent, and accuracy rate of 98 percent, but cannot provide detailed information about specific organ injury.[38] It is less useful to evaluate retroperitoneal injuries and hollow viscus injuries. At our institution we have found it to be most useful in hypotensive patients who are unstable to go to CT scan, but need a rapid test to assess for intra-abdominal hemorrhage that would require surgery.

CT scanning is the primary diagnostic modality in hemodynamically stable patients who have sustained blunt abdominal trauma. The current generation helical scanners provide rapid, high quality images that are very specific for organ injury and have an accuracy of around 95 percent. A CT scan can miss bowel injuries; therefore, there is still no substitute for comprehensive initial and serial physical examinations of the patient who has sustained blunt trauma. The CT scan is also useful for detecting injury to retroperitoneal organs, such as the kidney, pancreas, and duodenum.

The spleen is the most commonly injured abdominal organ following blunt trauma. Injury to the spleen is frequently associated with left lower chest trauma and lower rib fractures. Hemodynamically unstable patients with a positive FAST examination should go straight to the operating room for exploratory laparotomy and either splenectomy or splenorrhaphy. Stable patients undergo CT scanning, which enables one to grade the severity of the spleen injury, which, in turn, is predictive of the success of nonoperative management. A trend toward nonoperative management of spleen injuries in recent years is based on the known immunologic function of the intact spleen and the increased susceptibility to the overwhelming postsplenectomy infection (OPSI) syndrome in asplenic patients. The incidence of OPSI is estimated to be about 1–2 percent following splenectomy in adults, but the mortality may be as high as 50 percent. Infections from encapsulated organisms, such as Pneumococcus and Meningococcus, predominate in splenectomized patients, but there is also evidence for increased risk from viral illness and nonencapsulated bacteria. The nonoperative management of spleen

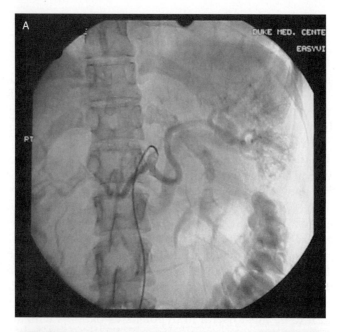

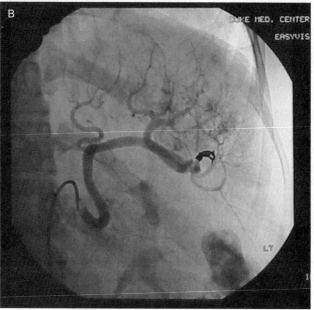

Figure 2-8 **(A) Pre- and (B) postangiographic embolization of a high-grade splenic laceration involving mainly the lower pole of the spleen. Embolization reduces the blood flow to the spleen, thereby reducing hemorrhage and increasing the success of nonoperative management of this injury.**

injuries is successful over 80 percent of the time; this success rate may be further enhanced by more recent angioembolization techniques by interventional radiologists (Fig. 2-8). It is important to conduct serial examinations and hematocrit determinations in patients who have sustained blunt splenic injury and are managed nonoperatively because some of these patients, particularly with higher-grade injuries, will develop delayed bleeding complications requiring surgery.[39,40]

Liver injuries are also common following abdominal trauma. As with spleen injuries, liver injuries due to blunt trauma are frequently managed nonoperatively, as long as concomitant bowel injuries are ruled out. CT scanning, again, is the diagnostic test of choice in stable patients because it allows one to grade the severity of the injury to the liver. Unstable patients with large liver lacerations may sustain large blood loss and transfusion requirements resulting in the lethal triad of hypothermia, acidosis, and coagulopathy. In these situations, a *damage control* laparotomy is frequently done in order to stop any *surgical* bleeding, stop any ongoing contamination from bowel injuries, and tamponade nonsurgical bleeding with laparotomy packs. The patient is then taken to the ICU for further resuscitation and correction of hypothermia, coagulopathy, and acidosis. The *open abdomen* also reduces the risk of abdominal compartment syndrome secondary to massive fluid resuscitation.[41] A definitive laparotomy procedure is then performed in 1 or 2 days. This approach to patients with massive liver injuries, or other intra-abdominal injuries resulting in massive fluid resuscitation and blood product transfusion, has yielded reduced mortality rates and improved outcomes in patients sustaining severe abdominal injuries.[42]

Gunshot wounds to the abdomen that traverse the peritoneum are generally best treated by expeditious exploratory laparotomy. Because of the large surface area of the bowel, intestinal injuries are commonly encountered following penetrating abdominal trauma. The overriding principle of the operative management of abdominal gunshot wounds is to thoroughly explore the entire abdomen, tracing the missile tract from entry to exit, examining the entire length of intestine, and inspecting the abdominal viscera and vasculature in proximity to the missile path.

Pelvic fractures are common injuries that are among the most challenging that a trauma surgeon will encounter. Although many pelvic fractures are relatively minor and may not even require specific treatment, disruption of the pelvic ring takes considerable force that may result in life-threatening hemorrhage and associated injuries. In fact, the main cause of death in patients with pelvic fractures is exsanguinating hemorrhage. Pelvic fractures may result from (1) AP compression, producing an *open book* type disruption of the pelvis; (2) lateral compression; and (3) vertical shear, resulting in Malgaigne fractures typically seen after a fall from heights and other mechanisms that produce a vertically oriented force applied to the anterior and posterior aspects of the pelvic ring (Fig. 2-9).

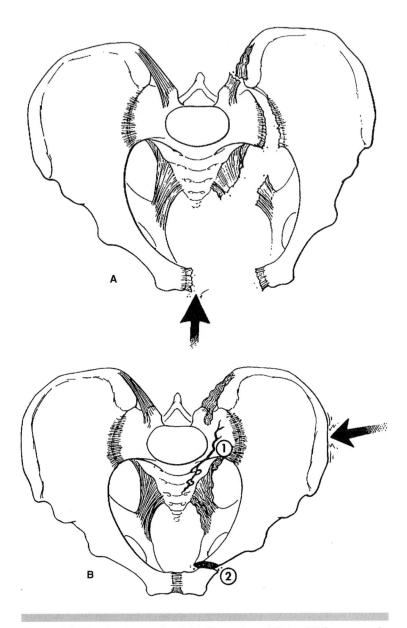

Figure 2-9 **Mechanisms of pelvic disruption. (A) An AP force resulting in an open book pelvis. (B) A lateral compressive force disrupting the pelvic ring. (C) A vertical shear force, or Malgaigne,
fracture.** (*Source:* Adapted from Wilson RF, Tyburski J, Georgiadis GM.
Pelvic fractures. In Wilson RF, Walt AJ, eds., *Management of Trauma:
Pitfalls and Practice,* 2nd ed. Baltimore, MD: Williams & Wilkins, 1996:
580–581.)

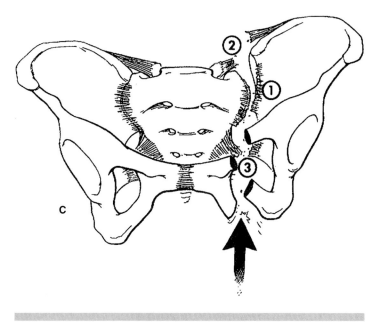

Figure 2-9 **(Continued)**

Goals of immediate evaluation and management of patients with pelvic fractures are to stabilize the bony pelvis, assess for intra-abdominal hemorrhage or other associated injuries that may require emergent surgery, control hemorrhage, and provide adequate resuscitation. An unstable pelvis, for instance one with a large open book component, should be stabilized initially with a pelvic binder or even a crossed bedsheet in order to reduce the increased pelvic volume and pelvic hemorrhage. Further stabilization with an external fixator device may also be expeditiously applied in the emergency department or operating room. Hypotensive patients with pelvic fractures undergo a FAST examination, specifically looking for fluid in the upper abdomen around the spleen and liver; such findings imply concomitant visceral injury requiring immediate surgery. If hemorrhage from extrapelvic sources has been ruled out and the patient remains hypotensive, an immediate arteriogram with angiographic embolization may be lifesaving. Pelvic bleeding is best approached by this method, rather than surgery, unless perineal, rectal, or vaginal lacerations are also present. Once stabilized, CT scan is done to rule out concomitant injuries, including bowel injuries or injuries to the urologic tract. Algorithm for the initial assessment and management of pelvic fractures is indicated in Fig. 2-10.

Management of pelvic fractures

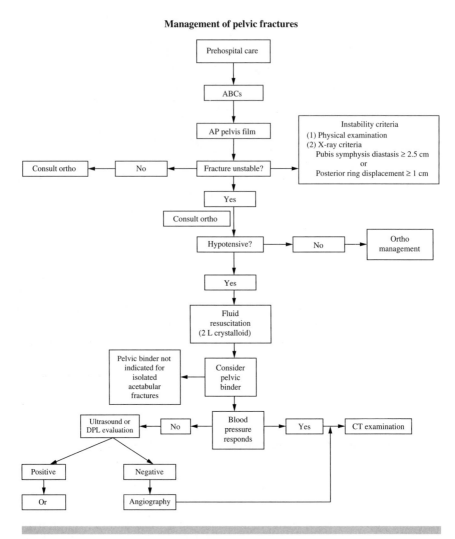

Figure 2-10 **Algorithm for management of pelvic fractures.**

Extremity Injury

Extremity injury may be associated with bony fracture, vascular disruption, nerve injury, and soft tissue crush, contusion, or avulsion. Broken extremities should be splinted after a thorough neurovascular examination. *Hard* signs of acute arterial injury include pulsatile bleeding, expanding hematoma, presence of a bruit or thrill, or frank ischemia associated with a pulse deficit or absence of Doppler signals. In such cases, irreversible nerve damage may occur as soon as 6 h following injury; therefore it is essential to make a quick diagnosis and revascularize the extremity as expeditiously as possible. Obtaining an arteriogram in these cases may only delay the time to revascularization. On the other hand, arteriogram is clearly indicated in instances where a limb is not frankly ischemic, but a pulse deficit is present. An ankle-brachial index, as determined by Doppler, of less than 0.9 compared to the contralateral side is a frequently used criterion for obtaining an arteriogram.[43] In cases of gunshot wounds or stab wounds to an extremity, proximity of the injury tract to a major extremity vessel is no longer considered an indication for arteriography.[44]

Compartment syndrome may be associated with vascular compromise or swelling of the muscle compartments due to crush, contusion, or associated fractures. Signs and symptoms of compartment syndrome include tense muscle compartment, paresthesias, neurologic deficit, paralysis, and diminished pulses or Doppler signals. Diagnosis can be easily confirmed by transducing a compartment pressure with a needle manometer or commercially available device. Compartment pressures exceeding 20–30 mmHg may be sufficient to obstruct capillary flow and produce a compartment syndrome. Treatment is immediate fasciotomy to release the involved muscle compartment. Sequelae of compartment syndrome or crush injury include rhabdomyolysis, hyperkalemia, and renal failure. Therapy is directed at adequate fluid resuscitation, diuresis with mannitol, which may enhance urine flow through its osmotic diuretic effect and also scavenge oxygen free radicals, and alkalinization of urine, which may prevent precipitation of myoglobin within the renal tubules.

REFERENCES

1. Available at: http://www.trauma.org/history/timeline.html.

2. McSwain N. Kinematics of trauma. In Mattox KL, Feliciano DV, Moore EE, eds., *Trauma*, 4th ed. New York: McGraw-Hill, 2000: 127–152.

3. American College of Surgeons Committee on Trauma: Initial Assessment and Management. In *Advanced Trauma Life Support Program for Doctors*, 7th ed. Chicago, IL: American College of Surgeons, 2004: 11–29.

4. McGahan J, Richards J, Gillen M. The focused abdominal sonography for trauma scan. *J Ultrasound Med* 21:789–800, 2002.

5. Guyot DR, McCarrol KA, Wilson RF. Diagnostic and interventional radiology in trauma. In Wilson RF, Walt AJ, eds., *Management of Trauma: Pitfalls and Practice*, 2nd ed. Baltimore, MD: Williams & Wilkins, 1996: 105–127.

6. Demetriades D, Velmahos G. Technology driven triage of abdominal trauma: the emerging era of nonoperative management. *Annu Rev Med* 54:1–15, 2003.

7. American College of Surgeons Committee on Trauma: Shock. In *Advanced Trauma Life Support Program for Doctors*, 7th ed. Chicago, IL: American College of Surgeons, 2004: 69–97.

8. Marino PL. Hemorrhage and hypovolemia. In *The ICU Book*, 2nd ed. Philadelphia, PA: Lippincott Williams & Wilkins, 1998: 207–227.

9. Shoemaker WC. Diagnosis and treatment of shock syndromes. In Ayres SM, Grenvik A, Holbrook PR, et al., eds., *Textbook of Critical Care*, 3rd ed. Philadelphia, PA: W.B. Saunders, 1995: 85–102.

10. Brain Injury Association of America. Available at: www.biausa.org.

11. Langlois JA, Rutland-Brown W, Thomas KE. *Traumatic Brain Injury in the United States: Emergency Department Visits, Hospitalizations, and Deaths*. Atlanta, GA: Centers for Disease Control and Prevention, National Center for Injury Prevention and Control, 2004.

12. Thurman DJ, Alverson C, Browne D, et al. *Traumatic Brain Injury in the United States: A Report to Congress*. Atlanta, GA: Centers for Disease Control and Prevention, National Center for Injury Prevention and Control, 1999.

13. Lewin ICF. *The Cost of Disorders of the Brain*. Washington, DC: The National Foundation for Brain Research, 1992.

14. Brain Trauma Foundation, Inc., American Association of Neurological Surgeons. *Management and Prognosis of Severe Traumatic Brain Injury*. New York, NY: Brain Trauma Foundation, Inc., 2000.

15. Roberts I, Yates D, Sandercock P, et al. Effect of intravenous corticosteroids on death within 14 days in 10008 adults with clinically significant head injury (MRC CRASH trial): randomized placebo-controlled trial. *Lancet* 364:1321–1328, 2004.

16. National Spinal Cord Injury Statistical Center. *Spinal Cord Injury: Facts and Figures at a Glance*. Birmingham, AL: The University of Alabama at Birmingham, 2004.

17. Diaz JJ Jr., Gillman C, Morris JA Jr., et al. Are five-view plain films of the cervical spine reliable? A prospective evaluation in blunt trauma patients with altered mental status. *J Trauma* 55:658–664, 2003.

18. Griffen MM, Frykberg ER, Kerwin AJ, et al. Radiographic clearance of blunt cervical spine injury: plain radiograph or computed tomography scan? *J Trauma* 55:222–227, 2003.

19. Hauser CJ, Visvikis G, Hinrichs C, et al. Prospective validation of computed tomographic screening of the thoracolumbar spine in trauma. *J Trauma* 55:228–235, 2003.

20. Bracken MB, Shepard MJ, Collins WF, et al. A randomized, controlled trial of methylprednisolone or naloxone in the treatment of acute spinal cord injury. Results of the Second National Acute Spinal Cord Injury Study. *N Engl J Med* 322:1405–1411, 1990.

21. Bracken MB, Shepard MJ, Holford TR, et al. Administration of methylprednisolone for 24 or 48 hours or tirilazad mesylate for 48 hours in the treatment of acute spinal cord injury. Results of the Third National Acute Spinal Cord Injury Randomized Controlled Trial. National Acute Spinal Cord Injury Study. *JAMA* 277:1597–1604, 1997.

22. Coleman WP, Benzel D, Cahill DW, et al. A critical appraisal of the reporting of the National Acute Spinal Cord Injury Studies (II and III) of methylprednisolone in acute spinal cord injury. *J Spinal Disord* 13:185–199, 2000.

23. Biffl WL, Moore EE, Offner PJ, et al. Blunt carotid and vertebral artery injuries. *World J Surg* 25:1036–1043, 2001.

24. Berne JD, Norwood SH, McAuley CE, et al. Helical computed tomographic angiography: an excellent screening test for blunt cerebrovascular injury. *J Trauma* 57:11–19, 2004.

25. Eachempati SR, Vaslef SN, Sebastian MW, et al. Blunt vascular injuries of the head and neck: Is heparinization necessary? *J Trauma* 45:997–1003, 1998.

26. Wilson RF, Diebel L. Injuries to the neck. In Wilson RF, Walt AJ, eds., *Management of Trauma: Pitfalls and Practice*, 2nd ed. Baltimore, MD: Williams & Wilkins, 1996: 270–287.

27. Saletta JD, Lowe RJ, Leonardo TL, et al. Penetrating injuries of the neck. *J Trauma* 16:579–587, 1976.

28. Obeid FN, Hadad GS, Horst HM, et al. A critical reappraisal of a mandatory exploration policy for penetrating wounds of the neck. *Surg Gynecol Obstet* 160:517–522, 1985.

29. LoCicero J, Mattox KL. Epidemiology of chest trauma. *Surg Clin North Am* 59:15, 1989.

30. Wilson RF, Stephenson LW. Thoracic trauma: heart. In Wilson RF, Walt AJ, eds., *Management of Trauma: Pitfalls and Practice*, 2nd ed. Baltimore, MD: Williams & Wilkins, 1996: 343–360.

31. Greendyke RM. Traumatic rupture of the aorta: special reference to automobile accidents. *JAMA* 195:527–530, 1966.

32. Wilson RF, Stephenson LW. Trauma to intrathoracic great vessels. In Wilson RF, Walt AJ, eds., *Management of Trauma: Pitfalls and Practice*, 2nd ed. Baltimore, MD: Williams & Wilkins, 1996: 361–387.

33. Fabian TC, Davis KA, Gavant ML, et al. Prospective study of blunt aortic injury: helical CT is diagnostic and antihypertensive therapy reduces rupture. *Ann Surg* 227:666–677, 1998.

34. Mirvis SE, Kathirkamuganathan S, Buell J, et al. Use of spiral computed tomography for the assessment of blunt trauma patients with potential aortic injury. *J Trauma* 45:922–930, 1998.

35. Dunham MB, Zygun D, Petrasek P, et al. Endovascular stent grafts for acute blunt aortic injury. *J Trauma* 56:1173–1178, 2004.

36. Fildes JJ, Betlej TM, Manglano R, et al. Limiting cardiac evaluation in patients with suspected myocardial contusion. *Am Surg* 61:832–835, 1995.

37. Stassen NA, Lukan JK, Spain DA, et al. Reevaluation of diagnostic procedures for transmediastinal gunshot wounds. *J Trauma* 53:635–638, 2002.

38. McKenney MG, Martin L, Lentz K, et al. 1000 consecutive ultrasounds for blunt abdominal trauma. *J Trauma* 40:607–612, 1996.

39. Peitzman AB, Heil B, Rivera L, et al. Blunt splenic injury in adults: multi-institutional study of the Eastern Association for the Surgery of Trauma. *J Trauma* 49:177–189, 2000.

40. Haan JM, Biffl W, Knudson MM, et al. Splenic embolization revisited: a multi-center review. *J Trauma* 56:542–547, 2004.

41. Ivatury RR, Sugarman HJ, Peitzman AB. Abdominal compartment syndrome: recognition and management. *Adv Surg* 35:251–269, 2001.

42. Vaslef SN, Knudsen NW, Neligan PJ, et al. Massive transfusion exceeding 50 units of blood products in trauma patients. *J Trauma* 53:291–296, 2002.

43. Lynch K, Johansen K. Can Doppler pressure measurement replace exclusion arteriography in the diagnosis of occult extremity arterial trauma? *Ann Surg* 214:737–741, 1991.

44. Frykberg ER, Crump JM, Vines FS, et al. A reassessment of the role of arteriography in penetrating proximity extremity trauma: a prospective study. *J Trauma* 29:1041–1052, 1989.

SURGICAL INFECTION

Wendy R. Cornett, MD

A *surgical infection* requires some physical intervention such as drainage, debridement, or correction of ongoing contamination, whereas a *medical infection* requires only antibiotics. In addition to specific knowledge about surgical infection, surgeons must be cognizant of any infection their patients may have, as well as wound factors and host factors, which may predispose to infection, and virulence factors of infecting pathogens.

DIAGNOSIS

Rubor, tumor, calor, and dolor—redness, swelling, heat, and pain—are the classic signs and symptoms of infection. A thorough history and physical examination of the patient will frequently reveal the source of infection.

Laboratory and radiologic evaluation should be targeted at the suspected source. Leukocytosis with a *left shift* or increased proportion of polymorphonuclear (PMN) leukocytes indicates acute infection. Eosinophilia may indicate allergy or parasitic infection. Leukopenia may occur in overwhelming sepsis. An immunocompromised patient may not have a change in white blood cell (WBC) count.

Culture results may confirm the diagnosis, and can be a useful adjunct for adjusting antibiotic therapy, but *pan-culturing* should not supplant a good bedside evaluation of the patient with infection. A Gram stain can provide rapid preliminary information about the pathogen to help guide antibiotic selection.

Aerobic, anaerobic, and fungal cultures should be obtained. Fungal culture, however, has a high false-negative rate, and empiric antifungal therapy should be considered in a septic patient with negative cultures.

Infection Versus Colonization

It is important to remember that a culture of your own *clean* hands will grow bacteria. Culturing an open, granulating wound on a quest for source of infection is likely to reveal bacteria due to colonization, but may not indicate infection. Hospital or chronic care facility inpatients may be colonized by more virulent bacteria including methicillin-resistant *Staphylococcus aureus* (MRSA) or vancomycin-resistant enterococcus (VRE). Wound culture is helpful only as a guide to adjusting antimicrobial therapy for an obviously infected wound, which does not respond to local measures. Positive cultures from a healthy appearing wound do not necessarily indicate infection or warrant additional treatment, but may require isolation precautions to prevent colonization or infection of other patients. Caution should be used in obtaining any cultures to assure that bacteria colonizing the skin do not contaminate the culture sample.

Pathogen Factors

The virulence of the organism may influence the development of infection. Gram-negative bacterial endotoxin contributes to sepsis syndrome. Exotoxin from *flesh eating bacteria* such as clostridia and streptococci allow rapid spread of infection through tissue. Postoperative fever should prompt a wound check to avoid dire consequences of missing such an infection. Encapsulated organisms such as *Klebsiella* and *Streptococcus pneumoniae* evade host defenses by inhibiting phagocytosis. Numerous mechanisms of antibiotic resistance continue to evolve.

Under the right circumstances, normally nonvirulent opportunistic organisms may cause infection.

Host Factors

Certain host factors significantly increase the ability of microorganisms to invade. Patients at extremes of age, using steroids, and with cancer, burns, trauma, diabetes, malnutrition, inherited or acquired immunocompromise, uremia, or obesity all have diminished humoral defenses putting them at risk for infection.

Patients with alteration of their normal flora are at risk for infection. Prior antibiotic use eliminates normal resident flora, opening the field for overgrowth of opportunistic pathogens. Patients on H_2-blockers may have bacterial colonization of the stomach, thus increasing the risk of pneumonia following aspiration of gastric contents.

Patients with peripheral vascular disease, hypovolemic shock, systemic hypoxemia, or vasoconstricting medications are at risk for infection due to decreased blood flow and decreased peripheral oxygen tension.

Wound Factors

The epithelium is the first line of defense. A break in the skin or mucus membrane, whether traumatic or surgical, opens a portal of entry for bacteria. Devitalized tissue and foreign material prevent circulating immune cells, antibodies, and antibiotics from reaching pathogens. Drains, sutures, and implantable devices are foreign bodies and increase the risk of infection.

Infection risk from high bacterial count can be reduced through irrigation of the wound. *The solution to pollution is dilution.*

PREVENTION

The lessons of Lister, Semmelweis, Pasteur, and other pioneers provide the basis for antisepsis and sterile technique. Hand washing before and after each patient remains the primary means of preventing infection. "The 10 most common causes of infection are the doctor's (or nurse's or student's) 10 fingers."

An important and avoidable cause of postoperative infection is contamination of the surgical field by the operating team. The operating team should wear clean scrubs and shoes or shoe covers, secure glasses with a strap, secure hair under a cap, wear a new mask, and remove rings and other jewelry. The team should avoid excess movement to decrease the risk of contamination. Short members of the team should use a step to keep the sterile portion of the gown at the appropriate level. Tall members should use caution to avoid touching the light handles with their head. Whenever contamination may have occurred, the team should assume that it did occur. While sneezing, particulate material exits from the sides of the mask and travels laterally and posteriorly; thus, it is preferable to face the field but step back slightly. Double gloving significantly reduces the rate of inner glove perforation by 70–78 percent in all types of surgery.[1] One pair of gloves will be a half size larger than usually worn. Sterile technique protects your patient. Universal precautions protect you and your patient.

Ultraviolet (UV) light and laminar flow/positive pressure ventilation systems decrease the overall bacterial numbers in the operating room.

Patient Prep

Mechanical bowel preparation decreases the bacterial content of the colon for cases in which entry into the bowel is anticipated. Numerous regimens are available. Magnesium citrate-based bowel cleansing is effective, but may cause electrolyte abnormalities. Agents such as polyethylene glycol (PEG) are associated with fewer electrolyte imbalances, but are sometimes difficult for the patient to tolerate due to the volume of liquid consumed. The Nichols-Condon prep is a nonabsorbed oral antibiotic regimen consisting of neomycin and erythromycin base, which further decreases the bacterial load in the prepped colon. Small studies have reopened the debate about the necessity of bowel preparation, and shown safety of colon surgery without bowel preparation in selected patients.[2,3]

If hair in the immediate area of the surgery is to be removed, it should be clipped with electric clippers at the time of the procedure. Shaving injures the skin and increases infection risk.

The patient's skin preparation typically consists of a 5–7-min scrub with detergent such as Betadine or chlorhexidine, followed by painting with antimicrobial solution such as povidone-iodine or chlorhexidine. Another method involves a 1-min scrub with 70 percent alcohol or 2 percent iodine in 90 percent alcohol instead of detergent. A drape is then applied directly to the skin, and an incision is made directly through the adherent drape. Alternatively, a single application agent such as DuraPrep® may be applied.

Prep the largest area that may possibly be needed. For example, the surgeon performing a thyroidectomy for a substernal goiter may prep the patient's chest, even though entry into the chest is not planned. Should unforeseen circumstances require it, access to the chest is quickly available.

Surgical Technique

Good surgical technique is essential to a good outcome. Tissue should be handled gently to preserve circulation, as crushed tissue may become devitalized. Debride devitalized tissue, remove foreign bodies, and limit amount of suture in the deep closure. Monofilament polypropylene or nylon suture is preferred over braided suture for contaminated wounds because it is less likely to serve as a nidus for infection. Gloves and instruments should be changed prior to closing a wound if a hollow viscus was entered during the case.

Seroma, hematoma, and dead space should be drained if the wound is already infected. However, the drain is a foreign body, and also increases the risk of infection. Closed suction drains decrease that risk over open drains such as Penrose drains.

Delayed primary closure can be used for infected or heavily contaminated wounds, with loose packing of the wound with gauze for about 5 days, followed by closure after the wound has developed capillary budding and the bloodstream can deliver phagocytic cells to the wound.

Antibiotic Prophylaxis

The risk of creating resistant organisms and inducing side effects such as anaphylaxis should be weighed against the benefit of prophylactic antibiotics.

The already low risk of developing an infection in a clean case is difficult to improve upon. The surgeon must also consider the consequences of infection. If infection would result in removal of implanted foreign body such as a hernia mesh, the low risk from side effects of antibiotics may be justified, even though the risk of infection is already low. Current standards of care favor the administration of prophylactic antibiotics in any case that is not classified as a clean case, any traumatic or emergency case, any case involving implantation of a foreign material, cardiac procedures performed through a median sternotomy, morbidly obese patients, and in patients with predisposition to infection as described above. Prophylactic antibiotics are ineffective and may lead to resistance in cases involving burns, open wounds, tracheostomy, chronic indwelling urinary catheter, or central venous catheter.[4]

If anaerobic flora are anticipated, a third-generation cephalosporin is appropriate. Otherwise, cefazolin is the most commonly chosen prophylactic antibiotic. In patients infected or colonized by MRSA, or those allergic to penicillin or cephalosporins, vancomycin is appropriate.

Ampicillin for endocarditis prevention should be given when indicated for patients at risk for bacterial endocarditis.

TREATMENT

The mainstay of surgical infection is to remove the source of bacteria. Incise and drain abscesses; irrigate and debride wounds to remove foreign bodies and dead tissue and decrease the bacterial load; remove a nidus of infection such as the gallbladder or perforated segment of colon; control ongoing bacterial contamination with diverting colostomy construction; and perform meticulous wound care.

A comprehensive description of antibiotic therapy is beyond the scope of this text. Briefly, antibiotics should be selected to cover the presumed or identified causative organisms. Prior to obtaining culture results, empiric therapy is chosen based on suspected organisms, and is usually broad spectrum. The antibiotic regimen can be revised as appropriate on review of culture results.

Axillary infections tend to have a significant anaerobic component. Infections of the oropharynx and below the waist tend to be mixed aerobic and anaerobic flora. Bacteroides species are obligate anaerobes and should be included in the treatment plan when the colon may be involved in the process. Hospital pharmacies review antibiotic resistance patterns specific to their institutions or even in individual intensive care units. These patterns can also help guide antibiotic choices.

In keeping track of antibiotic therapy, a reminder in each daily note of the number of days the patient has been on each antibiotic, total number of continuous antibiotic days if the antibiotics have been changed, and the planned duration of the antibiotic course is helpful.

SPECIFIC INFECTION REQUIRING SURGICAL INTERVENTION

Abscess

If there is pus, drain it is a relatively safe statement on a surgical service. An abscess cavity contains the liquefied debris center in which bacteria can grow unchecked. Antibiotics and host immune defenses cannot diffuse adequately into the center of an abscess from the capillaries at the periphery.

The body attempts to control or *wall off* infection by creating a fibrous wall around the source of infection. This confines the bacteria to a limited space, where they continue to multiply. As the volume of the abscess increases, the increasing pressure in the abscess cavity increases the likelihood of sepsis.

As a general rule, *an abscess will not heal without adequate incision and drainage (I&D)*. I&D can be accomplished by incising the skin over a palpable abscess and packing it with gauze, or percutaneously using ultrasound or computed tomography (CT) guidance and leaving a drain. The acidic environment of an abscess may decrease the effectiveness of local anesthesia.

Rarely, an abdominal abscess may be medically treated, such as salpingitis with tuboovarian abscess, pyelonephritis, amebic liver abscess, spontaneous bacterial peritonitis, *Shigella* or *Yersinia* enteritis, uncomplicated diverticulitis, and some cases of cholangitis.[5]

An abscess can occur anyplace in the body. General surgeons frequently encounter abscesses in sites including superficial skin and soft tissue, perirectal, thorax (empyema), intra-abdominal, pelvic, and retroperitoneal areas.

Necrotizing Fasciitis

Necrotizing fasciitis usually results from a mixed flora of aerobic and anaerobic organisms. Clostridial myonecrosis, also called gas gangrene due to the crepitus in the tissues, is often due to *Clostridium perfringens, C. novyi,* or *C. septicum.* Beta-hemolytic *Streptococcus pyogenes* may cause necrotizing fasciitis as a single organism.[6]

Due to the plane of necrotizing infections in the subcutaneous fascia between the skin and muscle, the skin may appear minimally involved, masking the severity of infection. Sepsis syndrome without evidence of other infectious source raises suspicion for necrotizing fasciitis. Similarly, rapid progression of or failure of antibiotic therapy for a *simple* soft tissue infection should prompt the clinician to investigate that possibility. The *mild* cellulitis may progress to include ecchymoses, severe edema, bullae, crepitus, or frank gangrene. Early operative intervention is critical.

Clostridial infections mandate removal of all involved tissue, and often require amputation of involved extremities. Nonclostridial infections may require only wide local incision and debridement without amputation, but will cause significant deformity.

Trauma

Traumatic wounds carry a high rate of infection. Care of the trauma patient includes minimizing the risk of infection by debriding all devitalized tissue, removing all foreign bodies, and thoroughly irrigating to remove dirt and decrease the bacterial load in the wound.

Tetanus diphtheria toxoid (Td) should be given to everyone every 10 years, and is adequate prophylaxis against tetanus for clean wounds such as surgical wounds. Following traumatic wounds, the risk of tetanus is higher, and the patient should receive Td vaccination if it has been more than 5 years since last immunization.

Tetanus immune globulin (TIG) is given only if the patient has not had the full childhood series or three doses of Td as an adult. TIG inactivates the *Clostridium tetani* toxin, but does not prevent infection. TIG is given as 250–500 U IM at a different site from the Td injection, and within 24 h of injury, with higher doses needed if the patient presents after 24 h.[5]

Diabetic Foot Infection

Care of the diabetic foot is a special case about which entire textbooks are published. Briefly, the clinician should be concerned that what appears to be a small ulcer on the plantar surface of the foot may indicate a severe midfoot infection hidden by a tremendous callus. The infection is usually polymicrobic, including *Pseudomonas, Staphylococcus, Streptococcus,* and both aerobes and anaerobes. The callus should be trimmed and the infection unroofed. All devitalized tissue should be removed and the infection adequately drained, but care must be taken to avoid removing viable tissue. Adequate drainage may require amputation.

Even minor infection in a diabetic foot must be watched closely and treated aggressively with bed rest, elevation of the foot, antibiotics, and I&D as necessary. Following resolution, the patient should have a podiatrist for routine toenail care, and should obtain appropriate footwear including extra-depth shoes with individually made shoe liners.

Central Venous Catheter

The surgical intervention for treatment of an infected central venous catheter is removal of that foreign body. When an infected catheter is suspected, either because of redness at the site, or lack of other source of infection, the catheter should be removed if at all possible. If the skin entry site appears clear of infection, the catheter may be exchanged using *Seldinger technique* (changing the catheter over a guide wire). If the site is red, or if the catheter is strongly suspected of being the source of infection, a new site should be chosen and a new catheter inserted.

Common sense applies, and all treatment teams should cooperate in the care of patients with tenuous IV access. For example, a patient in chronic renal failure with an infected dialysis catheter should have hemodialysis prior to removing the line, and a plan in place to reinsert a new catheter prior to the next dialysis session.

Whenever a line is removed in a septic appearing patient, the intracutaneous extravenous segment should be cultured. A culture of the tip of the catheter is effectively a blood culture. A culture of the extracutaneous portion would show colonization, not necessarily infection. A segment of catheter that resides in the patient's soft tissues prior to entering the vein will give a more accurate indication of whether the catheter was the source of the infection.

Silver impregnated catheters decrease the rate of infection compared to traditional catheters.

Other

Other infections requiring surgical intervention include cholecystitis, ascending cholangitis, splenic abscess, bacterial hepatic abscess, necrotizing pancreatitis, infected pancreatic pseudocyst, complicated diverticulitis, peritonitis due to perforated viscus, appendicitis, complicated tuboovarian abscess unresponsive to medical therapy, and postoperative intra-abdominal infectious complications.

ETIOLOGY OF POSTOPERATIVE FEVER AND INFECTION

Postoperative Fever

The etiology of fever occurring within 3 postoperative days is usually noninfectious. When thinking about a patient with postoperative fever, remember the 5 W's: wind, water, walk, wound, and wonder drug.

1. *Wind* refers to the respiratory system, and in the first 3 postoperative days fever is usually due to atelectasis.
2. *Water* refers to the urinary system. Especially in patients who undergo instrumentation of the urinary tract (such as cystoscopy or in-and-out catheterization) or have an indwelling urinary catheter, urinary tract infection should be considered. Urinalysis with culture and sensitivity should be obtained prior to starting empiric antibiotic therapy.
3. *Walk* refers to deep venous thrombosis. As history and physical examination are unreliable for diagnosis, the patient should undergo duplex ultrasonographic examination of the lower extremity venous system. In thinking about the venous system, central venous catheters and peripheral intravenous lines can be the source of postoperative fever, so the sites should be examined and lines removed or changed when prudent.
4. *Wound* refers, obviously, to wound infection. You will hear many surgeons say, "when the patient is sick, look where the doctor has been." This includes not only the skin incision, but also the body cavity in which the procedure was performed. After the fifth postoperative day, the most likely cause of fever is wound infection. Wound infection occurring within the first 24–48 h after surgery, however, can be caused by clostridial or streptococcal pathogens, and requires immediate diagnosis and treatment.
5. *Wonder drug* refers to the fever commonly associated with broad-spectrum antibiotics.

Postoperative Infection

Wound infection may occur as a result of a traumatic wound (see section Trauma) or as a result of a surgical wound. Surgical wound infection rates are

Table 3-1 **Wound Classification**

- *Clean*: Planned surgery (nontrauma, nonemergency), adequate preoperative surgical scrub, no break in technique, no entry into hollow viscera. Clean wounds have a 1.5–5% infection risk.
- *Clean/contaminated*: Otherwise clean case with controlled entry into the noninfected respiratory, biliary, gastrointestinal, or genitourinary tract, or a minor break in surgical technique. These cases carry a 7% infection risk with prophylactic antibiotics.
- *Contaminated*: Wounds involving penetrating trauma, entry into an infected viscus, or gross spillage of colon contents, or a major break in surgical technique have a 10–15% risk of infection.
- *Dirty/infected*: Wounds involving severe soiling from trauma-related debris, preoperative bowel perforation, gangrene, or gross pus have a 15–40% infection rate, even with antibiotics.

Source: Schwartz SI, Shires GT, Spencer FC, et al., eds. *Principles of Surgery*, 7th ed. New York: McGraw-Hill, 1999.

influenced by patient factors such as nutritional status and immunologic defenses and virulence factors of the pathogen, but depend largely on the type of operation.

Wounds are classified as clean, clean/contaminated, contaminated, or dirty/infected (Table 3-1).[6]

Distant infection doubles the rate of surgical site infection, and should be treated preoperatively in elective cases.

Bacteremia Versus Sepsis

Bacteremia is merely the presence of bacteria in the blood. A positive blood culture alone does not indicate sepsis. Transient bacteremia occurs in healthy people frequently after a bowel movement or after brushing the teeth, and is quickly cleared by the immune system. Sepsis is a syndrome including bacteremia, inappropriate vasodilation, hypotension, fever, and tachycardia in response to cytokine release.[6]

MEDICAL INFECTIONS IN SURGICAL PATIENTS

Nosocomial infections are those acquired in the hospital setting, and are therefore common in postoperative patients. Nosocomial infections generally involve more virulent and antibiotic-resistant organisms than community acquired infections.

Instrumentation of the respiratory tract such as bronchoscopy, tracheostomy or intubation, and mechanical ventilation increases the risk of nosocomial pneumonia. Nasotracheal intubation and to a lesser degree orotracheal intubation increase the risk of sinusitis. Lumbar puncture and both spinal and epidural anesthesia carry a small risk of meningitis. Instrumentation of the urinary tract increases the risk of cystitis and pyelonephritis. Patients with hemodialysis access or other implantable or temporary central venous access methods are at risk for bacterial endocarditis. Similarly, patients with preexisting valvular heart disease are at risk for seeding of the valves during invasive procedures. Patients receiving antibiotics, even those receiving only a prophylactic dose, are at risk for *Clostridium difficile* colitis. Patients receiving blood transfusions have a slight risk of hepatitis or HIV exposure, although transmission by transfusion continues to decrease with technological improvements.

Patients with cellulitis may be treated with oral antibiotics as an outpatient. If the patient has any confounding risk factors such as diabetes or immunosuppression, more aggressive medical treatment may be indicated, with vigilance to detect whether the infection progresses to a surgical infection.

Sepsis syndrome may result from a surgical infection, or may be unrelated, and involves a cascade of inflammatory mediators (including cytokines) and hemodynamic instability in response to infection.

Overwhelming postsplenectomy sepsis (OPSS) is a rare but potentially fatal syndrome caused by encapsulated organisms following splenectomy. Patients undergoing elective splenectomy are immunized in advance of the procedure. Optimal timing for immunization of patients undergoing splenectomy for trauma is debated. Immediate immunization decreases the risk losing a patient to follow up after discharge without immunization. Traditionally, however, the vaccines were given after normalization of the WBC count. Patients are immunized against encapsulated organisms, with Meningovax, Pneumovax, and *Haemophilus influenzae.*

REFERENCES

1. Tanner J, Parkinson H. Double gloving to reduce surgical cross-infection. *Cochrane Database Syst Rev* (3):CD003087, 2002.

2. Bucher P, Gervaz P, Soravia C, et al. Randomized clinical trial of mechanical bowel preparation versus no preparation before elective left-sided colorectal surgery. *Br J Surg* 92(4):409–414, 2005.

3. Jimenez JC, Wilson SE. Prophylaxis of infection for elective colorectal surgery. *Surg Infect* 4(3):273–280, 2003.

4. Greenfield LJ, ed. *Surgery: Scientific Principles and Practice*. Philadelphia, PA: J.B. Lippincott Co, 1993.

5. Sabiston DC, Lyerly HK, eds. *Textbook of Surgery*, 15th ed. Philadelphia, PA: W.B. Saunders, 1997.

6. Schwartz SI, Shires GT, Spencer FC, et al., eds. *Principles of Surgery*, 7th ed. New York: McGraw-Hill, 1999.

CHAPTER 4

THE ACUTE ABDOMEN

C. Denise Ching, MD
Aurora D. Pryor, MD

CLINICAL SCENARIO

An 18-year-old male with no past medical history presents to the acute care clinic complaining of a 1-day history of abdominal pain, nausea and vomiting. The pain initially began in his midepigastric region, waking him up in the morning. Throughout the course of the day the pain migrated to his right lower quadrant, settling two-thirds of the way from his navel to his right iliac crest. When he presents to the emergency department (ED), his temperature is 102°F. He has not been hungry all day. His blood gets drawn for a complete blood count (CBC) and it is seen that his white blood cell count is 12. What is causing his abdominal pain?

INTRODUCTION

The evaluation of the acute abdomen and early diagnosis of its etiology are some of the most important skills that should be learned by both surgical and medical professionals. The scenario described above is commonly seen in EDs, acute care clinics, and physicians' offices. In the case above, the teenager has presented with a case of appendicitis. Treatment is surgical resection. Delay in diagnosis and treatment could lead to rupture and eventual sepsis—processes associated with high morbidity and mortality. The phrase *acute abdomen* is often deceiving in that many people believe the term is pathognomonic with surgical therapy. However, it should be noted that optimal therapy for many people who present with an acute abdomen often involves nonsurgical management. This chapter will review the initial evaluation and management of the acute abdomen and discuss commonly encountered pathology and its diagnosis.

INITIAL EVALUATION

The initial evaluation of a patient with abdominal pain is extremely important. The physician's ability to collect a comprehensive medical history and perform a complete physical examination in a timely fashion is now often eclipsed and compromised by the facility of ordering a radiologic or serologic test and expecting that a single test will give the diagnosis. Although the sensitivity and specificity with which many tests can now aid in diagnosis often range in the upper 90th percentile, it is important to remember that these tests only serve as an *aid* to the physician. Nothing can replace a well-performed physical examination. For example, in the initial scenario, the patient is a young male who presents with classic signs and symptoms of acute appendicitis. Upon arrival to a medical treatment facility, some physicians may automatically start this patient on a care map where he gets laboratory tests drawn and then begins drinking his oral contrast for the inevitable computed tomography (CT) scan. However, many would argue that based on the strength of his physical examination and blood work, this patient could be taken to the operating room with confidence that the correct surgery was being performed.[1]

Key elements in the initial assessment include collecting a complete patient history. This includes the patient's past medical history including previous diagnoses, hospitalizations, or a history of trauma. Drug allergies and medications, including prescribed drugs and over-the-counter substances should also be noted. Family history and social history for any illegal substance, tobacco, or alcohol use as well as the patient's profession may also give clues to the diagnosis. One should ask about any recent sick contacts as well as recent travel history. The past surgical history will automatically rule out some diagnoses, that is, a patient cannot have appendicitis if the appendix is already out; and it will provide a clue as to some diagnoses that should be ranked higher on the list of differentials, that is, adhesions as a possible cause of small bowel obstruction in someone who has had abdominal surgery.

In addition to past medical history, a complete description of the patient's current problem should be elicited. This includes a description of the pain and symptoms. The time of onset, the length and duration of the pain, and whether it is constant or intermittent should all be recorded. One should inquire about the quality of the pain whether it is sharp and stabbing or more colicky. When initially asked about location of pain, patients may describe that their abdomen hurts diffusely. However, when probed further patients often can locate a single point where the pain is worst. Pain may also radiate to a different area, such as in cholecystitis, which can start in the right upper quadrant and then radiate up to the right shoulder, caused by diaphragmatic irritation from the inflamed gallbladder.

Along with the pain, there will be other symptoms that can help form a differential diagnosis. This includes a history of nausea and vomiting, diarrhea, constipation, and hematochezia. Nausea and vomiting may give clues to ileus or pancreatitis. Diarrhea can be secondary to an infectious etiology, food poisoning, acute mesenteric ischemia, or obstruction. Constipation from chronic dysmotility can cause abdominal pain significant enough to present as an acute abdomen. And people who present with hematochezia should always be worked up for potential malignancy. It can also be caused by infection or ischemia.

It is also important to look at the vital signs and the overall state of the patient. Before beginning the directed physical examination, look at the patient. Are they lying still because any movement causes extreme abdominal pain, implying peritoneal irritation? Or are they writhing around and rocking from side to side because they cannot seem to get comfortable, implying a more colicky pain caused by colonic distention or a kidney stone? Are they lying with their knees bent or in a slightly folded over position because it hurts to straighten out? Is the patient febrile, tachycardic, or hypotensive? Patients who present with the complaint of abdominal pain usually have been experiencing the pain for a substantial amount of time before they present to a physician. Patients will often believe that they have the flu, menstrual cramps, or some other more common etiology before they realize that the pain has not gone away and is actually worse. As a result, they often present late in the course of their illness. They may be dehydrated and potentially can be septic.

A thorough physical examination should include auscultation to listen for hypo or hyperactive bowel sounds. Palpation should be of the four main quadrants to look for guarding and rebound tenderness. Begin away from the quadrant to which the patient localizes the worst pain. A digital rectal examination should be performed in order to check for any blood in the stool, presence or absence of stool in the rectal vault, as well as to check for pelvic peritoneal signs. The patient should be examined for previous surgical scars and should be checked for any hernias, including inguinal and femoral, that could potentially be the source of pain secondary to incarceration. While performing the examination, keep in mind any recent pain medication the patient has received or if the patient is chronically immunosuppressed or on steroids, which could potentially dampen physical findings.

Resuscitation

During the initial period of assessment, it is important to assess whether the patient is dehydrated or intravascularly volume depleted secondary to sepsis. Intravenous fluids should be begun, because patients often have had decreased oral intake, vomiting, or diarrhea. It may be challenging to find intravenous access in the dehydrated patient. Fluid resuscitation requires a thorough knowledge of the patient's past medical history. An 86-year-old male with congestive heart failure and a cardiac ejection fraction of 15 percent will not be able to handle the same fluid load as a healthy 18-year-old male. A Foley catheter may need to be placed, to accurately measure urine output.

Urine output is an excellent way to monitor hydration status, with a minimum of $1/2$ cc/kg/h in a well-hydrated adult. A urinary catheter can also be helpful if the patient is too uncomfortable to use a bathroom. At times the patient may come in nauseated and vomiting, as often seen with small bowel obstruction. A nasogastric tube in these situations may assist with the patient's nausea and abdominal pain by suctioning out enteric contents and decompressing gastric dilatation. It can also be a diagnostic aid to diagnose an incarcerated paraesophageal hernia.

If the patient presents febrile, with a potential for infection or sepsis, it is appropriate to perform a thorough fever workup prior to identifying an exact diagnosis, drawing labs, blood cultures, sending off a urinalysis and urine culture and sensitivity, and checking a chest x-ray. Pneumonia, urinary tract infection, and kidney stones can all present as abdomen pain. If the chest x-ray and urinalysis rule out these sources of infection, then one should consider giving the patient an empiric dose of antibiotics with coverage of enteric bacteria, which can be later tailored to a specific organism or cause.

Laboratory and Radiologic Tests

After collecting the medical history and performing the physical examination, the next step will be to decide which blood work and radiologic tests would aid in diagnosis. When ordering blood work, one should begin to think about whether the patient may need to go to the operating room. If so, what laboratory and diagnostic tests should be done to prepare the patient for surgery? General blood work should be ordered, including a CBC to allow for assessment of leukocytosis or blood loss. An electrolyte panel (i.e., Chem 7, OP7) will give information regarding potential electrolyte abnormalities especially in vomiting and dehydrated patients, or those with medical comorbidities such as renal failure. If there is a question of hepatic compromise, a liver panel should be added. Checking a coagulation panel in older patients will help assess whether the patient is at risk for bleeding intraoperatively and also give an idea of the patient's hepatic synthetic function. If the patient presents with nausea and vomiting and there is a question of pancreatitis, amylase and lipase should be checked. Any concern for ischemic bowel should include a lactic acid level. Arterial blood gases should be drawn when there is a concern of respiratory status, as well as to assess if the patient is acidotic. A urinalysis may lead to the diagnosis of a renal stone as the source of pain, when blood is present in the urine. It also can identify a urinary tract infection. If the patient is in the age group where they are at risk for cardiac ischemia, a preoperative ECG should be obtained. And, if there is any question that abdominal pain could be due to a cardiac source, cardiac enzymes should be drawn.

Focused radiologic tests should be chosen. Different views of the abdomen can give information regarding bowel dilatation, the presence of an appendicolith, pneumatosis, air fluid levels consistent with obstruction, and perforation suggested by the presence of free air. Free air will not be easily seen on a flat plate kidney, ureter, and bladder (KUB). When one is concerned about free air, an upright chest x-ray should be ordered to evaluate for the presence of subdiaphragmatic air. Lateral decubitus films, with the patient either right or left side down, or upright films can also help delineate pathology.

Ultrasound is next in the arsenal of radiologic tests that can be used for diagnosis. Ultrasound is a relatively noninvasive, painless procedure that can be quickly performed, depending on the presence of an experienced ultrasonographer. Many EDs will carry their own ultrasound machines, which permit a quick examination of the abdomen. Ultrasound is based on the principal that sound waves (emitted from a transducer) will be conducted differently through objects of varying densities. When borders between substances of different densities are encountered, some sound waves are reflected back. It is those echoes that are detected and changed into a moving image displayed on a screen. Ultrasound waves pass easily through fluids and soft tissues and poorly though bone or gas.[2] Therefore, this technique is good for examining fluid-filled organs such as the liver and the gallbladder or the uterus, and can identify blood flow in vessels. Limitations include the patient's morphotype, being of limited value in obese people, and the skill of the ultrasonographer. In the setting of the acute abdomen, ultrasound provides a way to perform a quick examination to look for inflammation around the gallbladder or dilatation of the bile ducts (in the case of right upper quadrant pain) as well as the appendix. In the setting of lower quadrant pain, a transvaginal ultrasound can provide a look at the uterus as well as ovaries in women, and a regular ultrasound can rule out testicular pathologies such as epididymitis and torsion in males (which can cause referred pain to the lower quadrants).

CT scans are based on an x-ray tube and a detector being mounted on opposite sides of a circular, rotating frame. As the frame is rotated around the patient, a fan-shaped beam of x-rays is created. The opposite detector takes multiple snapshots in a single rotation. These profiles are then taken as a set, analyzed by a computer, and used to create cross-sectional slices of the patient's body. Spiral or helical scanning simply refers to the technology which allows the scanner to rotate continuously to take images of the human body, as opposed to rotating a complete 360° circle in one direction before having to rotate in the opposite direction to take the second slice (as was done in the earlier generation of CT scanners).[3] CT scans, with their high sensitivity and specificity for revealing disease processes have revolutionized medicine. However, it is also important to remember their limitations. CT scans are an image created of the patient at one brief moment in time. Patients who present early in a disease process often will not have obvious CT scan findings. Chronic processes such as abscesses and acute blunt trauma such as major organ rupture are more readily diagnosed by CT scan. Their use in the diagnosis of acute processes should be limited to extremely specific purposes, and not just ordered reflexively. In the appropriate clinical setting, CT scans are a great diagnostic aid.

HIDA scans, representing an example of cholescintigraphy, involve intravenous injection of hydroxy iminodiacetic acid, a radioactive chemical, which is taken up by the liver and secreted into bile. The dye then should disperse to where bile normally courses, that is, bile ducts, the gallbladder, and the intestine. Images are then taken of the patient's abdomen to detect where the radioactive dye has traveled. The presence or absence of radioactive dye in specific areas can help determine the presence or absence of obstruction in areas such as the cystic duct, which if obstructed will not permit the gallbladder to be visualized. This test is especially helpful for patients who present with right upper quadrant pain with normal ultrasound studies.

Although, all tests can be a great aid to the physician in disease diagnosis, when one becomes reliant on the results of a single radiologic test, they can also become the physician's handicap. Nothing can replace the physical examination. The abdomen itself can be divided into four different quadrants (six general areas). By carefully localizing the pain both by patient report and by physical examination, a focused differential diagnosis can be created (Table 4-1). It is after creating this differential diagnosis in your mind that one should *then* order blood work and radiographic tests in order to systematically go through your differential diagnosis to identify the specific disease process.

Table 4-1 **Differential Diagnosis of the Acute Abdomen by Location**

Right upper quadrant pain	Midepigastric pain	Left upper quadrant pain
Acute cholecystitis	Early appendicitis	Gastric ulcer
Leaking duodenal ulcer	Acute small bowel	Local peritonitis
Pulmonary process	obstrution	Acute pancreatitis
Biliary peritonitis	Intestinal colic	Inflamed jejunal
	Acute pancreatitis	diverticulum
	Exclude: coronary	Splenic artery
	thrombosis,	aneurysm
	hepes zoster	Rupture of the spleen
		Acute pyelonephritis
Right lower quadrant pain	Hypogastric pain	Left lower quadrant pain
Appendicitis	Early obstructed	Diverticulitis
Leaking duodenal ulcer	transverse colon	Cancer
Pyelonephritis	UTI	Pelvic peritonitis
Regional ileitis	Uterine irritation	Ovarian etiology
Inflamed Meckel	Perforated	Sigmoid volvulus
diverticulum	appendicitis	
Low gallbladder/	Perforated	
cholecystitis	diverticulum	
Diverticulitis		
Cecal volvulus		
Ovarian etiology		

Right Upper Quadrant Pain

Right upper quadrant pain can be caused by gallbladder disease including acute cholecystitis, biliary colic, biliary dyskinesia, cholangitis, and bile duct obstruction. Other sources of right upper quadrant pain include hepatic dysfunction or abscess, leaking duodenal ulcer, as well as processes outside of the peritoneal cavity, such as a right lower lobe pneumonia.

Hepatobiliary disease and gallbladder disease, depending on the severity, require different degrees of intervention. Emergent surgical intervention is rarely required. Most patients who present to the ED or doctor's office complaining of right upper quadrant pain can receive an outpatient workup for symptomatic cholelithiasis. If required, cholecystectomy can be elective in these patients. If, however, they have fever or unrelenting pain they may have acute cholecystitis requiring more urgent care. They usually require admission and cholecystectomy during that hospitalization. Cholangitis requires an inpatient admission for intravenous antibiotics and biliary decompression. Biliary obstruction will be evidenced by an elevated bilirubin and alkaline phosphatase and possibly CT scan or ultrasound findings showing intra or extrahepatic ductal dilatation. This can be due to both obstruction from a gallstone versus a more chronic process such as a malignant or benign mass originating from the bile duct, liver, or pancreas. Acute intervention requires drainage. This can be performed with endoscopic retrograde cholangiopancreatography, if the obstruction does not resolve, to remove an obstructing gallstone or to stent across an obstructing mass. Percutaneous transhepatic biliary drainage (PTC), or more rarely surgical intervention, can also be used. After the immediate obstruction has resolved and there are no signs of cholangitis, the patient can be evaluated for optimal surgical intervention depending on the disease process. Patients with perforated ulcers will be described under the section Midepigastric Pain. These patients will usually appear septic and require urgent care.

Left Upper Quadrant Pain

Left upper quadrant pain can be secondary to pancreatitis, peptic ulcer disease, subphrenic abscess, jejunal diverticulitis, splenic rupture or infarction, and left lower lobe pneumonia. Splenic infarction is commonly associated with sickle cell disease. This diagnosis does not always require surgical resection. Treatment should be considered if the patient exhibits clinical signs of infection such as a leukocytosis or has elevated temperatures. Refractory pain is also an indication for surgical resection.

Midepigastric Pain

Midepigastric pain is associated with early stages of acute appendicitis, acute small bowel obstruction, peptic ulcer disease, and acute pancreatitis. Pancreatitis, depending on the etiology of the inflammation, including gallstones, alcohol or idiopathic causes, requires different types of intervention. Gallstone pancreatitis is one of the few types of pancreatitis that require early surgical intervention.

It occurs when gallstones become lodged in the pancreatic duct causing obstruction and inflammation. Treatment involves admission for bowel rest and intravenous fluid hydration until the obstructing stone passes and the pancreatitis resolves. This is seen with cessation of clinical symptoms of pancreatitis and normalization of amylase and lipase serum levels. After resolution of the acute pancreatitic flare, the patient should undergo cholecystectomy during the same hospital admission as he or she will be at increased risk of having recurrent pancreatitis until the source of the gallstones is removed. Preoperative biliary decompression by ERCP or PTC may be required if the obstructing stone does not pass spontaneously. An intraoperative cholangiogram may be required in order to ensure no further gallstones are present in the biliary system.

Acute necrotizing pancreatitis is a severe form of pancreatitis that may require surgical intervention. It is seen in approximately 20 percent of all cases of pancreatitis. Necrosis alone is not an automatic indication for surgery. If the necrosis remains sterile, the patient should be treated with bowel rest until the pancreatitis resolves. The sequelae from the necrosis, including pancreatic pseudocysts and abscesses should be watched for and treated if the patient becomes symptomatic. The indication for operative intervention in necrotizing pancreatitis is hemodynamic instability. This is usually due to sepsis when the necrosis becomes infected. In these cases, mortality for untreated infected pancreatic necrosis approaches 90–100 percent. Many clinicians argue that pancreatic necrosis seen on CT scan should not be biopsied until the patient starts exhibiting clinical signs of sepsis as this could be a means of introducing infection into an otherwise sterile pancreatic phlegmon.

Other causes of midepigastric pain include gastroesophageal reflux disease (GERD), gastric and duodenal ulcer disease with or without perforation, and cardiac symptoms. All diseases should be ruled out per the risk factors seen in that patient. For example, if a 65-year-old gentleman with a known history of reflux presents to the ED complaining of midepigastric pain, even though the pain may be recurrent reflux, he should still get at the least an ECG to ensure that there is no cardiac ischemia occurring. GERD is treated surgically under specific criteria, including patients who are refractory to medical therapy, people who are noncompliant with their medications, and people with pathologic changes of dysplasia or malignancy secondary to reflux seen during esophagogastroduodenoscopy (EGD) evaluation. Reflux surgery is rarely done urgently. Ulcer disease has been seen to be highly correlated with *Helicobacter pylori* infection, which is treated initially with medical therapy. Patients with ulcer disease on initial diagnosis as well as when the disease is refractory to medical therapy should receive endoscopic evaluation with biopsies to rule out malignancy.

Perforated ulcers should be treated urgently. These patients often present with free air and sepsis. Specific surgical management is dependent on their previous history, so it is essential to ask some questions prior to induction of anesthesia. Patients should be asked about antacid therapy, including proton pump inhibitors, as well as nonsteroidal inflammatory agent use. Previous history of *H. pylori* infection and treatment is also important for surgical decision making. An assessment as to likely postoperative medical compliance should also be obtained. After this brief history, the patient should be resuscitated and taken to surgery.

Right Lower Quadrant Pain

Right lower quadrant pain is a common complaint. It is also one of the most difficult areas of the abdomen to evaluate because the differential diagnosis is widely varied. The resulting workup is dependent on the age and sex of the patient, as well as the clinical picture. The differential diagnosis can include appendicitis, diverticulitis, inflammatory bowel disease, cecal volvulus, inguinal or femoral hernias, urinary tract infections, renal stones, and pyelonephritis. In females, organs of the female reproductive tract must be evaluated as a possible source of the pain, including evaluation for mittelschmerz, endometriosis, and ectopic pregnancy.

Appendicitis is one of the most common causes of right lower quadrant pain, as outlined in the initial scenario. The peak incidence of appendicitis is between 10 and 12 years of age and slowly tapers over time. The incidence of perforated appendicitis is increased in young children and the elderly secondary to delayed or mistaken diagnosis. Healthy teenage males presenting with right lower quadrant pain, a history consistent with appendicitis, a low-grade fever, and moderate leukocytosis can be taken to the operating room without further tests.

In males in their 50s and 60s, other diseases should also be considered such as diverticulitis. In this population, as well as people with a history of inflammatory bowel disease, a CT scan should be used for further evaluation. Although this may lead to a slight delay in diagnosis, there is a much greater chance of having an incorrect diagnosis if one automatically assumes right lower quadrant pain is secondary to appendicitis.

Crohn's disease is a chronic disease not cured by surgical resection. Although the diseased portion of bowel may be resected with surgery, the disease can affect a previously unaffected portion of bowel at a later date. Surgical resection each time a portion of bowel is affected will eventually leave a patient with an inadequate length of bowel. With ulcerative colitis, the risk of cancer increases with the length of diagnosis. A patient has a 5 percent increased risk of colon cancer after the first 20 years of diagnosis, which increases 0.5 percent per year thereafter.[4] Total abdominal colectomy is the eventual recommendation for people diagnosed with ulcerative colitis. Toxic megacolon is the main reason for which patients with ulcerative colitis will require urgent surgery. Inflammatory bowel diseases can rarely be associated with toxic megacolon. This is a diagnosis that involves nonobstructive dilatation of the colon to greater than 6 cm accompanied by fever, tachycardia, leukocytosis, or other signs of hemodynamic instability. Patients will present with severe abdominal distention, hypoactive bowel sounds, and diffuse abdominal pain. Perforation is associated with a fivefold increase in mortality (normally approximately 5 percent) despite early resuscitation and surgical intervention. Surgical intervention is indicated by the presence of free air, worsening hemodynamic instability, progressive dilatation of the bowel, as well as nonresolution of the disease after 1–2 days. Further associations with toxic megacolon include infectious colitis and acute respiratory distress syndrome.

In ovulating females who present with right lower quadrant pain, the organs in the female reproductive system must be ruled out as a potential source of pathology. A complete pelvic examination should be performed on each female. A pregnancy test should be performed to rule out intrauterine or ectopic pregnancy. At times, a vaginal ultrasound may be required, as this provides a superior look at the ovaries and uterus, allowing for the assessment of torsion, abscesses, cysts, and tumors, as well as ectopic pregnancy.

Left Lower Quadrant Pain

Sources of left lower quadrant abdominal pain include diverticulitis, incarcerated hernia, and sigmoid volvulus. Incarcerated hernias and sigmoid volvulus will present with signs and symptoms of small bowel obstruction, which will be discussed later in this chapter. Diverticulitis is the inflammation of diverticula, small, thin-walled outpouchings in the bowel usually at points of inherent weakness, such as where the vasa recta enter into the colon wall. In Western populations, it is found more commonly in the descending colon, whereas in Asian populations, it is more commonly found in the ascending colon. Unless perforated, obstructed, or actively bleeding, it is treated medically during the initial diagnosis of the disease, with antibiotics and bowel rest being used until the patient's diverticulitis flare has resolved. Then special dietary recommendations, such as high fiber, low fat, and low-meat diets, are usually suggested. Surgical therapy is considered when the disease recurs multiple times, becomes refractory to medical therapy, or presents with frank perforation and abscesses. Even in the face of perforation, if the patient is hemodynamically stable and the abscess is contained, attempts for percutaneous drainage of the perforation site with antibiotics until the initial inflammation resolves (normally 4–6 weeks) is often recommended prior to surgical treatment. Hemodynamic instability and sepsis would be indications for immediate surgical therapy.

GENERALIZED ABDOMINAL PAIN

Generalized abdominal pain can be due to multiple etiologies, ranging from relatively benign sources such as food poisoning and infectious colitis to less benign processes including perforation. Four sources of generalized abdominal pain that warrant further discussion include bowel obstruction, perforation, mesenteric ischemia, and abdominal aortic aneurysms.

Small Bowel Obstruction

Small bowel obstruction presents with abdominal distention and crampy abdominal pain. Proximal small bowel obstruction can often present with nausea and vomiting. Patients may also have nausea and vomiting with distal small bowel and colonic obstruction, but it presents later in the course of the obstruction. Patients will report minimal flatus, and will describe a history of no bowel movements over a prolonged period of time. Patients will occasionally report small watery or mucus predominant bowel movements. There are functional and mechanical obstructions. A *mechanical obstruction* is when there is a physical blockage in the bowel. In the small bowel, this is most commonly due to adhesions from a prior surgery, but it can also be due to an intraluminal foreign body, incarcerated hernia, or intraluminal source such as intussusception or malignancy. In the large bowel, obstructions should be considered malignant until proven otherwise. Once this has been eliminated, less common causes such as diverticular stricture or volvulus should be ruled out. A *functional obstruction* is when dysmotility leads to bowel dilation such as in Ogilvie syndrome. These etiologies can usually be differentiated by careful history and appropriate diagnostic tests.

For the treatment of obstruction, the risk for ischemia and perforation secondary to compromised vascular supply, such as what can occur with a closed-loop obstruction, need to be assessed. If bowel is in jeopardy or necrotic, immediate surgical intervention is required in order to relieve the obstruction. Once these have been ruled out, attempts for symptomatic decompression and awaiting resolution of the small bowel obstruction may be made with nasogastric tube decompression, serial abdominal examinations, interval laboratory evaluations of the white blood cell count, and serial abdominal films. Many of these patients will resolve without surgery. Any signs of leukocytosis, peritoneal signs, fevers, or failure for the small bowel obstruction to resolve would be an indication for surgical intervention. Patients without prior surgery are more likely to have a surgical reason for bowel obstruction and prolonged management with nasogastric decompression is not recommended. CT scans during the initial diagnosis may help rule out closed loop obstruction that requires urgent surgery, as well as identify a transition point, hernia, or mass that would assist in surgical planning.

Perforation

Free perforation is an indication for immediate surgical intervention. Patients with perforation will often present with peritoneal signs secondary to leakage of enteric contents into the peritoneal cavity with resulting inflammation and abscesses. The most common reasons for perforation are peptic ulcer disease or diverticulitis. The history should be focused to help differentiate these. A change in bowel habits and frequent constipation can suggest a colonic source. Nonsteroidal drug use and tobacco abuse are associated with peptic ulcers. Perforation from either source can be contained or freed within the peritoneal cavity. Contained perforation may become walled off and develop into an abscess. These are often diagnosed by CT scans. Well-defined abscesses can be percutaneously drained with an interval resection of the perforated portion of bowel if indicated when the inflammation has resolved. This choice should be accompanied with antibiotics and careful follow-up to ensure that drainage is successful in controlling the infection and the patient remains hemodynamically stable. Generalized peritonitis with hemodynamic instability and free air on radiographs are indications for urgent surgical intervention following initial resuscitation.

Mesenteric Ischemia

Mesenteric ischemia is characterized by inadequate blood flow along mesenteric circulation, which when left untreated can lead to bowel ischemia, gangrene, and perforation. It can be acute or chronic, with acute mesenteric ischemia being a surgical emergency. Acute mesenteric ischemia can be due to acute arterial thrombosis, an acute arterial embolus, nonocclusive mesenteric ischemia, including systemic hypotension and hypoperfusion of the bowel, and mesenteric venous thrombosis.

The hallmark of mesenteric ischemia is pain out of proportion to physical examination findings. The pain will be moderate to severe, nonlocalized, colicky, and constant. Patients may have a history of abdominal angina including pain while during eating, weight loss, and anorexia. Acute arterial embolus is usually marked by an abrupt onset of sharp abdominal pain, vomiting, and diarrhea. Acute arterial and venous mesenteric thrombosis occurs over a longer period of time with acute and subacute abdominal symptoms spanning a longer period of time. These are typically the patients who complain of abdominal angina or intermittent colicky abdominal pain. Nonocclusive mesenteric ischemia can be accompanied with a prodrome of malaise and nonspecific abdominal pain, which then progresses to increased pain and nausea and even peritoneal signs with the progression of ischemia.

Mortality rates associated with acute mesenteric ischemia range from 70 percent during initial acute onset of disease to 90 percent when the disease has progressed to perforation. Vascular workup is indicated in the stable patient. Any question of ischemia should warrant exploratory laparotomy to check for bowel viability. The goal of resection should be to minimize the portion of bowel removed. Revascularization can be considered. A *second look* may be required, where nonviable bowel is removed in the first surgery and then a second look is scheduled the next day in order to see if any questionable bowel has recovered or progressed to necrosis, necessitating further resection.

Abdominal Aortic Aneurysm

Abdominal aortic aneurysms are focal dilations in the aorta often attributed to degeneration of an atherosclerotic aorta. Risk factors include gender (male), race (White), age (60–80 years), and smoking. If a patient with a known diagnosis of an abdominal aortic aneurysm presents with abdominal pain, ruling out rupture should always be considered. Without prior diagnosis, an aneurysm with the possibility of rupture should also be considered in patients with high-risk factors who present with a sudden drop in hematocrit and hemodynamic instability that transiently improves with fluid resuscitation. Patients will often present complaining of abdominal or back pain. A pulsatile abdominal mass can sometimes be palpated, depending on the girth of the patient. Mortality rates are at least 50 percent if the patient presents with rupture.

INDICATIONS FOR SURGERY

When should surgery be considered? For some disease processes, there is a clear indication, such as for appendicitis or perforated viscus. At other times, the patients become clinically symptomatic and begin to hemodynamically decompensate from their disease process and this can also be considered an indication for surgical therapy. However, sometimes there are certain disease processes that can potentially resolve, and it is elected to watch the patients and see if they improve with medical therapy and/or interventional radiology or endoscopic procedures. In these situations, there are no strict lines that determine when a patient should convert from medical therapy to surgical treatment. One factor that physicians should consider is when the patient begins to have a worsening physical examination. Peritoneal signs can develop. Peritoneal signs will be present as the inflammatory process in the abdomen causes first a localized irritation in the area and then progresses to a generalized irritation diffusely in the abdominal cavity as the peritoneal lining becomes inflamed. On initial presentation, patients can present complaining of pain in the car when they passed over bumps. Walking or small movements are extremely painful in peritonitis, and patients will be lying extremely still in bed. On physical examination, the patient's pain will be nondistractable. One must differentiate abdominal guarding of the patient based on anticipation of pain versus the actual presence of pain causing guarding. Lightly shaking the patients' bed, or tapping the patients' heels when they are lying supine in bed will at times elicit abdominal pain, especially when there is peritoneal inflammation. An exception to this is when a patient has a history of being chronically on steroids. Steroids, with their anti-inflammatory effects, can mask symptoms so that a patient's physical examination can be more benign than the underlying disease process. This, in addition to a rising white blood cell count, new onset of elevated temperature, and the development of acidemia are all signs of worsening infection that would be an indication for surgery. Finally, there are certain times where patients fail medical therapy, such as a small bowel obstruction that does not resolve with time, that should also be considered for surgical treatment.

The diagnosis and management of the patient with an acute abdomen is a surgical art. Physicians need to focus on the appropriate resuscitation and workup, guided by the nature and location of the abdominal pain in order to determine the right treatment. Try your skills at this with a final clinical case.

CLINICAL SCENARIO

A 25-year-old White male presents to the ED complaining of sharp onset of abdominal pain in the middle of the night. He was *hanging out* with friends when the pain started. He went home and lay in bed that night, but his pain continued to worsen. He describes the pain as having started off in his epigastrium but now his abdomen diffusely hurts. By the time he presents to the ED, his temperature is 39°C, his blood pressure is 95/45, pulse 135, respiratory rate 28, O_2 saturation on room air 99 percent. What do you do next?

Elicit a Medical History

The patient reports no past medical history. He has not seen a doctor since he was a child and has had no hospitalizations and no history of past surgeries. He reports smoking a half of a pack of cigarettes per day, moderate alcohol use, and occasional drug use, including marijuana and cocaine. He takes no medications except for an over-the-counter multivitamin daily and ibuprofen for the occasional headache and muscle pain. He has no known drug allergies. At the same time that you have been learning the medical history, a nurse has been putting in two large bore IVs and starting intravenous fluids for resuscitation. What next?

Elicit a More Thorough History of the Current Complaint

The patient has told you already that his pain started off in the midepigastrium and then moved diffusely all over his abdomen. But how about other symptoms and the timing of events? When asked, he reports that the pain initially started after dinner. He states that he had been out with his friends. When asked directly, he reports some drug use and drinking, consisting of a couple of beers, some mixed cocktails, marijuana, and a small amount of crack cocaine. Later in the evening, he noticed that he had some slight, sharp abdominal pain that he attributed to reflux from the dinner. The pain seemed to go away. He stayed out for about an hour more and then went home where he again noticed the abdominal pain. He slept poorly throughout the night and then in the morning, noticing that his pain was much worse, presented to the ED.

He now has had some nausea but no vomiting. He had no fevers initially, but noticed when he got out of bed in the morning that his temperature was 101.5°F. He had a normal bowel movement yesterday morning, with no blood seen in the stool. Since then his abdominal pain has worsened, he has passed no flatus and has had no bowel movement. Driving over in the car to the ED caused him extreme pain, especially when the car would go over any small bumps in the road. He has not eaten anything since last night, before the abdominal pain started. He has had no recent sick contacts. He has not urinated today and is feeling dehydrated.

Now you have collected an entire medical history on him and feel that you have collected an accurate review of the events. What is your next step?

Perform the Physical Examination

When you initially approach the patient you notice that he is lying on his back with his knees bent, and he is lying still on the hospital gurney. The patient is thin, and his abdomen is slightly distended. When asked, the patient reports that the pain is everywhere. His pain, however, started at a single area underneath his rib cage. He has barely audible, slowed bowel sounds on auscultation. You notice that the patient has a rigid abdomen, and that he is severely guarding. Gently shaking the gurney reproduces the same type of abdominal pain. What labs and radiology tests do you want?

Labs

The complete blood count (CBC) shows that the white blood cell count is 17; hematocrit and platelets are within normal limits. The chemistry panel shows that labs are normal except for a blood urea nitrogen (BUN) of 17 and creatinine of 1.4. Amylase and lipase are normal. Urinalysis and coagulation labs are still pending.

Radiology Tests

A flat plate kidney, ureter, and bladder (KUB) shows normal caliber, nondilated loops of bowel. Secondary to the history of cocaine use and the acute onset of the abdominal pain, you elect to get an upright chest x-ray that shows a large amount of free air underneath the left diaphragm. What is your next step?

Treatment

No further radiologic tests are necessary as the free air underneath the diaphragm tell us that there is a perforation. You give him broad-spectrum antibiotics. Make sure he has received at least 2 L of lactated ringers or normal saline intravenously. A CT scan is not necessary, as this is most likely an acute process, with the onset of symptoms the evening before. A CT scan will most likely give no further information regarding the location of the perforation. The coagulation panel at this point in time has come back normal, and the young man is scheduled to go immediately to the operating room for exploratory laparotomy. Intraoperatively, the patient is found to have a duodenal perforation next to the pylorus, commonly associated with crack cocaine use.[5]

REFERENCES

1. Ruggieri P. *Medical Crossfire*. 2001;3(11).
2. Available at: http://yourmedicalsource.com/library/ultrasound/US_work.html.
3. Available at: http://www.yourmedicalsource.com/library/ctscan/CTS_after.html.
4. Gyde SN, Prior P, Allan RN, et al. Colorectal cancer in ulcerative colitis: a cohort study of primary referrals from three centers. Gut 29:206–217, 1988.
5. Feliciano DV, Ojukwu JC, Rozycki GS, et al. The epidemic of cocaine-related juxtapyloric perforations: with a comment on the importance of testing for helicobacter pylori. *Ann Surg* 229(6):801, 1999.

THE OPERATING ROOM

L. Scott Levin, MD, FACS

In modern medicine, surgical procedures are now being conducted in endoscopy suites (gastrointestinal evaluation and biopsy of lesions), catheterization laboratories (cardiac aberrant pathway ablation), and in vascular radiology suites, where stents and angioplasties are performed.[1] In all of these procedures, there are physicians who carry out these procedures, as well as support staff who facilitate patient care and performance of surgical procedures.

Traditionally, the *operating room* has been the hospital location where open surgery is performed, and in the modern day practice, even minimally invasive surgery is still performed in the operating room. This includes robotic surgery and endoscopic surgery. In all operating rooms, there is a common technology and common protocols that allow patients to be safely treated. The operating room is a concert of *care providers*, which includes surgeons, anesthesiologists, nurses, technical support staff, and occasionally, corporate representatives who facilitate the transition of new technology into surgical practice. In addition, there may be observers, medical students, or observers from other institutions, and surgical residents that participate in the operating room experience. The most critical individual in the operating room, of course, is the patient (Table 5-1).

Continued efforts have focused on patient safety, both from an anesthesia perspective and from a surgical standpoint, in terms of decreasing morbidity and mortality. The hospital support staff have been instrumental in facilitating safe care for the patient. An example of this is a patient being marked preoperatively either by the surgeon or his/her designee by the physician and usually both, indicating the correct site of surgery.[2,3] The policy of creating a *time-out*, which has all members of the surgical team concurring that the procedure, the equipment, appropriate x-rays and studies, appropriate prepping techniques, appropriate perioperative medications and appropriate scheduled surgery, and actual surgery to be performed are all *in sync* before the operation begins, is critically important.

Patient safety must be kept at the forefront of surgical practice, to improve care and to avoid mishaps that lead to morbidity or death. Prior to

Table 5-1 **OR Principles**

1. Patient focused
2. Safety
3. Communication
4. Proficiency
5. Teamwork

the patient entering the operating room, a series of events have taken place that ultimately lead to surgery. The patient may have been referred to a health-care system for evaluation by a surgeon or internal medicine physician. Certain studies were made to obtain a diagnosis, ordered either by the surgeon or other members of the health-care team. A diagnosis is then made, preoperative consultation is obtained, and the operation to be performed is discussed with the patient and family.[4] Informed consent has been obtained, the surgery has been scheduled and matched to the patient's unique hospital identification number, and any special equipment needed has been ordered and procured. Informed consent should indicate to patients and their families the indication for surgery, the surgical procedure, and the complications that can occur such as bleeding, infection, nerve injury, and even death. Informed consent is very important to assure good communication among surgeons, patients, and families. The equipment needed, the surgeon and assistants are designated, the anesthesiologist and choice of anesthesia designated, and other notations that clarify the procedure are listed.

The surgeon should meet the patient and, if needed, the family before operation. This usually takes place in the induction area after the patients have been registered by the health-care system. The surgeon has a responsibility to put the patient at ease, reassure him or her that a certain operation will be performed, indicate that safety is paramount by marking the site of surgery, and answer any last minute questions that the patient or family may have. The patient is then escorted to the operating room and undergoes anesthesia either with general anesthesia or a variety of techniques including regional blockade that allow the patient to be aware or sedated and have appropriate analgesia so that surgery can be performed.

After the patient enters the operating room the patient will be addressed by several members of the health-care team. Attendants may help position the patient. It is the surgeon's responsibility to ensure that all extremities are padded, and that pressure points such as the heels, sacrum, and occiput are all well padded to avoid pressure sores, particularly for a long operation. All peripheral nerves such as the ulnar nerve and peroneal nerve should be well padded to avoid pressure phenomena that can lead to postoperative paresthesias or neuropraxia.[5] While the surgeon is preparing for surgery, the nurses and other personnel are preparing the operating table with the necessary equipments. It is also a good practice for the surgeon to discuss the procedure to be performed with the operating room team, the anticipated difficult areas of the dissection or surgery, and anticipated length of time that it will take to perform the operation. After anesthesia is obtained, the patient is prepped by the surgical team. Occasionally in different hospitals, the nursing staff will be responsible for prepping the patient with a variety of topical solutions that decrease microbial colonization and clean the skin in preparation for applying drapes in order to begin surgery. The *prepping of patients* is done on the abdomen and thorax actions starting at the middle of a wound and proceeding outward. Prep solutions such as Zeferan and a variety of soaps, betadine solution and scrub, and alcohol may be used. While prepping patients, it is imperative to assure that the prep solution does not pool, because of the risk of maceration or chemical burn to the skin. A surgical time-out is performed prior to prepping which includes agreement of the health-care team on equipment, studies, preoperative pharmacology, procedure to be performed, identification of the patient with history number, and to be assure the surgical procedure coincides with operative permit and the posting of the daily operative schedule. Almost always the patient will be grounded so that electrocautery can be used to control bleeding.

It is a good practice for the surgeon to announce when he or she is about to begin so that all members of the team are aware. Continued communication between the anesthesia service and surgery, and surgeon and nursing will assure smooth surgery. Before beginning, it is important to have cautery and suction available if they will be needed. Blood products should also be readily available if transfusion is anticipated.

The operating team includes the surgeon, who serves as leader, surgical assistants, physician assistants (PAs), medical students, and residents. The anesthesia team consists of an attending anesthesiologist, residents, perhaps a certified resident nurse and anesthesiologist, and anesthesia technicians. The nursing team consists of a scrub nurse, who is responsible for passing instruments, and a circulating nurse, who may be called upon to provide additional supplies during the course of the operation. It is vitally important that everybody in the operating room be identified and it is a good practice to list the people who are participating in the operating room including attending surgeon, surgical assistants, anesthesiologists, students, and observers. These can be posted on a grease board or chalkboard so that patient privacy is respected and disclosure of participating individuals is also designated.

Instrumentation and equipment in the operating room will include an instrument table, cautery, anesthesia machine, and additional technology that would include devices such as surgical navigation systems, x-ray imaging systems, robotic systems, blood recirculation systems, heart and lung machines, and other equipments that facilitate the operation. Personnel should be aware of wires, cords, and hoses and try to position them to avoid interference with staff walking through the operating room.

To decrease the risk of surgical wound infection, it is good practice to limit the flow of traffic through the operating room.[6] Hospital personnel and surgeons should be cognizant of ongoing procedures and only enter rooms when their presence is needed. One should not *cut through* rooms to get to another place in the facility but proceed along sterile corridors that are designated in all operating rooms.

Communication is important. At times, it may be necessary to temporarily stop surgery to wait for equipment or correct physiologic parameters that are not optimal. This includes points where there may be excessive bleeding. Surgery should be stopped to allow transfusion and fluid resuscitation to occur by the anesthesiologist. The procedure may be temporarily suspended while x-ray studies are reviewed. It is important to have all diagnostic tests that may be critical for intraoperative decision making present and immediately available in the operating room. This is part of preoperative planning and x-rays should be displayed if they are needed for the initial stages of the procedure. These may need to be changed during the operation.

The maintenance of sterile technique is one of the hallmarks of surgery.[7,8] Prior to entering the operating room all surgical personnel are to use a decontamination solution or scrub based on Joint Commission on Accreditation of Health Care Organizations (JCAHO) guidelines. Members of the operating team are gowned and gloved by the scrub nurse and, at all times, sterility must be maintained which involves placement of hands above the waist and in the midline. Any question of sterile technique being violated should be acknowledged by the surgical team. Gowns and gloves should be appropriately changed as needed. Surgeons or their assistants may need to rescrub before reentering the operating room.

Distractions must be avoided in the operating room. Cellular phones and pagers must be turned over or signed out so that the operation can proceed without interruption. Conversation in the operating room should only be pertinent to the procedure. This assures that the health-care team in the operating room can concentrate on the needs of the patient.

It is the responsibility of the operating surgeon and nursing personnel to keep families informed of the progress of surgery. There are instances in which decision making may require the surgeon to exit the operating room to speak with the family directly. The surgeon must be available immediately and the patient should be attended to by another surgeon of the chief operating surgeon's designation. This could be a resident but there must be an appropriate assistant scrubbed at the operating table at all times. Under no circumstances should a patient be left to the operating room nurses and the anesthesia team alone.

Surgery is accomplished by instruments being passed back and forth between the scrub nurse and the surgeon. Universal precautions must be taken at all times for patients. Universal precautions imply that all patients, until proven otherwise, may be infected with a communicable disease. For this reason, it is imperative that the location of all sharp instruments be designated and the passage between the nurse and the surgeon in a highly technical procedure be respected. The surgeon or the assistants should calmly communicate to the nurse and other assistants as to what the requirements are, and it should be understood that usually there is only one nurse and perhaps two or three operating surgeons and, therefore, patience and respect are important for normal and safe conduct in the operating room. There is no place for raised tones of voice or disrespect of any nature because any degree of anxiety or urgency on the part of an operating surgeon can be translated to anxiety on the part of the other members of the health-care team which creates an unsafe environment, may affect the quality of service rendered thereby doing the patient a disservice.

In terms of universal precautions, communication should indicate to the nurse that a knife or needle has been placed in a particular place outside the operating field so that the nurse can pick up or handle these sharp instruments and avoid any sharps coming in contact with the operating surgeon, the nurse, or any other member of the health-care team. If the patient is known to have any communicable disease, such as HIV, then it is appropriate for the surgeon to pick up the instrument from the tray rather than directly from the nurse's hands to avoid mishaps such as a puncture. Any time a glove or gown is punctured inadvertently with a sharp instrument, the gown, the instrument or the suture, and the like should be discarded. A new gown and gloves should be applied to the person who has had a mishap and any break of the surgeon skin, assistant's skin, or nursing skin should be noted and an incident report should be filed indicating not only the breach of sterility, but the fact that an injury has occurred. This should be an incident report that is documented.

After the operation is completed, a sterile dressing is applied. In most cases, this should be discussed before the end of the procedure so that the necessary materials are available. At the conclusion of a case, the patient, based on the preference of the anesthesiologist, may remain intubated and is transported out of the operating room. It is the responsibility of the operating surgeon to escort the patient, with the anesthesiologist, to the recovery room or, as the case may be, to the intensive care unit. Prior to departure from the operating room, the instruments, sponge, and needle count must be correct and if there is any question about a missing instrument, missing needle, or sponge, the wound should either be reexplored or an x-ray should be obtained to assure that no foreign body has inadvertently been left in the patient.[9]

After the patient has been transported to the recovery area and is stable, an operative note should be dictated at that time by the operating surgeon and a brief operative note should be place in the medical record in the patient's chart indicating the preoperative diagnosis, the postoperative diagnosis, the procedure performed, the key members of the operation team, whether there were any specimens sent (including cultures, blood loss, the fluids given, whether drains were placed), and a brief note of the pertinent operative findings. Any complications that occurred should be documented in the medical record as a complication and should be dictated as such. Any surgical mishap that occurs, such as the transection of a nerve or blood vessel, should be noted (a repair presumably is accomplished) in the record. Any adverse event that occurs should be disclosed to the family and, ultimately, to the patient.

On occasion, intraoperative deaths occur. If this takes place, a formal operative note should be dictated indicating the demise of the patient. The medical examiner should be notified and it is appropriate that support personnel such as the Chaplin or social workers be informed that a death has occurred. The hallmark of the operating room is an environment where patients are cared for in a true sanctuary, where continued learning and education occur, and where there is compassion for all members of the healthcare team. It is always a privilege for a surgeon to be in that environment and it should be treated with respect and compassion.

REFERENCES

1. Khaitan L, Chekan E, Brennan EJ Jr, et al. Diagnostic laparoscopy outside the operating room. *Semin Laparosc Surg* 6(1):32–40, 1999.

2. Cronen G, Ringus V, Sigle G, et al. Sterility of surgical site marking. *J Bone Joint Surg Am* 87(10):2193–2195, 2005.

3. Levin LS. Clinical orthopaedics and related research. Editorial comment. 2005:(433).

4. Wallace LM. Informed consent to elective surgery: the 'therapeutic' value? *Soc Sci Med* 22(1):29–33, 1986.

5. Winfree CJ, Kline DG. Intraoperative positioning nerve injuries. *Surg Neurol* 63(1):5–18, 2005; discussion 18.

6. Pryor F, Messmer PR. The effect of traffic patterns in the OR on surgical site infections. *AORN J* 68(4):649–660, 1998.

7. Mangram AJ, Horan TC, Pearson ML, et al. Hospital Infection Control Practices Advisory Committee. *Am J Infect Control* 27(2):97–132, 1999; quiz 133–134; discussion 96.

8. McCoy KD, Beekmann SE, Ferguson KJ, et al. Monitoring adherence to standard precautions. *Am J Infect Control* 29(1):24–31, 2001.

9. Gawande AA, Studdert DM, Orav EJ, et al. Risk factors for retained instruments and sponges after surgery. *N Engl J Med* 16;348(3):229–235, 2003.

THE POSTOPERATIVE

CARE OF THE

SURGICAL PATIENT

Philip Y. Wai, MD
Paul C. Kuo, MD, MBA
Rebecca A. Schroeder, MD

INTRODUCTION

Postoperative care of surgical patients has evolved as a distinct specialty care area as surgical procedures have increased in number and complexity. Although one of the first descriptions of postsurgical care was offered by Florence Nightingale in 1863, the very earliest physical postoperative care areas appeared in the 1920s and 1930s as part of critical care areas in selected academic hospitals. Prior to that time, surgical patients were cared for on general medicine wards or in private homes. Interestingly, it was only with the intense nursing shortage during and following World War II that the astoundingly high early postoperative mortality rates were recognized and *postanesthesia recovery units* (PACU) and specialized surgical wards resembling modern units began to appear.

The Postanesthesia Care Unit (PACU)

The PACU is a standard fixture in all facilities that perform invasive procedures of any kind. It is essentially a critical care unit adapted to place less emphasis on ventilator services and more on rapid patient turnover. As such, it must be able to handle invasive hemodynamic monitoring including arterial, central venous, pulmonary arterial, and even intracerebral pressure or spinal drainage catheters. Nursing care ratios are as intensive as in any critical care unit, and a consulting physician must be immediately available.

The amount of time each patient spends in the PACU depends on the surgical procedure, other medical conditions the patient may have, and complications that may develop during the recovery period. One large trial from 1992 showed an overall complication rate of 24 percent for a general surgical adult population in an academic hospital. The most common of these was nausea and vomiting (9.8 percent), followed by the need for airway support (6.9 percent), hypotension (2.7 percent), arrhythmia (1.4 percent), and hypertension (1.1 percent). The development of problems was highest in patients who were ASA (American Society of Anesthesiologists) Classification II, had undergone emergency, abdominal, or orthopedic procedures, cases of 2–4 h duration, had a history of smoking or had developed intraoperative hypothermia. However, it is important to know that the patients in this study are most likely to develop serious or life-threatening complications would have gone to the intensive care unit and were not included in the analysis. In the current practice environment, many of these patients will not go to a critical care area, or will go to a step-down unit and spend some time in a PACU in the interim. Also, poor pain control was not listed as a complication.

Standard guidelines have been established to help define when patients are ready to be discharged from the PACU. While there are many variations on these in different institutions, a general list is provided in Table 6-1. Broadly speaking, a patient must be stable, able to seek assistance should a problem arise, and free from any significant, ongoing process such as nausea and vomiting or severe pain prior to being moved to a less monitored environment.

Table 6-1 **PACU Discharge Criteria**

Patient must be/have:
Fully awake and alert
Able to maintain airway
Stable vital signs × 30–60 min
Ability to call for help as needed
No obvious surgical complications
Pain controlled
Nausea/vomiting controlled
Normothermia
Resolution of block (unless of upper extremity)

INPATIENT CARE

The postoperative care of the surgical ward patient is directed at providing the appropriate level of support to facilitate recovery and a return to normal daily function. Organ systems are addressed in a systematic and comprehensive fashion to avoid unnecessary complications. Prophylactic therapy is administered when there is a high risk for clinical disease. The caveat to adequate ward management is the early recognition of a patient who is becoming acutely or critically ill and who may no longer be appropriately managed in a nonintensive setting.

Pain Control

Postoperative pain control has become a topic of great interest to the general public in recent years. In fact, regulatory agencies have become involved, with The Joint Commission of Accreditation of Health Care Organizations that recently issued a challenge to improve pain control. Pain is a determinant in patient recovery outcomes and satisfaction for inpatient and outpatient surgical procedures. Studies have shown that 50–75 percent of all patients have inadequate pain relief, and it seems to be the most severe in thoracic, head and neck, orthopedic and upper abdominal procedures. Inadequate pain relief leads to increased sympathetic tone, cardiac work, systemic vascular resistance, and more frequent myocardial ischemia. It also leads to decreased functional residual capacity (FRC) and vital capacity (VC), increased atelectasis, impairment of normal respiratory muscle function and cough, and higher rates of pneumonia. Pain impairs neuroendocrine and metabolic function, increases postoperative nausea and vomiting, and decreases patient movement leading to deep venous thrombosis (DVT). Inadequately managed acute pain may actually increase the risk of developing chronic disabling pain syndromes. And it greatly prolongs hospitalization and decreases patient satisfaction. It is no surprise that pain is the focus of so much attention during the perioperative period.

Appropriate management of postoperative pain must account for a variety of issues. These include not only the site and type of surgery and the patient's other medical conditions and medications, but also the nursing staff level and type of unit where care is being provided, the patient's anticipated length of stay, and possibly even the patient's home situation. For example, an epidural catheter may be routine practice on a regular surgical floor at one hospital but not at another. One patient may be a good candidate for a regional block but another patient may be on oral anticoagulation and unable to receive a block. And, a specific patient may be a particularly ideal candidate for a specific procedure, but a language barrier precludes informed consent.

A variety of techniques for pain control are available to the physicians caring for postoperative patients and may be viewed as an ascending hierarchy of invasiveness and risk. The oldest and least satisfactory is intramuscular (IM) injection of narcotics on a scheduled or as-needed (prn) basis. This is rarely done in today's environment. It is plagued by problems of variable onset and delayed respiratory depression, as well as pain at the injection site and lack of ability to titrate the needed dose. The most common and probably the standard to which other methods are compared is intravenous (IV) injection of a variety of narcotics, most often via a pump activated by a button controlled by the patient (*PCA* or *patient-controlled analgesia*). When the patient pushes the button, a small dose of narcotic is administered directly into the patient's IV. The pump is programmed to limit the dose to a maximum bolus per *button-push*, with a time lockout, and a maximum dose per 4-h period. A basal rate may also be programmed as a background, although this is reserved for special situations such as severe cancer pain or patients on chronic opiates. The idea is that the risk of respiratory depression is minimized as the patient will not push the button if he or she is too sleepy. This is completely dependent; however, on the basic concept that *no one* pushes the button other than the patient. Family members or helpful friends who think that patients *look like they are in pain* have caused respiratory arrest by attempting to help out and pushing the button for sleeping patients.

Peripheral nerve blocks have been performed for many years and are safe and effective. These are extremely diverse in description, but the most common encountered in postsurgical patients are interscalene, axillary, supraclavicular and infraclavicular for the upper extremity, and femoral, sciatic, popliteal, and lumbar plexus for the lower extremity. Catheters may also be placed in any of these locations for continuous infusion of local anesthetic in special situations. If done as single-shot blocks, they must be monitored for regression, although patients may be intentionally discharged from the recovery room or an ambulatory surgery center with long-acting blocks in place for extended pain control. This is possible only when the patient is deemed reliable to report any problems, and has appropriate assistance at home or on the surgical floor. More peripheral blocks, such as ankle, median nerve, ulnar nerve, and digital nerve blocks are single-shot blocks of the foot and hand or even a single digit. These areas may be difficult to assess as they are usually hidden under dressings but carry a very low risk of any neurologic injury.

A step beyond peripheral nerve blocks is central neuraxial blocks (i.e., spinal, caudal, or epidural blocks). All of these techniques may be used as a primary anesthetic technique for the surgical procedure, and extended by use of some combination or single use of narcotics and local anesthetics, depending on the clinical indication. For example, if a spinal anesthetic is planned for a lower extremity amputation, a narcotic may be added to the intrathecal mixture to provide analgesia for up to 18 h postoperatively, or an epidural catheter may be placed at the same time and while not used intraoperatively, is available for use for several days postoperatively. Although epidural catheters are routine, intrathecal catheters for continuous infusion of any medication are rarely used and require a much higher degree of vigilance to prevent potentially catastrophic complications. A caudal block is similar to an epidural block, but placed via the sacral hiatus and is used almost exclusively in very young children for urologic, perineal, or lower extremity surgery. *Continuous epidural analgesia* (CEA) with a mixture of low-dose local anesthetic and narcotic, most often fentanyl, is ideal for those procedures that are associated with intense postoperative pain, specifically thoracotomy, upper abdominal procedures with flank or subcostal incisions, and some major orthopedic procedures. There may also be other benefits to CEA including improved patency of vascular grafts, decreased incidence of DVT in orthopedic patients, and modulation of the neuroendocrine response to surgical stress, especially with thoracic-level catheters. In general, the catheter must be placed near the dermatomal level of the incision in order for optimal benefit. That is, for a thoracotomy, a catheter must be placed at a T4 to T6 level, whereas a lumbar catheter will suffice for a total hip replacement. Furthermore, the risk of placement of a lumbar catheter is much lower as they are actually placed below the level of the adult spinal cord. In most hospitals, an acute pain service is responsible for management of any invasive catheter placed for postoperative pain management.

Recent research into pain management has emphasized that optimal success in relieving pain occurs by exploiting a variety of modalities. As such, much importance has been placed on use of nonsteroidal anti-inflammatory agents, especially with the release of *ketorolac*, the only injectable agent currently available in the United States. In addition, a variety of agents used intraoperatively have been reported to have a *drug-sparing* effect in postoperative pain control such as α_2 agonists (clonidine and dexmedetomidine) and ketamine, although their impact is not well-defined.

Nausea and Vomiting

Interestingly, in patient surveys, postoperative pain is not what patients rate as the worst thing about their experience. It is nausea, with or without vomiting that they rate as the most unpleasant thing, the single factor they would pay the most to eliminate when asked about paying money out of pocket. If untreated, more than one-third of all patients will develop nausea with or without vomiting (N/V) at a cost to the health-care system of several hundred million dollars annually. It may be more common after general anesthetics than regional ones, but not necessarily so. Patients after some procedures are without doubt more prone to develop nausea or vomiting, including all laparoscopic procedures, strabismus surgeries, certain breast and gynecologic procedures, and those that involve use of nitrous oxide and opioids. Young women also seem to be at higher risk, as do nonsmokers. Certainly, those with a history of postoperative N/V or motion sickness are at very high risk. Moreover, patients who are experiencing pain, dizziness, as well as those who are relatively dehydrated and those who prematurely attempt oral intake are vulnerable.

Nausea with or without vomiting is a serious issue regardless of patient satisfaction. Vomiting puts patients at risk of aspiration, esophageal rupture, suture dehiscence, or disruption of the surgical site. Also, increases in intrathoracic pressure that accompany retching can cause elevations in intracerebral pressure, or venous bleeding in proximal surgical wounds such as carotid endarterectomies or other head and neck sites, possibly resulting in catastrophic airway compromise. The excessive motion of vomiting can even disrupt cervical spine repairs and threaten the cord itself. Although, these severe outcomes are rare, prolonged stays in the PACU are commonly result, as do unplanned admissions to the hospital in ambulatory surgery centers. Also, a significant number of patients, especially those undergoing outpatient procedures, continue to experience N/V after they are discharged and are unable to receive adequate pharmacologic treatment, resulting in days lost from work, continued morbidity, and dissatisfaction.

A Herculean effort has been put forth in an effort to find a solution to this problem. More than 1000 randomized, controlled trials have been published evaluating pharmacologic treatment for N/V, not counting nonpharmacologic approaches. These have compared a variety of drugs including droperidol, dexamethasone, serotonin antagonists (ondansetron, dolasetron), Phenergan, metoclopramide, hydroxyzine, as well as intraoperative interventions such as using propofol for induction of general anesthesia, avoidance of opioids and nitrous oxide, generous rehydration, and avoiding general anesthesia. In general, it has been found that combination therapy is better than therapy with a single agent. Prophylaxis is only indicated for high-risk patients, specifically those undergoing high-risk procedures and those with a history of postoperative N/V or motion sickness. Some literature also supports treating female nonsmokers prophylactically.

The most recent notable large trial involved 5199 patients and 6 strategies (including intraoperative intervention) in increasing numbers of combinations. The conclusions in a simplified form are as follows: (1) ondansetron, dexamethasone, and droperidol all decreased N/V by about the same amount when used as a single agent (26 percent) for prophylaxis in high-risk patients, (2) dexamethasone did not work well as a rescue dose in the PACU, (3) ondansetron was best as rescue drug in PACU, and (4) rescue treatment worked best if it was not the same drug as was used for prophylaxis.

It is important to consider other causes of N/V. For example, increases in gastric distention or intracerebral pressure could present as N/V, but could herald the presence of serious surgical complications. Involving the surgeons in evaluating changes in the patient's condition is always advisable. One interesting development in the treatment of postoperative N/V is the incorporation of the alternative method of acupressure. Stimulation of the *meridian P6* point bilaterally (a point near the palmaris longus tendon approximately 3 cm proximal to the wrist crease), either by manual pressure with application of cotton elastic bands, or by extremely low-level electric stimulation may decrease the incidence of postoperative N/V. While the evidence for efficacy is not absolutely clear, the risk of these alternative treatments is extraordinarily low.

Delirium

Postoperative delirium is becoming recognized as a marker for greater risk of morbidity and mortality following all kinds of surgical procedures, especially in elderly patients. Its incidence is greatest in those with predisposing factors, such as dementia and preexisting cognitive deficits, but is also high after specific procedures, such as some orthopedic procedures, and those involving prolonged intensive care unit stays. Severity of delirium can range from *mild confusion* that is barely detectable by staff and family, to *wild delusional* and *near-violent behavior* in which the patient is a danger to himself or herself and others. In addition, episodes of delirium can lead to other complications, such as episodes of tachycardia and hypertension resulting in myocardial infarction (MI). In all delirious patients, it is important to rule out metabolic causes of delirium, including drug and alcohol withdrawal, electrolyte abnormalities, and hypoglycemia. Strategies to decrease the incidence of delirium such as cycling the lights in the critical care unit to simulate night and day have met with limited success. Treatment of postoperative delirium is most successful with butyrophenones, most commonly haloperidol, although use of other sedatives, such as dexmedetomidine have shown some promise.

Agitation

Agitation is not uncommon in the postoperative population, particularly in the first few hours following surgery and can look very much like delirium except that patients are generally still alert and oriented. However, it can herald the presence of some serious complications, including hypoxia, hypercarbia, and acidosis. Alternatively, it may simply be the result of pain or bladder distention, especially in patients unable to effectively communicate. Agitation may be associated with use of certain intraoperative medications, especially atropine, ketamine, and scopolamine. However, the presence of this alteration in mental status should not be dismissed without due consideration in vulnerable patients. General agitation has been reported as the only presenting complaint in some cases of postoperative intra-abdominal and intracerebral hemorrhage.

Hyperthermia

Fever in the postoperative patient is probably the most common complication noted on a surgical floor. The majority of patients who develop a fever in the postoperative period do not harbor an infection. Within the first 3 postoperative days, fever suggests atelectasis from chronic *hypoventilation,* a common occurrence in the postoperative patient, causing low-grade fever in the absence of active infection. Other noninfections causes include febrile reactions to medications and DVT. However, a measured core temperature greater than 38.5°C should be regarded with a high index of suspicion for an infectious process and warrants a focused history, physical examination, and a targeted diagnostic workup that may consist of blood, urine, or sputum cultures, chest x-rays, and cultures of relevant surgical drains or indwelling lines. Common infectious causes are discussed under the section Infectious Disease. There is little evidence to support empiric antibiotics except in immunosuppressed patients. Generally, antibiotic therapy should be guided by culture data. Febrile patients without clinical evidence of active infection should be treated with antipyretics.

THE PULMONARY SYSTEM

The most urgent pulmonary complications include *airway obstruction, pneumothorax*, and *pulmonary embolus* (PE). However, the most common changes in pulmonary function in the postoperative setting are related to hypoventilation, decreases in VC and FRC resulting in atelectasis, and hypoxemia and pneumonia. Respiratory failure (sustained tachypnea, respiratory acidosis, and hypercarbia) necessitates immediate respiratory support with supplemental oxygen and if necessary, endotracheal intubation with positive pressure ventilation or mask bilevel positive airway pressure support. An appropriate workup for an inciting cause must follow (Table 6-2).

Airway Obstruction

Obstruction of the airway is one of the most urgent complications that can develop in the postoperative patient, and is all the more likely due to the manipulation of the airway that occurs as part of general endotracheal anesthesia. Although the majority of the risk occurs in a highly monitored environment of the PACU, a significant number of cases of airway obstruction occur in delayed settings on surgical wards. This is also becoming a more recognized phenomenon as obstructive sleep apnea and obesity have become more common in the general and surgical populations.

Potential causes of airway obstruction are diverse. It is critically important to determine whether the cause of obstruction is in the upper or lower airway. In the somnolent or unconscious patient, the most common cause is the tongue or pharyngeal soft tissue. A physical examination is mandatory to document presence or absence of breath sounds. Placing the stethoscope over the larynx is a good place to listen to determine if any air is actually moving when breath sounds in the chest are difficult to hear. A squeaking sound would indicate laryngospasm with movement of a tiny amount of air, whereas no sound would mean complete spasm with no air movement, or

Table 6-2 **Common Causes of Respiratory Failure in Postoperative Patients**

Hypoventilation
Secondary to medications, obesity, pain, decreased level of consciousness,
  diaphragmatic dysfunction following thoracic or upper abdominal surgery,
  surgical dressings, poor patient positioning, postoperative delirium, weakness
Airway obstruction
Upper airway vs. lower airway, laryngospasm, bronchospasm, foreign bodies
Pulmonary edema
Pneumonia
Aspiration
Pulmonary embolism
Pleural effusion
Pneumothorax
Tension vs. stable
Exacerbation of preexisting disease
COPD
Bronchospastic disease
Interstitial or restrictive disease

obstruction somewhere else. Observation of respiratory efforts of the chest is
also important. There should be coordinated movement of the abdomen and
the chest outward and inward together, without retraction of the intercostal or
supraclavicular regions. An obstructed pattern would be *bucket-breathing*,
that is, paradoxical movement of the abdomen outward with the chest
inward, followed by the chest going outward while the abdomen pushed
inward, and so forth. This pattern is especially prominent in children who
have compliant chest cavities. Retractions are very important, although more
difficult to see in obese patients. The best places to look are above the clavicle and in the sternal notch. Another factor to note is how much muscular
effort is used by the abdomen to exhale. Great exhalation effort, taking a prolonged period of time, is indicative of lower airway obstruction, for example
wheezing.

When determining the cause of airway obstruction, the setting is important to consider. What type of surgery did the patient have? How long ago
was it? What drugs did the patient receive and when? What type of medical
problems does the patient have? What other medications does the patient
take? Does the patient have any allergies? The issue of *latex allergy* is of special importance for this last issue. With the dramatic increase in use of latex
gloves in the last few decades, the incidence of latex allergy has increased
dramatically in some populations. One specific manifestation of latex allergy

is profound bronchospasm, and one particular at-risk population is health-care workers. If this is suspected, all latex products must be removed from the area and the allergy must be aggressively treated with epinephrine in order for the bronchospasm to be adequately treated.

Regardless of when or where airway obstruction occurs, it must be treated simultaneously with its workup. The patient's mental status must be ascertained, the airway positioned with a jaw lift, and the patient encouraged to take deep breaths. Supplemental oxygen is applied. Oral or nasal airways may be used if necessary, keeping in mind that in awake patients, they may stimulate vomiting. If the patient has recently undergone head and neck or carotid surgery, a quick check for wound hematoma or retained throat packs or sponges is made. A quick physical examination to assess for air movement, breath sounds, and respiratory efforts is essential. The responsible surgeons must be notified immediately. Gentle suctioning of the pharynx may be appropriate if there are secretions or vomitus, and the patient may need to be placed in the lateral position if vomiting. If continued support of the airway is required, positive pressure with a *bag-valve-mask* should be applied. If laryngospasm is suspected, it can usually be broken with continuous pressure, although a small dose of succinylcholine (20 mg) may be used. If all these efforts are unsuccessful, or if the patient is unresponsive or hypoxemia is severe, immediate endotracheal intubation should be performed with cricoid pressure to help protect the lower respiratory tract from aspiration as quickly as possible. If the recent surgery involved the neck, however, it should be remember that the anatomy may have been radically altered, and direct laryngoscopy may be impossible. In that catastrophic case, emergent cricothyroidostomy may be needed.

Hypoventilation

Hypoventilation in postsurgical patients is extremely common but is most often mild and not noticed. Specifically, it is defined as a $PaCO_2$ less than 45 mmHg on an arterial blood gas measurement, although the test is not often done and the patient's baseline measurement must be taken into account. Clinical signs of mild-to-moderate hypercarbia and respiratory acidosis include *tachycardia, hypertension,* and *ventricular ectopy.* Neurologic depression and circulatory collapse may result if the hypercarbia is severe and untreated. In a review of 13,000 postoperative patients, 0.02 percent developed serious respiratory failure, 77 percent in the first hour. Most of the cases were identified primarily by pulse oximetry or by alert nurses and were attributed to upper airway obstruction, excessive fluid administration, and residual drug effects, mostly sedatives, anesthetics, and muscle relaxants. Other contributing factors included hypothermia, electrolyte abnormalities, magnesium therapy (especially in obstetric patients), and other drug interactions. Obese patients, those with tight dressings around the chest or abdomen, or those splinting due to postoperative pain are also at risk.

Upper abdominal and thoracic incisions can cause diaphragmatic dysfunction even in patients with good pain control. Patients in poor position in hospital beds who are unable to straighten themselves properly can develop hypercarbia and respiratory acidosis. Those with preexisting lung disease are at particularly high risk of respiratory failure, being much more susceptible to respiratory depression from anesthetics, narcotics, and benzodiazepines used perioperatively. And finally, those with excessive carbon dioxide production from hyperthermia, shivering or sepsis may develop hypercarbia exacerbating a perioperative respiratory acidosis in an already compromised patient.

It is important to evaluate the patient's mental status, strength, complaints of pain, medical history including recent surgical procedure and current complaints, recent drug administration, and any change in physical status or recent events as reported by the patient or nurse. Treatment of hypoventilation and respiratory acidosis depends on the cause. For example, judicious pain medication is appropriate if splinting is the problem, repositioning of the patient into the sitting position as tolerated, incentive spirometry, pharmacologic reversal of narcotics, benzodiazepines, and muscle relaxants as appropriate, correction of electrolyte abnormalities as indicated, and assisted ventilation up to endotracheal intubation as required.

Hypoxemia

The list of possible causes of hypoxemia in the postsurgical patient is long and complex. For this reason, diagnosis and treatment must proceed systematically. *Hypoxemia* is defined as PaO_2 less than 60 mmHg, and is usually diagnosed by pulse oximetry or less often, arterial blood gas measurement. Clinically, hypoxic patients appear restless, tachycardic, and cyanotic, although cyanosis may not be apparent in severely anemic patients. At more advanced stages, however, patients become somnolent, and will eventually suffer respiratory arrest. Patients at highest risk for postoperative hypoxia are those at the extremes of age, those with a history of obesity, obstructive sleep apnea, or a high ASA Classification status, or those who have undergone a lengthy surgical procedure. Also, at risk are those with particularly high-oxygen consumption rates, for example, those shivering or those with sepsis or other hypermetabolic state.

Hypoxia in postoperative patients is most often due to hypoventilation (as discussed earlier) or pulmonary shunting and mismatch of ventilation and blood flow. However, as with airway obstruction, hypoxemia must be treated at the same time or even prior to the confirmation of a diagnosis. Supplemental oxygen is applied as a first treatment, and is often adequate by itself. Ventilatory support is provided in increasing degrees, depending on the patient's presentation. Patients must be evaluated and treated for airway obstruction and hypoventilation as mentioned earlier. If these are not the cause, attention must be turned elsewhere. If hypoxia becomes profound and does not respond to supplemental oxygen, positive pressure ventilation must be initiated, up to and including endotracheal intubation and mechanical ventilation if necessary. Additional workup would include arterial blood gas measurement, chest radiograph, electrocardiogram, and possibly transthoracic echocardiogram if a cardiac cause of respiratory failure was suspected.

The most common cause of intrapulmonary shunting after general anesthesia is decreased FRC. This is most severe after upper abdominal procedures but accompanies almost all surgical procedures and is secondary to microatelectasis. Other causes of shunt/mismatch are macroatelectasis secondary to hypoventilation, as well as aspiration, pulmonary edema, and PE. *Pneumothorax* is a particular risk after any surgical procedure during which a central line has been placed in the great veins of the neck or any procedure in the neck, thorax, upper abdomen, or retroperitoneum, including nephrectomy. Patients with *bullous emphysema* have an especially high risk of rupturing blebs during periods of positive pressure ventilation, which may result in tension pneumothorax. Definitive treatment of clinically significant pneumothorax is through placement of a chest thoracostomy tube. Patients with a history of reactive airway disease or tobacco use may benefit from bronchodilator therapy. This may be true even if no active wheezing is heard, as severe spasm may preclude adequate air movement needed to detect wheezing on clinical examination. It should also be remembered that all causes of wheezing are not pulmonary.

Pulmonary Aspiration and Pneumonia

The physiologic gastroesophageal and pharyngoesophageal sphincters normally prevent aspiration of oropharyngeal and gastric contents. However, depressed consciousness, poor positioning of the patient, presence of gastrointestinal (GI) obstruction, and interruption of normal barrier function with nasogastric or endotracheal tubes are responsible for most cases of aspiration pneumonia. Mortality from aspiration pneumonia is exceedingly high and appropriate attention and care is required to reduce this risk in the postoperative patient. The *chemical pneumonitis* that develops causes local inflammation and edema, increases the risk for secondary infection, and can produce a systemic inflammatory response.

Lower respiratory tract pneumonia is one of the most common complications contributing to mortality in the postoperative patient. Clinical manifestations of pneumonia include fever, tachypnea, increased secretions, and sputum production. Typically, chest radiography does not correlate with either progression or resolution, most often lagging behind the clinical course. However, it often shows pulmonary consolidation or infiltrate. Appropriate prevention includes early mobilization, use of incentive spirometry, respiratory exercises, and deep breathing and coughing. Treatment involves administering antibiotics and adequate pulmonary toilet based on culture results.

THE CARDIOVASCULAR SYSTEM

Postoperative cardiovascular complications may be life threatening and should be promptly addressed. The management of cardiovascular disease following surgery should ideally be part of a regimen of comprehensive care that begins in the preoperative phase and extends not only into the operating room but also throughout the entire hospital stay and the rehabilitation period.

Hypotension

Hypotension can be a devastating complication in any patient, but is especially common in the perioperative period. Causes of hypotension can be divided into four basic groups: those arising from problems with: (1) cardiac preload, (2) cardiac afterload, (3) left ventricular function, and (4) cardiac rate and rhythm (Table 6-3). Any hypotensive patient must be assessed for

Table 6-3 **Common Causes of Hypotension during the Postoperative Period**

Preload
Inadequate oral intake or intra/postoperative volume replacement
  (vomiting, diarrhea, fistulas, drains)
Blood loss/hemorrhage
Diuresis
Third space losses of fluid
Pulmonary embolism
Pneumothorax
Pericardial tamponade
Afterload
Medications (antihypertensives, negative inotropes, and so on)
Shock (septic, neurogenic, anaphylactic)
Liver failure
Inotropy
Myocardial ischemia/infarction
Medications (beta-blockers, calcium channel blockers)
Cardiomyopathy
Hypocalcemia
Acidosis
Hypothermia
Rate/rhythm
Bradycardia
Supraventricular tachycardia (especially atrial fibrillation/flutter with rapid
  ventricular response)
VT/VF
Heart block

the severity of the problem and treated accordingly. For a blood pressure 20–30 percent less than the patient's baseline, or a mean arterial blood pressure less than 55 mmHg, a fluid bolus of 250–500 mL crystalloid or colloid, or administration of a vasopressor is appropriate. Also, placing the patient either flat and raising the legs, or in the Trendelenburg position (30° head down) may be helpful. The patient's volume status must be evaluated, clinically by physical signs and symptoms, and historically by collecting data on recent volume infusions, blood loss, drain, chest tube, urine output (UOP), and so forth. If the patient is hemodynamically unstable, assistance should immediately be called for and the patient managed according to advanced cardiac life support (ACLS) protocols.

Fortunately, the vast majority of patients who develop hypotension in the recovery room or in a surgical ward do not require invasive measures for evaluation or treatment. By far, the most common cause of hypotension in the postoperative patient is *decreased preload* due to relative or absolute hypovolemia. This is usually due to inadequate fluid replacement in the operating room, ongoing blood loss or drainage, continuing sequestration of hypotonic fluid (so-called *third-spacing*), redistribution of blood with rewarming or regression of a neuraxial block after surgery, diuresis, or capillary leakage secondary to a systemic or regional inflammatory process. Appropriate treatment is replacement of fluid with either crystalloid or colloid, although the choice of which fluid and the appropriate amount remains highly controversial. This is likely to continue due to the intense nature of competing priorities. Certain organs such as the kidney are better preserved by aggressively resuscitating preload with volume infusion. However, the lung survives much better by limiting volume resuscitation and maintaining perfusion pressure of peripheral organs with inotropes and vasopressors. Also, colloids are expensive and tend to cause delayed peripheral edema, as they will continue to hold edema fluid in the interstitial tissues once they have migrated out of the vascular space. Use of large amounts of crystalloid may cause tremendous immediate peripheral edema, and impairs tissue oxygen delivery. However, this edema often resolves. Assessing patients for decreased preload includes looking for tachycardia, orthostasis, dizziness, poor UOP, concentrated urine, poor jugular venous pulses, and a lack of jugular venous distention in the supine position. Also, new sources of blood and fluid loss, vomiting, diarrhea, diuresis, or poor oral intake are clues. Changes in clinical status such as chest pain, evolving infection, respiratory distress, fever, and changes in mental status should all prompt further investigation.

Changes in cardiac afterload can certainly manifest as hypotension. This most commonly accompanies inflammatory and infectious conditions such as shock and sepsis. These would also be encountered in patients suffering allergic responses to medications or latex, and more severe transfusion reactions to blood products. These are not subtle conditions and are due to excessive vasodilation. Often more intensive interventions are required with movement to a critical care unit, invasive monitoring, and vasopressor support.

Left ventricular dysfunction and cardiac rate and rhythm are the last two major causes of hypotension. Hypotension due to decreased cardiac output may be a result of myocardial ischemia, metabolic acidosis, moderate or severe hypothermia, sepsis, mechanical compression as from pericardial tamponade or large or tension pneumothorax, valvular dysfunction, pulmonary embolism, electrolyte abnormalities, or drug toxicity. Likewise, the causes of the spectrum of dysrhythmias encountered in postoperative patients are diverse. They include life-threatening conditions such as hypoxia, hypercarbia, acidosis, and myocardial ischemia, but also alkalosis, hypothermia, anemia, and electrolyte abnormalities, most often hypokalemia. Again, for any hemodynamically unstable patient, ACLS care should be instituted immediately. For patients in ventricular fibrillation (VF) and for those in pulseless ventricular tachycardia (VT), ACLS care would include immediate electrical defibrillation. Simultaneous with treatment of all hypotensive episodes should be efforts at diagnosis and treatment of the underlying cause. This may include arterial blood gas analysis, blood counts and chemistries, chest radiography, electrocardiogram, possible echocardiography if available, as well as immediate and serial physical examinations.

Hypertension

The most common cause of hypertension in the postoperative population is failure to restart regular medications, most often due to inability to take oral medications or tolerate a regular diet. Patients may be nauseated or in pain, or suffering from postoperative ileus. However, it is important to rule out other important causes of hypertension, including hypoxia, hypercarbia, acidosis, bladder distention, or even intracranial hypertension in the neurosurgical patient. Unusual conditions including malignant hyperthermia, pheochromocytoma, and thyroid storm may also present as hypertension. It is rare that the degree of hypertension reaches dangerous levels, although anything more than 20–30 percent greater than a patient's baseline blood pressure level should be treated aggressively because untreated hypertension is associated with myocardial ischemia, congestive heart failure, and increased surgical bleeding. The most often used agents include beta-blockers, alpha-blockers, calcium channel blockers, direct vasodilators, and nitrates.

Myocardial Infarction

The incidence of postoperative MI varies from 0.4 to 12 percent depending on the patient population and the manner studied. Patients at highest risk include those with preoperative congestive heart failure, ischemia, who are over 70 years of age, those with other comorbidities such as diabetes mellitus, renal insufficiency, or other atherosclerotic disease (e.g., carotid artery stenosis and peripheral vascular disease). The most recent data on perioperative MI show that those at the highest risk of MI develop tachycardia and hypertension, not only intraoperatively, but even more importantly, during the postoperative period. What may happen is that precipitating factors, including but not limited to poor pain control, periods of delirium and confusion, anxiety, dysrhythmias, episodes of hypoxemia related to intermittent airway obstruction during sleep or medication-related sedation, untoward events such as hemorrhage or vomiting, and so forth, combine to cause repeated episodes of myocardial ischemia. These repeated episodes affect vulnerable areas of subendocardium and an infarction results.

The majority of these infarctions are of the non-Q-wave type, are asymptomatic, and remain undiagnosed. Many of these patients cannot complain of chest pain or dyspnea due to a variety of factors. In other patients, presentation may be very subtle. For example, a change in mental status may herald a perioperative MI. A postoperative workup may identify an ongoing MI in the absence of clinical symptoms in high-risk patients. Diagnosis is best confirmed by electrocardiogram and serial-elevated creatine kinase-MB enzyme and troponin levels.

However in some patients, perhaps due to the hypercoagulable state associated with surgery, acute coronary syndromes will occur and present dramatically with extreme ST-elevation infarctions and even abrupt cardiac arrest. Treatment includes moving the patient to a monitored setting, and following ACLS protocols as indicated. In all cases, pain control, oxygenation, nitroglycerin, and aspirin therapy should be addressed or considered. Unless contraindicated, all patients should receive beta-blockers. Also, use of heparin and other thrombolytic therapy may be considered and cardiology consultation is appropriate.

Arrhythmia

The majority of postoperative dysrhythmias are benign and take the form of unifocal primary ventricular contractions, caused primarily by alterations in electrolytes or mild hypothermia. In addition, many patients have this at baseline without previous documentation. Other more concerning dysrhythmias include new-onset atrial fibrillation/flutter and other supraventricular tachycardias. Atrial fibrillation is of great concern in patients with known structural heart disease and should initiate immediate rate control. Patients should be moved to a highly monitored setting. Myocardial ischemia or infarction should be ruled out in these patients. For all patients, immediate identification of the rhythm should be accomplished with a 12-lead ECG, and electrolyte levels, including calcium, magnesium, and acid-base status should be checked. At the same time, relevant history should be obtained and physical examination performed, to assess factors such as pain control, underlying infection, the development of congestive heart failure and pulmonary edema, and the possibility of pulmonary embolism. ACLS protocols should be followed for patients with more malignant rhythms such as VT or VF with synchronized cardioversion or defibrillation as required. Carotid sinus massage should be used with care in postoperative patients following any procedures near the head or neck.

THE GASTROINTESTINAL SYSTEM

After surgery of the GI tract, normal peristalsis is depressed, otherwise known as ileus. Resolution of the ileus occurs in an organ-specific manner with function returning to the small intestine within hours, the stomach within 24–48 h, and the colon within 2–4 days. Electrolyte abnormalities, use of opioids, and pain and underlying infection or inflammation can prolong the course of postoperative ileus. Treatment consists of supportive therapy with suspension of oral intake, administration of IV fluids, and treatment of exacerbating conditions.

Gastric distention represents a significant postoperative complication that can interfere with oral feeding, result in mucosal engorgement and ischemia, and predisposes to gastric volvulus. Treatment of distention with nasogastric tubes allows gastric decompression and minimizes vomiting and aspiration. However, routine use of these devices is unnecessary and may contribute to development of atelectasis and pneumonia.

Enteral feeding of the GI system should be instituted as soon as there is an adequate level of consciousness, return of protective airway reflexes adequate to protect against aspiration, and resolution of any postoperative ileus for a variety of reasons. Nutrition absorbed via the intestinal lining has been demonstrated to preserve the integrity of the mucosa, may reduce bacterial translocation rates, and decrease the incidence of opportunistic infection. In addition, a subset of postoperative patients who remain without oral intake for extended periods of time are at high risk of development of stress gastritis and ulcer formation. Results from a Canadian critical care trials group showed that routine prophylaxis against stress ulcers (e.g., with H_2-blockers) in mechanically ventilated patients who were also coagulopathic decreased the risk of GI bleeding. However, routine use of these agents is unnecessary in the majority of patients.

Patients who do not resume bowel function within the expected time frame may have developed mechanical obstruction. Causes include postoperative adhesions, mesenteric hernias, and surgical error. Obstructive symptoms are sometimes indistinguishable from ileus and may require further imaging to confirm the diagnosis. Appropriate management includes an initial trial of nasogastric decompression although operative management exploration is appropriate if workup suggests mechanical obstruction.

FLUIDS, ELECTROLYTES, AND NUTRITION
Volume Status

The management of fluids in the surgical patient addresses the requirements for end-organ perfusion (e.g., kidneys) without precipitating cardiac failure, pulmonary edema, and detrimental electrolyte disturbances. Entire textbooks have been written on the subject of intravascular fluid regulation, electrolyte physiology, and acid-base control. Furthermore, recommendations and guidelines for management of the wide variety of patients found in critical care areas including the operating room and PACU, as well as the general surgical wards, have populated journals for decades. Although no consensus has been reached on the ideal manner in which to manage any specific subset of patients, most probably due to the unimaginable variation found within any *defined* subset, some general guiding principles exist. The following summarizes these principles. One is referred to the relevant published literature for more detailed discussion.

Surgical stress is one important factor contributing to the hormone-mediated changes in a postoperative patient's volume status. Amongst the tremendously complex neuroendocrine response to surgical stress is activation of the renin-angiotensin system, stimulating conversion of angiotensin I to angiotensin II and release of aldosterone. These hormones have potent vasoconstrictive properties, and also renal-tubular sodium reabsorption and subsequent shifts in fluid balance. Subsequent release of antidiuretic hormone in a response to surgical stimulation and anesthesia also contributes to fluid retention and further vasoconstriction. These effects subside around postoperative day 3 and a prompt diuresis of excess fluid may be seen.

The goals of IV fluid therapy are to: (1) replace fluids lost preoperatively and intraoperatively, (2) fulfill routine maintenance requirements, and (3) prevent deficits from ongoing pathologic losses during the postoperative period. Estimating a patient's perioperative deficit is done by calculating the preoperative fluid deficit, and accounting for blood and other fluid losses. Insensible losses through evaporation both from the respiratory tract and especially from the operative field must be taken into account as they may be massive during some procedures, particularly pancreatic cases, burns, and in febrile or septic patients. Maintenance needs based on body weight can be calculated using the summation of the *10-5-2* rule with 100 mL/kg/day administered for the first 0–10 kg of body weight, 50 mL/kg/day for each kg of body weight between 11 and 20 kg, and finally 20 mL/kg/day for each kg of body weight greater than 20 kg. The hourly IV maintenance fluid infusion rate is the total divided by 24. Other fluid losses may be large and should not be overlooked. These might include nasogastric, fistula, abdominal, or other drain output.

Clinical findings associated with hypovolemia include decreased skin turgor, weight loss, oliguria, orthostatic hypotension, tachycardia, and hypotension. Laboratory variables that may be measured include increases in serum creatinine and blood urea nitrogen (BUN) with intravascular depletion suggested by an increase in BUN/creatinine ratio greater than 20. The use of Foley catheters and measurement of hourly UOP can provide a relatively noninvasive means of assessing intravascular volume status. UOP corresponding to adequate renal perfusion for an average adult is approximately 0.5 mL/kg/h. The risk of urinary tract infection (UTI) is higher in the presence of indwelling urinary catheters and the benefits and risks of catheter placement should be carefully considered. When UOP decreases below the accepted threshold, overall volume status and other causes of decreased UOP should be considered (see Endocrine and Renal Systems) in the fractional excretion of sodium (FENA) may help differentiate hypovolemia from other causes of low UOP. A value of less than 1 in an oliguric patient suggests prerenal intravascular depletion and should be managed by fluid resuscitation. Invasive methods of evaluating cardiac preload in an acute or intensive care setting include the measurements of central venous pressure and pulmonary artery capillary wedge pressure as well as assessment of cardiac output.

Common parenteral fluids used in IV replacement include crystalloid such as the various saline and lactated Ringer's (LR) solutions. Isotonic saline contains 154 meq/L of both sodium and chloride ions but does not contain potassium or bicarbonate ion. When these solutions are given in large quantities, they may overload the kidney's ability to excrete chloride ion, resulting in a dilutional metabolic acidosis. LR is a *physiologic* solution containing 130 meq/L of sodium, 4 meq/L of potassium, 109 meq/L of chloride, and 28 meq/L of bicarbonate. It is appropriate for replacing fluid losses from GI sources as well as extracellular deficits. Hypertonic saline and colloid solutions are not routinely outside the intensive care unit.

Most cases of volume deficiency surgical patients are due to preoperative fasting in preparation for elective cases, anorexia associated with underlying surgical pathology, and ongoing fluid losses consistently underestimated by clinicians. A common but less visible cause of fluid overload is *fluid sequestration* in the extravascular spaces secondary to surgery, trauma, or other disease process such as liver failure. Intravascular volume excess is best treated by fluid restriction, patient mobilization, and appropriate use of loop diuretics.

Electrolytes

Electrolyte abnormalities accompany fluid shifts and adversely affect the recovering patient by affecting multiple-organ systems. Hyponatremia can result from a primary sodium loss or excess free water with normal levels of sodium. In the surgical patient, hyponatremia is most commonly caused by excess water secondary to infusion of hypotonic solutions, by renal reabsorption of excess free water, or excess oral intake of free water (Table 6-4). During

Table 6-4 **Differential Diagnosis of Hyponatremia**

Hypovolemic hyponatremia
Diuresis (especially with loop diuretics)
Diarrhea
Excessive sweating (as with fever, hyperthyroidism)
Hypervolemic hyponatremia
Congestive heart failure
Cirrhosis
Hypoproteinemia (e.g., secondary to nephrotic syndrome or malnutrition)
Euvolemic hyponatremia
SIADH
Paraneoplastic syndromes/CNS lesions
Hypothyroidism
Adrenal insufficiency
Medications

the perioperative period, release of antidiuretic hormone (ADH) increases reabsorption of free water in the renal collecting tubules. A systematic approach to the diagnosis and management of hyponatremia requires an assessment of the effective circulating volume. *Hypovolemic hyponatremia* can be caused by direct sodium losses through the GI tract, skin, or renal systems. In surgical patients, the replacement of solute and fluid with hypotonic solutions exacerbates this form of hyponatremia. Loop diuretics also produce hypovolemic hyponatremia. *Hypervolemic hyponatremia* results from congestive heart failure, cirrhotic states, and other hypoproteinemic conditions such as malnutrition. Hyponatremia with euvolemia can result from the syndrome of inappropriate ADH secretion (SIADH), pulmonary or central nervous system (CNS) lesions, hypothyroidism, adrenal insufficiency, or a wide variety of medications including narcotics and some antineoplastic agents. In these states, the underlying condition should be treated in conjunction with water restriction. Hypovolemic hyponatremia should be treated with free water restriction and isotonic fluid replacement. Treatment of hypervolemic hyponatremia requires water restriction, sodium restriction, and judicious use of loop diuretics. Excessively rapid normalization of serum sodium can lead to irreversible central pontine myelinolysis. The rate of replacement should not exceed 0.5 meq/L/h. This phenomenon is of great concern in patients receiving transfusion with massive amounts of fresh frozen plasma (FFP), which has a high sodium content.

Hypernatremia is less common than hyponatremia in the postoperative patient and is associated with free water loss, hypovolemia, and oliguria.

Treatment requires the replacement of free water according to the calculated water deficit. Rapid correction of severe hypernatremia can result in severe neurologic symptoms, cerebral edema, and brain stem herniation.

Postoperatively, hyperkalemia can result from diminished renal function, administration of exogenous potassium, crush injuries, ischemia-reperfusion syndromes, massive blood transfusion, and tumor lysis. The complications of hyperkalemia are primarily related to cardiac dysrhythmia and an electrocardiogram may demonstrate peaked T-waves, flattened P-waves, prolongation of the QRS complex, or a variety of ectopic ventricular rhythms. Left untreated, patients can develop VF or cardiac arrest. First-line therapy consists of administering calcium gluconate to reduce cardiac membrane instability. Thereafter, insulin administered with glucose (causing potassium to shift intracellularly), exchange resins such as sodium polystyrene sulfonate, sodium bicarbonate, or dialysis maybe effective treatments for hyperkalemia. It is important to remember that glucose and insulin therapy do not actually reduce total body potassium.

Hypokalemia results from decreased dietary intake, GI losses, increased renal losses, metabolic alkalosis, or redistribution within the intracellular space from glucose insulin or bicarbonate administration. Severe hypokalemia can cause muscle fatigue, ileus, and cardiac arrhythmias. Treatment involves potassium replacement.

Other important electrolytes that require attention in the postoperative patient include magnesium, calcium, and phosphate. Hypomagnesemia is common and most often secondary to GI loss, hypercalcemia due to primary hyperparathyroidism, and hypophosphatemia from increased renal or GI losses or after major liver resections. Treatment involves oral replacement of magnesium and phosphate, and fluid rehydration in hypercalcemic states. After restoring intravascular volume, loop diuretics may be administered to lower serum calcium. New-onset hypercalcemia requires a diagnostic workup.

Nutrition

Adequate nutritional support is increasingly recognized to be integral in the care of every surgical patient. The optimal strategy for caring for these patients depends on the underlying diagnosis and metabolic state. While many patients are malnourished due to their primary disease, fasting usually accompanies inpatient diagnostic testing and therapeutic interventions and may further exacerbate preexisting catabolic conditions.

Preoperatively, a patient's nutritional status is evaluated with a history addressing recent weight loss, dietary intake, and preexisting medical conditions such as cirrhosis or cancer that cause rapid weight loss. On physical examination, findings of muscle wasting and loss of subcutaneous fat may be present. Other objective assessments may include daily weight measurements and serial laboratory tests including prealbumin and transferrin, although these are nonspecific.

The caloric needs of a patient can be estimated by assessing the *basal energy expenditure* (BEE) using the *Harris-Benedict equation*. Most patients require approximately 20–25 kcal/kg/day although these needs may be tremendously increased in times of stress such fever, sepsis, burn injury, and trauma. Although rarely used in clinical practice, the *respiratory quotient* (RQ; defined as $RQ = CO_2$ produced per O_2 consumed) may yield information on the primary metabolic substrate and insight into the catabolic state of the patient ($RQ < 0.7$, starvation; $RQ = 0.7$, fat metabolism; $RQ = 1.0$, carbohydrate metabolism; $RQ > 1.0$, lipogenesis/overfeeding). Refeeding syndrome occurs when essential electrolytes (e.g., potassium, magnesium, and phosphorus) are transported intracellularly secondary to glucose administration in a patient who has undergone prolonged fasting or is chronically malnourished. This potentially fatal metabolic derangement can be avoided by correcting electrolyte abnormalities prior to and during the administration of nutrition.

Necessary calories may be derived from protein (4 kcal/g), carbohydrate (3.4–4 kcal/g), and fat (9 kcal/g). Up to 30 percent of daily caloric requirements can be supplied by fat. Higher proportions of fat-derived calories may impair cellular immunity and reticuloendothelial function. Certain medical conditions produce specific metabolic demands and the balance of proteins, carbohydrates, and fat needed by individual patients will vary. For example, while 0.8–1.0 g/kg/day of protein may be adequate in healthy patients, amounts of 1.0–1.6 g/kg/day may be necessary in septic or burn patients, and restricted amounts of 0.6 g/kg/day may be appropriate in patients with hepatic cirrhosis and encephalopathy. A key parameter to consider is the patient's *nitrogen balance* (the difference between the amount of nitrogen ingested and nitrogen excreted). A minimum of 100 g/day of carbohydrate are required for the brain and red blood cells, and at least 3–5 percent of calories are required as essential fatty acid to prevent fatty acid deficiency. Excess administration of carbohydrate can lead to lipogenesis while excess lipid administration can adversely affect immunity, gas exchange, and increase the risk of sepsis.

For patients who are unable to take oral feedings or unable to tolerate enteral feedings of any kind, IV nutrition becomes necessary. Central catheters are preferred for concentrated (e.g., greater than 7% dextrose) parenteral feeding solutions although peripheral sites may be used for more dilute solutions. Complications associated with parenteral feeding include catheter-related sepsis, pneumothorax, venous thrombosis, hepatic transaminitis, hepatic steatosis, and acalculous cholecystitis. Direct enteral nutrition (oral, or nasogastric, gastric or jejunal feeding tubes) avoids many of these risks and cumulative evidence has shown that enteral feeding more effectively maintains the integrity of the gut mucosa, and may decrease bacterial translocation into the bloodstream. Recently, studies have even suggested that some patients may benefit from early feeding after bowel surgery.

ENDOCRINE AND RENAL SYSTEMS

Patients with diabetes mellitus, whether taking oral hypoglycemic therapy or insulin, are commonly found among the surgical population and frequently suffer from its complications, including renal insufficiency, widespread atherosclerosis, coronary artery disease, and hypertension. Tight control of hyperglycemia has been shown to improve surgical outcomes, especially in the neurosurgical, cardiac, and intensive care populations. On the morning of elective surgery, according to current recommendation, half the normal morning dose of long-acting insulin is given subcutaneously along with a 5 percent glucose IV solution as an IV maintenance infusion. Surgical stress, concurrent medications (especially steroids), and complicating infection exacerbate hyperglycemic control. The goal of treatment depends on the care setting, with tighter control being possible in a more critical care unit with more frequent blood glucose monitoring availability. In the immediate perioperative period, when patients are still not tolerating oral intake and are dependent on IV fluids, it is generally considered more advisable to err on the side of slightly higher blood glucose levels, with target levels of 150–200 mg/dL. This is to protect the patients against the devastating complications of hypoglycemia that may not be detected or show the typical symptoms, that is, decreased levels of consciousness, somnolence, tremor, and confusion. While still recovering from the effects of anesthesia, the effects of their pain medication, mild forms of postoperative delirium or agitation may all mimic hypoglycemia and diagnosis may be delayed. Blood glucose measurements on a regular surgical floor are performed every 4 h and insulin provided on a sliding scale (Table 6-5). However, once the patient is protected from hypoglycemia by a regular supply of glucose calories, either internally or parenterally, tighter glucose control is the goal. On the other hand, in an intensive care unit, patients are

Table 6-5 **Insulin Sliding Scale**

Finger Stick Glucose (mg/dL)	Units
120–150	2 (regular insulin subcutaneously)
150–200	4
200–250	6
250–300	8
>300	10 (call house officer immediately for evaluation of patient)

managed with continuous insulin infusions, with blood glucose measurements performed regularly, sometimes on an hourly basis. Hyperglycemia should be treated with the aim of maintaining glucose levels between 100 and 120 mg/dL. As glucose levels normalize, the daily insulin requirements can be used to calculate the amount of long- or intermediate-acting insulin required for postoperative coverage with short-acting regular insulin used for supplementation according to a sliding scale. While a patient is receiving insulin but not receiving nutrition, maintenance fluids should always contain at least 5 percent dextrose.

Adrenal insufficiency is a life-threatening condition that can occur in selected patients during the postoperative period. Patients who are receiving chronic steroids or who have been recently treated with steroid therapy are at increased risk for developing adrenal insufficiency. Clinical findings include hypotension unresponsive to fluid resuscitation, and minimally responsive to vasopressors. Although the syndrome is rare, clinical studies have shown an increased mortality rate in those in whom it occurs. Treatment involves the IV administration methylprednisolone or hydrocortisone, as well as resuscitation with fluids and vasopressors and inotropes as required.

Causes of postoperative renal insufficiency are generally divided into three general etiologic groups: *prerenal*, *intrinsic*, and *postrenal*. *Prerenal* causes of acute renal failure include intravascular depletion for any reason. The most common, although not the only, intrinsic cause is acute tubular necrosis (ATN). *Postrenal* causes are obstructive in nature and involve conditions such as prostatic hypertrophy, nephrolithiasis, or extrinsic compression of the ureter. Identifying which of these is responsible for the decrement in renal function is of the utmost importance prior to choosing a therapy. After identification, therapy can be directed at the underlying causes. For example, intravascular depletion should be corrected with fluid replacement. Postrenal obstruction can be relieved by bladder catheterization, stone removal, nephrostomy, or other appropriate maneuvers. Treatment of ATN involves appropriate fluid management, use of diuretics and, if necessary, and dialysis.

THE HEMATOLOGIC SYSTEM

Postoperative decreases in hematocrit can result from a variety of processes including hemorrhage, preoperative anemia, or the dilutional effects of fluid administration. While transfusion of blood products is common practice, it is becoming increasingly recognized that mild to moderate anemia maybe well tolerated and blood product transfusion is not benign. Complications associated with transfusion of blood products include, but are not limited to, transfusion-related acute lung injury, transmission of blood-borne pathogens (including the possibility of prions—an issue not well-defined at this time), fever, back pain, bronchospasm, hypotension, development of a variety of antibodies precluding later transfusion or transplantation, rash, urticaria, hemolysis, and anaphylaxis. These risks can lead to critical illness or death in an otherwise healthy patient and underscore the need for clinical judgment prior to every decision to transfusion. The current standard for administering blood to a patient includes an assessment made on a case-by-case basis. Strict adherence to arbitrary and universal transfusion triggers without consideration of the individual clinical situation and bleeding risk is inappropriate. Patients with no evidence of heart disease and no postoperative complications have been shown to tolerate a hemoglobin of 6 g/dL, whereas a patient with myocardial ischemia and ongoing blood loss may benefit from transfusion that maintains a higher circulating hemoglobin level. In many instances, even a careful examination may not detect ongoing bleeding, and a low threshold for diagnostic workup is required for serial, decreasing hematocrits that cannot be otherwise explained.

In many surgical patients, ongoing blood loss is caused by abnormal hemostasis, most often caused by acidosis, hypothermia, sepsis, or significant trauma. Such patients require exogenous clotting factors provided in FFP or cryoprecipitate. In rare instances, bleeding will be due to an unrelated underlying genetic conditions that will require targeted therapy. Patients with hemophilia A (Factor VIII deficiency), hemophilia B (Factor IX deficiency), von Willebrand disease (von Willebrand factor and Factor VIII:C deficiency), protein C, S, or antithrombin III deficiency, Factor V Leiden deficiency, require careful pre- and postoperative management, and hematology consultation is indicated. Other patients with conditions including systemic lupus erythematosus (lupus anticoagulant), or who are taking medications such as warfarin, platelet inhibitors, or other anticoagulants will be at risk for abnormal bleeding, in the perioperative period.

It is also important to remember that many surgical patients with chronic diseases such as cancer, renal failure, a history of previous gastric surgery or resection of the terminal ileum, or a variety of other illnesses of long duration may suffer from anemia of chronic disease. Other patients might be deficient in iron, folic acid, or vitamin B_{12} and require appropriate supplementation during the perioperative period when blood loss exacerbates their baseline anemia and cannot be physiologically restored in the context of these deficiencies. Therapy with erythropoietin may be beneficial in these cases.

Almost all patients are at risk for developing deep venous thrombosis (DVT) from immobilization on the operating table. Patients with limited mobility secondary to fractures, physical traction, fatigue, or pain associated with large incisions may benefit from subcutaneous heparin to prevent the complications of DVT. The risk of DVT and fatal pulmonary embolism is so high in the orthopedic population that patients are anticoagulated with warfarin immediately following total joint replacement and it is continued well into the rehabilitation period. The physical findings of Homan's sign, unilateral edema, calf pain, or venous distention is present in less than one-third of patients with DVT and the diagnosis is best confirmed using bilateral venous-Doppler examination of the lower extremities. An increasingly common alternative or supplement to the use of heparin is the application of pneumatic compression devices, a type of stocking placed most often on the calves to prevent stasis, beginning prior to induction of anesthesia in the operating room. In certain patients, the use of an intracaval filter is indicated for the prevention of PE.

The patient who has developed any kind of hemodynamic or respiratory insufficiency as a result of coagulopathy, be it bleeding or reaction to transfusion, should receive immediate attention, and consideration should be given to diagnostic workup, the need for an intensive care setting, and even operative exploration.

Infectious Disease

Fever in the postoperative patient does not by itself always herald the onset of an infectious process. Hypoventilation leading to atelectasis is a common cause of fever and should be treated with pulmonary toilet and not antibiotics. Patients with signs and symptoms consistent with infection require a history and targeted physical examination. This is especially true of those at increased risk such as those with contaminated surgical wounds, trauma patients, cancer patients, or those on chronic steroids or immunosuppressed for another reason. A diagnostic workup can consist of blood, urine, sputum or wound cultures, chest radiographs, and cultures of indwelling lines or surgical drains. The most common nonsurgical source is the urinary tract although lower respiratory tract infections are the leading cause of nosocomial infection leading to death in the surgical population. Treatment of infection involves removing potential sources (indwelling devices or lines), administering specific antibiotic therapy based on culture data, and modulating host factors (e.g., correcting hyperglycemia and opening wounds) that contribute to infection (Table 6-6).

As discussed earlier, *pneumonia* is a serious, life-threatening complication in the surgical patient. Laboratory information guiding therapy includes Gram's stain and culture of sputum, bronchial washings, and even sometimes, bronchial biopsies. While broad-spectrum coverage against gram-negative species is often started empirically, it should be noted that gram-positive *Staphylococcus aureus* is a frequent cause of pneumonia. In addition, aspiration pneumonia must be considered in all patients who are intubated or who have depressed levels of consciousness, even for brief periods of time. Postoperative pneumonia should be treated for 14–21 days.

The majority of UTIs result from underlying genitourinary disease or seeding from indwelling bladder catheters. For this reason, these catheters should be removed as soon as possible. Diagnosis requires the presence of more than 100,000 colony forming units (CFU)/mL on a sterile urine culture.

Table 6-6 **Antibiotic Recommendations**

Suspected Source	Antibiotic Agent
Simple wound infection	Cephazolin or other first-generation cephalosporin
Intra-abdominal infection	Quinolone + metronidazole or piperacillin/tazobactam (Zosyn)
UTI	Quinolone or third-generation cephalosporin or ampicillin + gentamycin
Pneumonia (gram-negative bacteria)	Aminoglycoside + cefuroxime or TMP-SMZ or aminoglycoside + antipseudomonal penicillin or ceftazidime
Pneumonia (gram-positive bacteria)	Vancomycin
Pneumonic (mixed flora)	Imipenem

The most common organisms include *Escherichia coli, E. faecalis,* and *E. faecium,* but a wide variety of organisms are seen. Unlike more benign outpatient UTIs, catheter-related infections require a longer course of treatment of 10–14 days.

Administration of preoperative antibiotics immediately prior to skin incision has recently been shown to decrease the rate of wound infection, although there is no evidence that there is a benefit from continuing them into the postoperative period. The development of a wound infection depends on four critical factors: *pathogenicity of the organism, host defense, local environment,* and *surgical technique.* Factors that alter host defense include comorbid diseases such as diabetes, cancer, trauma, malnutrition, acquired or inherited immunodeficiency, and immunosuppressive medications. Foreign bodies including suture material, hematomas, and seromas provide a nidus of infection in the local wound environment and are associated with an increased risk of infection. In these instances, removal of foreign material and drainage of these collections is the standard of care. Meticulous, aseptic surgical technique decreases the risk of postoperative wound infection. Traumatic handling of tissue, placement of tight, strangulating sutures, excessive use of electrocautery, and use of polyfilament or silk sutures contributes to tissue necrosis and bacterial growth and should be avoided. The incidence of wound infection varies among clean (less than 1.5 percent), clean-contaminated (less than 3 percent), or contaminated (less than 5 percent) surgical wounds. Suspicion of cellulitis at the surgical site should prompt an examination for the cardinal signs of infection, including blanching erythema, warmth, local tenderness, and edema. Fluid collections in a wound that has developed cellulitis should prompt removal of the sutures, opening of the wound, drainage, irrigation, and open packing. This can often be performed at the bedside.

Wound infections can harbor a variety of organisms. *S. aureus* is a frequent culprit in wound infections and is treated with penicillinase-resistant antibiotics. Infection with methicillin-resistant *S. aureus* requires IV administration of vancomycin. Gram-negative species that can produce surgical infections include *Escherichia, Proteus, Klebsiella,* and *Pseudomonas. Pseudomonas* is particularly difficult to treat due to multidrug resistance. Although a variety of third-generation cephalosporins and extended-spectrum penicillins have been used to treat these infections, the appropriate use of antibiotic should ideally be based on cultures and specific sensitivity data to achieve success. Anaerobic organisms found in wounds include *Bacteroides fragilis* and typically signals a known or unknown break in the anatomic integrity of the GI tract or the onset of tissue necrosis. *B. fragilis* is typically treated with metronidazole or clindamycin.

Clostridium difficile is a common cause of colitis in the postoperative patient resulting from overgrowth with this organism and alterations in the host flora secondary to antibiotic use. A high index of suspicion is required for diagnosis and is confirmed with culture, biochemical assays, or direct visualization of pseudomembranes on endoscopic examination. Typically, discontinuation of current antibiotics and administration of oral vancomycin or metronidazole is adequate and appropriate therapy.

Other important surgical infections include necrotizing soft-tissue infections by *Clostridium* or other gram-positive species. These microbes produce a rapidly progressive destruction of tissue leading to sepsis and multiorgan failure. Wide surgical resection and debridement are the mainstay of initial therapy supplemented with broad-spectrum antibiotic coverage until specific culture data are available. Less dramatic but also important is sinusitis, a special problem in patients with nasogastric or nasal endotracheal tubes. Treatment includes removal of the tube if possible, and administration of amoxicillin-clavulanic acid or trimethoprim-sulfamethoxazole (TMP-SMZ). Gram-negative species including *E. coli, Klebsiella,* or *Proteus,* or other organisms such as *Enterococcus, Clostridium,* and *Bacteroides* are usually the agents responsible for acute cholecystitis and are treated with third-generation cephalosporins and metronidazole. Finally, patients who have undergone splenectomy for any reason are susceptible to infection by encapsulated organisms such as *Streptococcus pneumoniae, Haemophilus influenzae,* and *Neisseria meningitidis.* In these patients, administration of vaccines against pneumococcus, *H. influenzae,* and meningococcus should be given preoperatively if possible.

Wound Care, Drains, and Tubes

Epithelialization over a closed surgical site is generally complete after 24–48 h and sterile dressings applied in the operating room can be removed at this time.

Findings that warrant earlier examination include copious drainage, wet dressings, fever, or signs of cellulitis. Sudden discharge of serosanguineous fluid from the wound is pathognomonic for fascial wound dehiscence and usually requires operative intervention. In wounds that remain dry, continue to be well approximated, and show signs of healing, abdominal staples or skin sutures can generally be removed after 5–7 days. In healthy patients, wound remodeling and contraction becomes optimal by 6–8 weeks and can be subjected to the stresses of normal activities. It should be noted that wounds only achieve 70–80 percent of the tensile strength of normal skin for months after the incision is closed. Preoperative steroids, immunosuppression, and malnutrition delay wound closure and healing. Patients with deficiencies of vitamin C and A develop poorly healed wounds due to inappropriate hydroxylation and cross-linking of collagen. In these patients nutritional supplementation may be beneficial.

In contaminated cases, where gross spillage from a nonsterile cavity has infiltrated the surgical site, the skin and subcutaneous layers should be left open to allow for adequate drainage. Reapproximation of these incisions can be performed later through delayed primary (sutured after a few days) or secondary (allowing the would to heal by itself) closure. Wound care of open skin incisions typically involves loosely packing wet-to-dry dressings into a wound, and changing them twice a day.

Surgical drains prevent accumulation of fluid at surgical sites, reduce stasis associated with microbial growth, and provide clues regarding the integrity of a surgical anastomosis. Examples of open drainage systems include the Penrose drain, a simple rubber tube that drains fluids onto surgical packing. Closed systems include the Jackson-Pratt and Duvall drains. These drains are placed with sterile technique in the operating room and drain fluids into closed containers such as plastic bulbs that are usually under gentle vacuum suction. These can be opened and emptied on the ward, the drainage measured and sampled, and the suction replaced. As these outlets can provide mechanisms for both fluid evacuation and pathogen entry, they should be removed as soon as they are no longer necessary and must be handled carefully. Postoperatively, appropriate drain care involves daily inspection for the amount and quality of fluid returned. Acute and sustained increases in the rate of fluid accumulating in a drain require further examination of the surgical site. Changes in character of the fluid may herald bleeding, infection, or anastomotic leak. In addition to proper inspection, closed drainage systems should also be *milked* to ensure that the lumens are patent and not contributing to stasis at the surgical site.

The nasogastric tube is typically a sump drain that is placed through the nasal cavity and into the stomach. In certain instances, a postpyloric position is desired. Drainage and decompression help protect some GI anastomoses and decrease complications from prolonged ileus. Complications associated with nasogastric tubes include nasal erosion and necrosis, sinusitis, hypokalemia, hypochloremia, metabolic alkalosis, reflux gastritis, and aspiration pneumonia. The nasogastric tube should be connected to low-intermittent suction and irrigated frequently to ensure patency. In certain cases, the nasogastric tube or a Dobhoff feeding tube placed in the postpyloric position can be used for early resumption of postoperative feeding in a patient who cannot take oral feeds due to a depressed level of consciousness, or dysphagia, or in patients who have a high-GI anastomosis with no other contraindication to oral feeding.

RECOMMENDED READING

1. Norton JA, Bollinger RR, Chang AE, et al. *Surgery: Basic Science and Clinical Evidence*. New York: Springer-Verlag, 2001.

2. Greenfield LJ, Mulholland MW, Oldham KT, et al. *Surgery: Scientific Principles and Practice*, 3rd ed. Philadelphia, PA: Lippincott Williams and Wilkins, 2001.

3. Way LW. *Current Surgical Diagnosis and Treatment*, 10th ed. Norwalk, CA: Appleton and Lange, 1994.

WOUND HEALING AND

WOUND MANAGEMENT

Detlev Erdmann, MD, PhD
Tracey H. Stokes, MD

INTRODUCTION

According to the Merriam-Webster Dictionary, a *wound* is a noun of Old English etymology meaning "an injury to the body (as from violence, accident, or surgery) that involves laceration or breaking of a membrane (as the skin) and usually damage to underlying tissues." The definition, however, is far more complex. Wounds can be superficial, affecting only the skin, or can be deep with damage to underlying structures, such as muscle, bone, tendon, nerve, blood vessels, and others (Fig. 7-1). Wounds can be acute or chronic. Chronic wounds persist for weeks or even years without complete healing (Fig. 7-2). Wounds can be life threatening, can inhibit function, and can compromise appearance. The ability to heal a wound is essential for survival in higher species. Improving spontaneous wound healing and intervening with certain operative techniques are fundamental aspects of plastic surgery.

HISTORICAL BACKGROUND

Wounds and their management are described in the medical literature as early as 1700 B.C. Until the midsixteenth century, surgeons treated war wounds (amputations) with boiling oil, hot cautery, and by means of scalding water with disastrous results. Less aggressive methods of wound care with more rapid healing and fewer complications were introduced by the French surgeon Ambroise Paré (1517–1590).

The complex process of wound healing on a cellular level was not clarified until the twentieth century, and research is still ongoing. Modern scientific

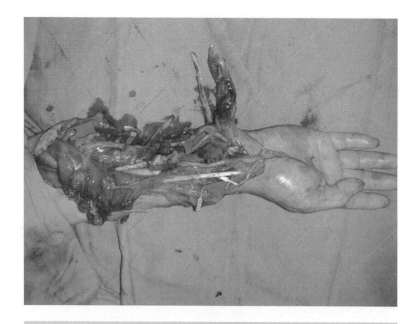

Figure 7-1 **Deep wound to the forearm with damage to underlying structures, including muscle, tendons, nerves, and blood vessels.**

trends such as *tissue engineering* would not be possible without our improved understanding of wounds and their healing.

PHASES OF WOUND HEALING

There are three classic phases of wound healing: *inflammation, fibroplasia*, and *maturation* (Fig. 7-3).[1]

Inflammatory Phase

The *inflammatory phase* occurs during days 0–4 after injury. The initial changes are vascular including a vasoconstriction phase leading to reduced blood flow to aid hemostasis. Vasoconstriction is followed by a period of vasodilation with a simultaneous increase in endothelial cell permeability secondary to histamine. Hemostatic factors, such as kinin components and prostaglandins, initiate local inflammation. Fibronectin, a major component of granulation tissue, attracts neutrophil granulocytes, fibroblasts, monocytes, and endothelial cells culminating in a dynamic cellular milieu and local substances at the injury site. The precise role of each type of inflammatory cell remains unclear. Both polymorphonuclear (PMN) granulocytes and mononuclear leucocytes (MONO) migrate into the wound in numbers

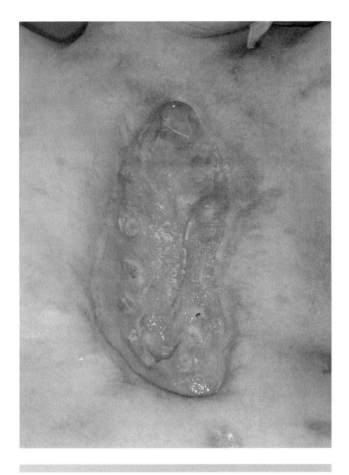

Figure 7-2 **Chronic wound of the sternum with granulation tissue.**

directly proportional to the concentration of local factors. Studies have demonstrated that monocytes must be present during the inflammatory phase to trigger fibroblast production and subsequent migration into the wound.

Proliferative (Fibroblastic) Phase

During the *proliferative phase* of wound healing, fibroblasts move into the wound bed along a framework of fibrin fibers. Fibroblasts produce several essential substances, including glycosaminoglycans such as hyaluronic acid, chondroitin-4 sulfate, dermatan sulfate, and heparin sulfate which are all hydrated into ground substance. Fibroblasts also produce tropocollagen, a precursor of collagen. Collagen is responsible for the increasing tensile strength of the wound. The proliferative phase lasts from day 4 to approximately 2–4 weeks (Fig. 7-4).

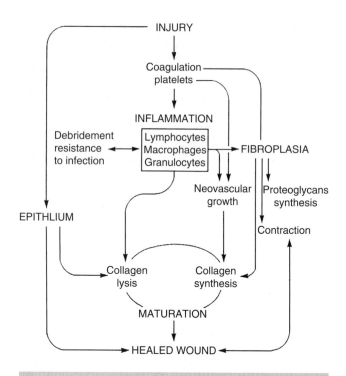

Figure 7-3 **Schematic of three classic phases of wound healing: inflammatory phase, proliferative phase, and remodeling phase.**

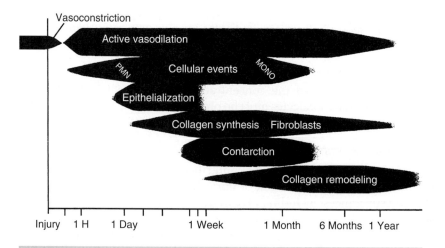

Figure 7-4 **Time sequence of classic wound healing.**

Remodeling (Maturation) Phase

The *remodeling phase* begins approximately 3 weeks after injury and is characterized by an increase in tensile strength.[2] Collagen is at the same time produced, degraded, and reorganized. Most of the immature type III collagen deposited during the initial phase of healing is replaced by type I collagen, until the normal ratio of 4:1 (type I to type III) in skin is achieved. Glycosaminoglycans are degraded, and the water content of the wound slowly returns to normal. More stable and permanent cross-linking of the collagen is established. The length of the remodeling phase is variable and dependent on patient age, genetic background, wound location, and chronicity.

CELLULAR SYSTEM

Various cells have a specific role during wound healing and are briefly described in the following section.

Myofibroblast

Contraction is an active and essential part of the repair process to close the gap in soft tissues. A *contracture*, on the other hand, is an undesirable result of healing due to contraction, fibrosis, or other type of tissue damage.[3] *Myofibroblasts* are responsible for wound contraction. These cells differ from regular fibroblasts due to their cytoplasmic microfilaments similar to those of smooth muscle cells. Within the filamentous system are areas of dense bodies that serve as attachments for contraction. Myofibroblasts have well-formed intercellular attachments, such as desmosomes and maculae adherens.

Epithelial Cell

Epithelial repair always follows the same sequence of events: mobilization, migration, mitosis, and differentiation. During *mobilization* epithelial cells enlarge, flatten, and detach from neighboring cells and the basement membrane. During *migration* cells flow across the gap in the wound. In *mitosis*, migrating cells start to divide and multiply. Increasing cell numbers thicken the new epithelium. Once the wound gap has been closed, cellular *differentiation* from basal to surface layers resumes.

Macrophage

The inflammatory phase of wound healing is characterized by the presence of PMN granulocytes and MONO/macrophages. *Macrophages* appear within 48–96 h after injury and mainly participate in the inflammatory process and debridement. Macrophages release at least two important substances, known as cytokines: interleukin 1 (IL-1) and tumor necrosis factor α (TNF-α)[4]. IL-1 stimulates angiogenesis, fibroblast proliferation, and collagen synthesis. TNF-α stimulates angiogenesis and collagen synthesis.

Lymphocyte

T lymphocytes migrate into the wound after macrophages and produce substances known as lymphokines that induce fibroblast proliferation, angiogenesis, and collagen synthesis.

Factors in Wound Healing

Many intrinsic and extrinsic factors influence wound healing. Medical treatment relies on the manipulation of these factors in order to achieve wound closure. The search for mechanical, pharmacologic, and organic agents to stimulate cells for collagen synthesis, cytokine production, angiogenesis, and many others is of major interest. Such research has been ongoing for decades until today.

Oxygen

At a PO_2 of 30–40 mmHg, fibroblasts are stimulated. Collagen synthesis cannot take place unless the PO_2 is higher than 40 mmHg. Oxygen stimulates epithelial cells, and insufficient oxygen remains the most common cause of wound infections and improper wound healing.[5]

Hyperbaric oxygen therapy can increase the PO_2 in wounds as long as blood vessels are present, but cannot alter wound ischemia in case of impaired perfusion (blood supply).

Certain underlying conditions, such as peripheral vascular disease, diabetes mellitus, and others, are associated with impaired tissue perfusion due to damaged large and small blood vessels. Such comorbid conditions often set the stage for tissue ischemia and subsequent impaired wound healing.

Hematocrit

The *hematocrit* reflects the body's ability to transport O_2 to the wound. However, data regarding decreased hematocrit and impaired wound healing remain inconclusive.

Corticosteroids

Corticosteroids have been shown to inhibit macrophages, collagen production, angiogenesis, and wound contraction.

Vitamin A has been shown to counteract the inhibitory effects of steroids on wound healing.[6] It increases collagen deposition and wound breaking strength as well as reepithelialization.

Vitamins

Vitamin C (ascorbic acid) is an essential cofactor in collagen synthesis and wound healing. Even healed wounds deprived of vitamin C exhibit diminished tensile strength.

Vitamin E serves as a membrane stabilizer and antioxidant, therefore limiting free radicals and cellular damage.

Zinc

Zinc is a common constituent of enzymes and essential for enzyme function. Zinc promotes proliferation of epithelial cells and fibroblasts.

Growth Factors

Growth factors are polypeptides produced by various cells, such as epithelial cells, platelets, macrophages, fibroblasts, and others, and are named accordingly. Growth factors act as mitogens by promoting cell proliferation and as chemoattractants by inducing cell migration. The family of fibroblast growth factors (FGF) has been shown to have the most profound effect on the wound healing process (Table 7-1).[7]

Nicotine

Smoking and *nicotine* ingestion produce vasoconstriction, engender tissue hypoxia, and cause increased local carboxyhemoglobin levels.[8]

Age

Aging is associated with delayed and prolonged phases of wound healing, which is less quantitative than qualitative. Impairment of wound healing in the elderly may also be attributed to intolerance to ischemia and associated comorbidities.

Malnutrition

Malnutrition and low protein levels below 2 g/dL in humans are associated with decreased wound tensile strength, a prolonged inflammatory phase, and decreased collagen production.

Infection

Open wounds are colonized with bacteria. If the bacterial load exceeds 10^5/g tissue, local defense mechanisms become insufficient, and the wound becomes infected.[9] *Wound infection* engenders decreased PO_2 and increased collagenolysis prolonging the inflammatory phase. Leukocyte chemotaxis and migration, phagocytosis, and killing of pathogens are all impaired. Angiogenesis is compromised and wound epithelialization delayed leading to a chronic, nonhealing wound.

Chemotherapy

Chemotherapeutic agents generally lead to decreased fibroblast proliferation and wound contraction.[10] However, when chemotherapy is started 2 weeks after wound repair, little effect is noted on long-term wound healing.

Table 7-1 **Growth Factor Signals at the Wound Site**

Growth Factor	Sources	Primary Target Cells and Effect
EGF	Platelets	Keratinocyte motogen and mitogen
TGF-α	Macrophages Keratinocytes	Keratinocyte motogen and mitogen
HB-EGF	Macrophages	Keratinocyte and fibroblast mitogen
FGFs 1, 2, and 4	Macrophages Damaged endothelial cells	Angiogenic and fibroblast mitogen
FGF7 (KGF)	Dermal fibroblasts	Keratinocyte motogen and mitogen
PDGF	Platelets Macrophages Keratinocytes	Chemotactic for macrophages and fibroblasts Macrophage activation Fibroblast mitogen and matrix production
IGF-1	Plasma Platelets	Endothelial cell and fibroblast mitogen
VEGF	Keratinocytes Macrophages	Angiogenesis
TGF-β1 and -β2	Platelets Macrophages	Keratinocyte migration Chemotactic for macrophages and fibroblasts Fibroblast matrix synthesis and remodeling
TGF-β3	Macrophages	Antiscarring
CTGF	Fibroblasts Endothelia	Fibroblasts Downstream of TGF-β1
Activin	Fibroblasts Keratinocytes	Currently unknown
IL-1α and β	Neutrophils	Early activators of growth factor expression in macrophages, keratinocytes, and fibroblasts
TNF-α	Neutrophils	Similar to IL-1α and β

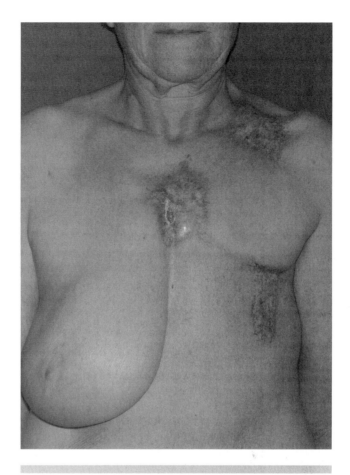

Figure 7-5 **Female patient with chest wall wound after radiation (left breast removed due to breast cancer).**

Radiotherapy

Acute effects of *radiation* on tissues include stasis and occlusion of small blood vessels. In addition, there is a direct effect of radiation on fibroblast proliferation leading to both decreased collagen production and decreased wound tensile strength.[11] Radiation may lead to chronic, nonhealing wounds with a potentially devastating impact for the patient (Fig. 7-5).

FETAL WOUND HEALING

Fetal wound healing differs fundamentally from normal postnatal healing. Adult wound healing is characterized by collagen deposition, collagen remodeling, and scar formation. Fetal wound healing resembles a regenerative process with minimal amounts or even lack of scar formation.[12] This may be due to an absence of the inflammatory phase of normal healing and due to a different wound matrix composition consisting of a high concentration of hyaluronic acid. Additionally, the collagen laid down in fetal wounds is in a structural orientation rather than as scar tissue.

KELOIDS AND HYPERTROPHIC SCARS

Hypertrophic scars are characteristically elevated but remain within the limits of the initial injury and regress spontaneously. *Keloids* extend beyond the original wound and do not regress (Fig. 7-6).[13] Even though they are

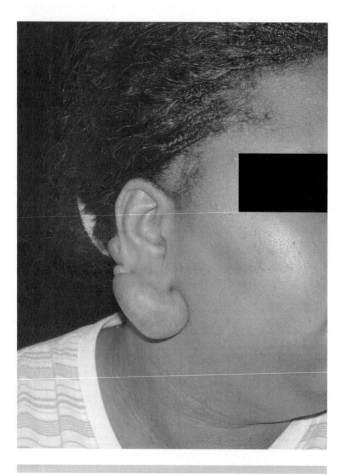

Figure 7-6 **Typical earlobe keloid after piercing. Notice that the keloid extends well beyond the original wound (ear pierce).**

most prevalent in patients between 10 and 30 years of age, keloids can occur at any age. Keloids are far more common in African-Americans than in other races. The underlying mechanism of hypertrophic scar and keloid formation is excessive collagen production with concomitant decreased collagen degradation. Although keloids have been shown to have an underlying genetic basis, various other contributing factors, such as androgens/estrogens, immunologic alterations, and others have been implicated as well.

WOUND MANAGEMENT

Wounds can be managed either *nonoperatively* or *operatively* depending on the individual clinical situation.

Nonoperative Wound Management

Adequate dressings may convert an initially nonhealing wound into a healing wound. A well-hydrated wound will epithelialize more rapidly than a dry wound, which explains why wet dressings promote wound healing.

Occlusive dressings are associated with increased angiogenesis, improved dermal repair, and accelerated wound epithelialization, due to thermal insulation, alterations in pH, PO_2, and PCO_2, and the maintenance of growth factors in the wound environment.[14] Skin maceration is the major downside of occlusive dressings, which is why many modern occlusive dressings are semipermeable. A newly developed and recently popularized type of occlusive dressing is the vacuum-assisted wound closure (VAC). The VAC system combines an occlusive dressing with suction thus creating a wound vacuum (Fig. 7-7). The system is placed on a clean wound bed to promote granulation tissue growth, fluid removal, and wound contraction, as well as to provide a moist healing environment, to enhance blood flow and to protect the wound from outside contaminants.[15,16] The subatmospheric pressure is set to 125 mmHg below ambient pressure and changed every other day. This is an appropriate, manageable, and efficacious therapy for both inpatients and outpatients.

Operative Wound Management

There are certain fundamentals of wound closure which apply to any operative management of a skin wound:

- The incision lines should be placed in the natural skin folds, especially in the face so that the final scar lies in relaxed skin tension lines.
- Tissues should be handled gently, including using appropriate surgical instruments and suture material of the proper thickness.
- Hemostasis should be ensured and iatrogenic contamination avoided.

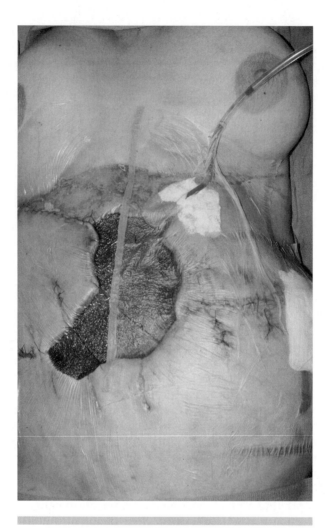

Figure 7-7 **Vacuum-assisted wound closure; the VAC system combines an occlusive dressing with suction creating the ideal environment to promote wound healing while providing temporary wound closure.**

- Tension at the wound edges should be avoided.
- Suture material should be kept in place as long as necessary but should be removed as early as possible.

The *reconstructive ladder* represents a generally accepted principle in the operative management of wounds. A wound itself can either be *simple* or *complex*. Therefore, its management can encompass various types of reconstructive strategies from simple wound closure to closure using a local flap to wound reconstruction with a pedicled flap and finally to microvascular free tissue transfer. The principles of *simple wound closure* are discussed earlier. A *local flap* can include skin, muscle, fascia, or a combination of such tissues randomly rotated or advanced into the nearby defect or wound (Fig. 7-8A and 8B). Z-plasties, and VY-plasties are examples of local, random pattern flaps without a defined blood supply. A *pedicled flap* is a regional transfer of skin, muscle, fascia, or a combination of the tissues based on a defined axial blood supply with a pedicle containing a named artery and its venae

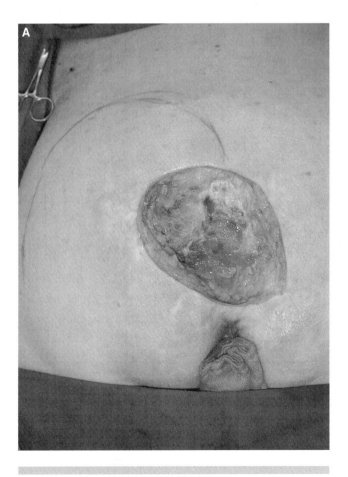

Figure 7-8 **Myocutaneous (muscle/skin) flap rotated into a nearby defect (wound), in this case a sacral decubitus ulcer after debridement.**

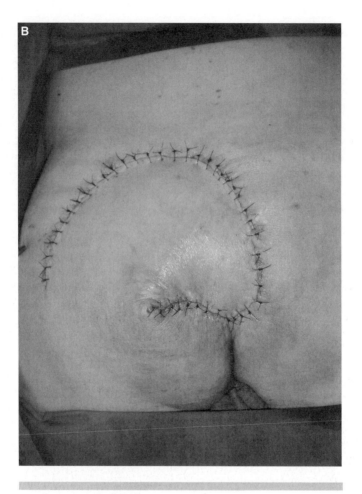

Figure 7-8 **(Continued)**

comitantes (associated veins). *Microvascular free tissue transfer* represents the
transplantation of an axial pattern flap to a distant location, for example, the
transfer of the latissimus dorsi muscle and its cutaneous paddle from the
back to cover a large forearm wound (Fig. 7-9A and 9B). Such transfer is
performed by temporarily interrupting the blood supply of the muscle and
subsequently restoring blood flow via anastomosis to vessels at the new
location.

Split thickness skin grafts (STSG) and *full thickness skin grafts* (FTSG)
represent a simple form of free tissue transfer. However, the initial nutritional and oxygen supply of a graft is maintained by diffusion from the
host bed.

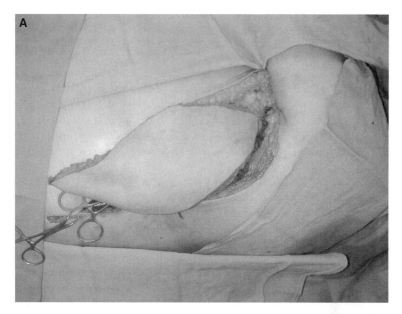

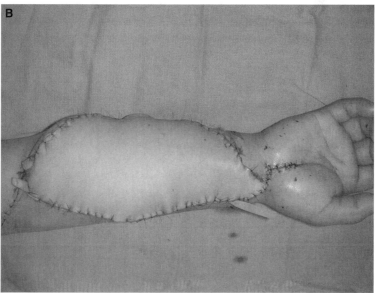

Figure 7-9 **Microvascular free tissue transfer; transplantation of an axial pattern flap to a distant location by temporary interrupting the blood supply; in this case a myocutaneous latissimus dorsi flap to a forearm wound (same patient as in Fig. 7-1).**

REFERENCES

1. Hunt TK, Heppenstall RB, Pines E, et al., eds. *Soft and Hard Tissue Repair: Biological and Clinical Aspects*. New York: Praeger, 1984.

2. Madden JW, Peacock EE. Studies on the biology of collagen during wound healing. III. Dynamic metabolism of scar collagen and remodeling of dermal wounds. *Ann Surg* 174:511, 1971.

3. Peacock EE. *Wound Repair*. Philadelphia, PA: W.B. Saunders, 1984.

4. Wahl SM. Host immune factors regulating fibrosis. *Ciba Found Symp* 14:175, 1985.

5. Hunt TK. Disorders of wound healing. *World J Surg* 4:271, 1980.

6. Hunt TK. Vitamin A and wound healing. *J Am Acad Dermatol* 15:817, 1986.

7. Martin P. Wound healing: aiming for perfect skin regeneration. *Science* 276:75, 1997.

8. Forrest CR, Pang CY, Lindsay WK. Dose and time effects of nicotine treatment on the capillary blood flow and viability of random pattern skin flaps in the rat. *Br J Plast Surg* 40:295, 1987.

9. Robson MC, Stenberg BD, Heggers JP. Wound healing alterations caused by infection. *Clin Plast Surg* 17:485, 1990.

10. Falcone RE, Nappi JF. Chemotherapy and wound healing. *Surg Clin North Am* 64:779, 1984.

11. Miller SH, Rudolph R. Healing in the irradiated wound. *Clin Plast Surg* 17:503, 1990.

12. Mast BA, Diegelmann RF, Krummel TM, et al. Scarless wound healing in the mammalian fetus. *Surg Gynecol Obstet* 174:441, 1992.

13. Goldwyn RM. Keloid. *Plast Reconstr Surg* 68:640, 1981.

14. Carver N, Leigh IM. Synthetic dressings. *Int J Dermatol* 31:10, 1992.

15. Morykwas MJ, Argenta LC, Shelton-Brown EI, et al. Vacuum-assisted closure: a new method for wound control and treatment: animal studies and basic foundation. *Ann Plast Surg* 38:553, 1997.

16. Argenta LC, Morykwas MJ. Vacuum-assisted closure: a new method for wound control and treatment: clinical experience. *Ann Plast Surg* 38:563, 1997.

COMMON

SURGICAL

DISEASES

ESOPHAGUS

Shu S. Lin, MD, PhD

ANATOMY AND PHYSIOLOGY[1,6,7,8]

Relationship to Other Structures

The *esophagus* is the portion of the digestive tract between the pharynx and stomach. It is approximately 25 cm in length. It is normally a collapsed muscular tube that lies anterior to the spine. Other key adjacent structures are the trachea and pericardium anteriorly, azygos vein and the thoracic duct to its right, and the descending aorta to its left for most of its length within the thoracic cavity. In reference to the spine, the esophagus extends from the level of about C6 to T12.

Layers of the Esophageal Wall

Starting from the outermost layer, the esophagus is composed of the adventitia, muscularis, submucosa, and mucosa. Unlike most other parts of the gastrointestinal tract, the esophagus has no serosal covering. The *adventitia* is a loose fibroareolar tissue that separates the esophagus from the other vital structures within the mediastinum. The *muscularis* consists of an outer, longitudinal and an inner, circular layer; these muscle layers are striated in the upper third of the esophagus and nonstriated in the lower two-thirds. This transition of striated to smooth muscle composition allows voluntary control of the esophagus during the early phases of swallowing action. The *submucosa* contains a rich network of blood vessels and lymphatics among collagenous and elastic tissue; it also contains mucus-secreting glands that help lubricate the esophageal lumen. Throughout most of the length of the esophagus, the *mucosa* is characterized by a thin layer of muscularis mucosa onto which stratified squamous epithelium rests on the luminal surface; only in the most distal 1–2 cm of the esophagus is the mucosa lined by junctional columnar epithelium.

Anatomic Segments of the Esophagus

The esophagus is typically divided into four segments:[7] pharyngoesophageal, cervical, thoracic, and abdominal. The *pharyngoesophageal segment* is a relatively short segment between the laryngopharynx and the cricopharyngeus muscle, the lowest part of the inferior pharyngeal constrictor that defines the upper esophageal sphincter (UES). The *cervical esophagus* begins when the fibers of the cricopharyngeus muscle form the outer longitudinal and inner circular layers of the muscularis, and it extends down to the level of the first thoracic vertebra. The cervical esophagus is about 5 cm long and tends to run more on the left side of the trachea, making it easier to surgically access this structure through a left neck incision. The *thoracic segment* starts once it is in the posterior mediastinum, and it deviates slightly to the left as it passes behind the great vessels and the aortic arch. After coursing behind the left mainstem bronchus, it then curves to the right in the subcarinal region; this is the reason that surgical exposure of the midesophagus is best approached through a right chest incision. Just before going through the diaphragmatic hiatus near the level of T11, the esophagus returns to a slightly left-sided position. The *abdominal esophagus*, which varies from one to several centimeters in normal individuals, constitutes the segment between the esophageal hiatus at the level of the diaphragm and the esophagogastric junction. The lower thoracic esophagus and the abdominal esophagus are most approachable through a left-sided chest incision or an upper midline abdominal incision.

Normal Anatomic Constrictions

The esophagus has three points of naturally occurring constrictions (Fig. 8-1). The cricopharyngeus sphincter makes up the *cervical or cricopharyngeal constriction*, which is considered the narrowest point of the entire gastrointestinal tract. The next area of constriction is the *bronchoaortic or aortic constriction*, where the left mainstem bronchus and the aortic arch cross the esophagus. As the name implies, the *diaphragmatic or hiatal constriction* is located at a point where the esophagus passes the diaphragmatic hiatus, and it therefore defines the transition point between the thoracic esophagus and the abdominal esophagus.

Vascular Supply

The arterial blood supply to the esophagus is provided by a number of sources, with abundant collateral communications within each segment. The *superior thyroid arteries* and the *inferior thyroid arteries* both supply the cervical esophagus. In the thoracic esophagus, direct branches from the *aorta*, as well as the *inferior thyroid arteries, intercostals, bronchial arteries, inferior phrenic arteries*, and *left gastric artery*, all contribute to forming a network of capillaries before penetrating the muscularis layer. The distal portion of the esophagus, including the abdominal segment, has its arterial supply based mainly on the *left gastric artery*. The network of venous return generally follows the arterial system and drains into the inferior thyroid vein in the cervical segment; the bronchial, azygous, and hemiazygos veins in the thoracic segment; and the coronary vein in the abdominal segment.

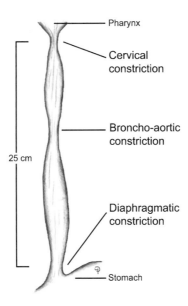

Figure 8-1 **Three points of naturally occurring constrictions of the esophagus. Because of various normal anatomic factors, the esophageal lumen is narrowed in three distinct areas: cervical (or cricopharyngeal) constriction, bronchoaortic (or aortic) constriction, and diaphragmatic (or hiatal) constriction. The cervical constriction is typically the narrowest point of the entire gastrointestinal tract, and the diaphragmatic constriction defines the transition point between the thoracic esophagus and the abdominal esophagus.** (*Source: Illustration by William Parker, PhD.*)

Lymphatic Drainage

Learning the anatomy of the lymphatic system is important to understand some of the principles of esophageal oncology. The lymphatic drainage of the esophagus occurs in the submucosal plexus in a longitudinal fashion, such that lymph can travel along the esophagus over a long distance along the submucosal layer before going through the muscularis and entering a set of regional lymph nodes. The direction of the lymph flow typically is cephalad in the upper two-thirds of the esophagus and caudad in the lower one-third. Groups of regional lymph nodes draining the esophagus include the cervical, paratracheal, hilar, subcarinal, paraesophageal, and paraaortic nodes in the upper two-thirds, and paraesophageal, paraaortic, left gastric, and celiac nodes in the lower third.

Autonomic Innervations

The autonomic innervation provides the esophagus with various motor, sensory, and secretory functions. The parasympathetic innervation comes predominantly from the *vagus nerve*, which is present on the right and the left side of the esophagus throughout the majority of its length but coalesces to form anterior and posterior trunks distally. The *superior laryngeal nerve* that arises from the vagus nerve in the cervical segment divides into the *external* laryngeal branch, which innervates the *motor* function of the cricothyroid muscle and inferior pharyngeal constrictor, and *internal* laryngeal branch, which provides the *sensory* nerves to the pharyngeal surface and the base of the tongue. The *recurrent laryngeal nerve* emanating from the vagus nerve also provides parasympathetic innervation to the cervical esophagus and the UES; injury to this structure might lead not only to hoarseness but also to secondary tracheobronchial aspiration during swallowing. Within the esophageal wall, *Meissner's plexus* provides the intrinsic autonomic innervation in the submucosal layer and *Auerbach's plexus* in between the longitudinal and circular muscle layers.

Upper and Lower Esophageal Sphincters

The UES is a true anatomic structure created by the function of cricopharyngeus muscle. The basal resting pressure ranges widely from about 20 to 120 mmHg, with a mean pressure of approximately 40 mmHg. The *lower esophageal sphincter* (LES), on the other hand, is only a functional sphincter, in that a high-pressure zone (HPZ) in a 3- to 5-cm segment of the distal esophagus has been demonstrated manometrically but no true anatomic sphincter is known to exist; it is therefore, often referred to as the LES mechanism or the distal esophageal HPZ. The resting pressure of this HPZ typically ranges from 10 to 20 mmHg. Although the absolute value of the HPZ resting pressure does not define competence or incompetence of the LES mechanism, mean resting pressures of less than 6 mmHg or overall LES mechanism length of less than 2 cm are more apt to be associated with gastroesophageal (GE) reflux. Furthermore, the resting pressure of HPZ may be affected by a wide variety of factors such as hormones (increased by gastrin, motilin, prostaglandin $F_{2\alpha}$, and bombesin; decreased by secretin, cholecystokinin, glucagons, progesterone, estrogen, and prostaglandins E_1, E_2, A_1), drugs (increased by caffeine, norepinephrine, phenylephrine, edrophonium, bethanechol, methacholine, and metoclopramide; decreased by phentolamine, atropine, theophylline, isoproterenol, ethanol, epinephrine, nicotine, and nitroglycerin), foods (increased by protein; decreased by fat and chocolate), and environmental conditions (increased by gastric alkalinization and gastric distention; decreased by gastric acidification, gastrectomy, hypoglycemia, hypothyroidism, amyloidosis, pernicious anemia, and epidermolysis bullosa).

Contractions of the Esophageal Body

The motor function of the esophagus is physiologically driven by three different types of contractions or waveforms. *Primary waves* describe the cranial-to-caudal, sequential contractions (peristalsis) that send the food bolus down to the stomach with swallowing. *Secondary waves* then clear the esophagus of any residual debris by providing another set of sequential, peristaltic contractions, but only after the original food bolus has passed into the stomach. *Tertiary waves*, on the other hand, are nonsequential, monophasic, or multiphasic contractions that often occur in older individuals and have no known true functions.

PATHOLOGY OF THE ESOPHAGUS[2,3,4,6,9,10,11,13,14]

Motility Disorders

Esophageal motility disorders are functional pathology in which the primary etiology cannot be a structural obstruction from within the lumen or an extrinsic compression from outside the wall of the esophagus. Various methods of evaluating esophageal motility disorders include esophagogram, endoscopy, esophageal manometry, and intraesophageal pH testing. Although radiographic studies such as esophagogram may provide some structural information about the pathologic process, esophageal manometry is the method of choice in distinguishing the different types of motility disorders (Table 8-1).[9]

UPPER ESOPHAGEAL SPHINCTER DYSFUNCTION

Definition and Clinical Presentations

UES dysfunction is characterized by difficulty in propelling liquid or solid food from the oropharynx to the upper esophagus. It is variably known as oropharyngeal dysphagia, cricopharyngeal dysfunction, or cricopharyngeal achalasia. Classic presentation include dysphagia felt between the thyroid cartilage and suprasternal notch; expectoration of excessive saliva, due to the patient's inability to swallow the 1–1.5 L of saliva normally produced each day; intermittent hoarseness, through mechanisms affecting the inferior pharyngeal constrictor muscle; and weight loss, from the lack of nutritional intake as a result of the dysphagia.

Diagnostic Tests

Because of the asymmetric nature of the UES, which also changes position during swallowing, it is difficult to characterize this disorder with a standard manometry. Fortunately, newer manometries, including those with circumferential sphincter microtransducer catheter, are able to document either the abnormal tones in the UES or the lack of coordinated peristalsis between the oropharynx and the upper esophagus in these patients. Manometric studies may further demonstrate abnormal peristalsis of the thoracic esophagus in one-third of patients with UES dysfunction. A high degree of suspicion should be kept based on the classic clinical symptoms described earlier, supplemented by information from various studies. Other nonmotor causes of upper esophageal dysphagia, such as carcinoma, stricture, and trauma, should be ruled out. A barium esophagogram may be helpful in demonstrating structural abnormalities in the upper esophagus (such as Zenker

Normal Findings

LES pressure 15–25 mmHg (never >45 mmHg) with normal relaxation with swallowing

Mean amplitude of distal esophageal peristaltic wave 30–100 mmHg (never > 190 mmHg)

Simultaneous contractions occurring after <10% of wet swallows

Monophasic waveforms (with not more than two peaks)

Duration of distal esophageal peristaltic wave: 2–6 s

No repetitive contractions

Primary Motility Disorders

Achalasia

Aperistalsis in esophageal body

Partial or absent LES relaxation with swallowing

LES pressure normal or >45 mmHg

Intraesophageal basal pressure > intragastric

DES

Simultaneous (nonperistaltic) contractions

   Repetitive (at least three peaks)

   Increased duration (>6 s)

Spontaneous contractions

Intermittent normal peristalsis

Contractions may be of increased amplitude

Nutcracker esophagus

Mean peristaltic amplitude (10 wet swallows) in distal esophagus > 180 mmHg

Increased duration of contractions (>6 s) frequent

Normal peristaltic sequences

Hypertensive LES

LES pressure >45 mmHg but with normal relaxation

Normal esophageal peristalsis

Nonspecific esophageal motility disorders

No or decreased amplitude of peristalsis

   Normal LES pressure

   Normal LES relaxation

Abnormal peristalsis, including any of the following:

   Abnormal waveforms

   Isolated simultaneous contractions

   Isolated spontaneous contractions

   Normal peristalsis sequence maintained

   LES normal

Vigorous achalasia

Repetitive simultaneous contractions in body of esophagus (as with DES)

Partial or absent LES relaxation (as with achalasia)

Source: Reprinted with permission from Orringer MB. The esophagus: part III, disorders of esophageal motility. In Sabiston DC, Lyerly HK, eds., *Textbook of Surgery: The Biological Basis of Modern Surgical Practice*, 15th ed. Philadelphia, PA: W.B. Saunders, 1997: 722.

diverticulum or cricopharyngeal bar) and in the rest of the esophagus causing referred symptoms to the neck (such as distal esophageal tumor or GE
reflux disease). Esophageal pH studies will also provide some information
about the status of GE reflux and thus help guide the management of these
patients. Endoscopy will not give the diagnosis of UES dysfunction, but it is
important in ruling out the presence of tumor and esophagitis.

Treatment

Since there are many potential causes, including neurogenic, myogenic,
structural, mechanical, and iatrogenic etiologies, the management of UES
dysfunction depends of the individual case. In appropriate situations, a cervical
esophagomyotomy is performed—an oblique, left neck incision is made, and
a longitudinal incision of the muscularis layer, but not the submucosal and
mucosal layers, of the proximal esophagus is made on the posterolateral
aspect, from the level of the superior cornu of the thyroid cartilage to 1–2 cm
behind the clavicle. Symptomatic relief has been obtained in 65–85 percent
of the patients undergoing this procedure.

ACHALASIA

Definition and Clinical Presentations

The Greek translation of achalasia is *failure of relaxation*, and, in medical
terms, achalasia refers to an inability of the LES to properly relax during the
swallowing motion. The histopathologic basis of achalasia is that there is
degeneration of the ganglion cells of Aurebach's plexus in the esophageal
body and the LES. In South America, a parasitic infection by *Trypanosoma
cruzi* (Chagas disease) is often the cause of the destruction of these ganglion
cells; in Europe and North America, the etiology is less clear. The classic triad
of symptoms includes dysphagia, regurgitation, and weight loss.
Regurgitation of residual esophageal contents may lead to recurrent pneumonia and/or tracheobronchitis. Only a third of the patients will have
substernal or epigastric pain, which is more typical of esophageal spasm.
Esophageal cancer, characteristically a midesophageal squamous cell carcinoma, may be a late complication of achalasia, as one-tenth of patients with
achalasia will develop this after 15–25 years.

Diagnostic Tests

The finding of *bird's beak* tapering of the distal esophagus on barium
esophagogram is the classic hallmark of achalasia (Fig. 8-2). However, this
radiographic appearance may vary depending on the chronicity of the disorder, from only a mild dilatation of the mid and proximal esophagus in
early stage disease to sigmoid-shaped megaesophagus in advanced disease.
Manometry typically shows an increased baseline LES pressure, the absence
of LES relaxation normally seen with swallowing, and the lack of appropriate peristalsis throughout the rest of the esophagus. Endoscopy is performed

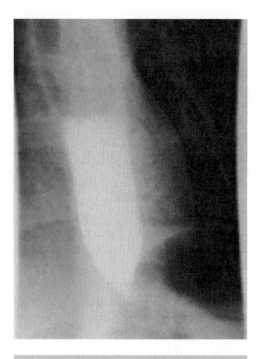

Figure 8-2 **As shown in this barium esophagogram, achalasia is classically characterized radiographically by the smooth tapering of the distal esophagus, resembling
the shape of a birdís beak.** (Source: Courtesy
of Caroline Carrico, MD, and Anamaria Gaca,
MD, Department of Radiology, Duke University
Medical Center.)

to rule out carcinoma (both in the distal esophagus and in the cardia of the
stomach) and to evaluate the presence of any esophagitis or stricture.

Treatment

The goal of the treatment is to provide symptomatic palliation by relieving the functional obstruction at the LES. Medical therapy includes nitrates
and calcium channel blockers. Balloon dilatation can be used in those who
fail medical management and is a good first-line treatment, as the majority
of patients (65–77 percent) obtain symptomatic relief, with only 1–5 percent
risk of perforation.[9] Repeat dilation procedures may be performed, but if
the symptoms persist, then a distal esophagomyotomy (modified Heller
myotomy) can be considered in appropriate situations. Approximately 15–20
percent of patients will require this operation,[14] in which a longitudinal
myotomy is performed, beginning from the level of the inferior pulmonary

vein down across the LES and typically 1 cm onto the stomach. This operation can be performed through a left thoracotomy or an abdominal incision; it can also be done thoracoscopically or laparoscopically. Some surgeons favor performing an antireflux procedure with the myotomy to prevent problems with GE reflux. The risk of perforation in this operation is about 1 percent.[9,14] In cases of sigmoid-shaped megaesophagus, symptoms of dysphagia and regurgitation can be relieved by esophageal resection, which would also effectively eliminate any possible risk of developing esophageal cancer.

DIFFUSE ESOPHAGEAL SPASM

Definition and Clinical Presentations

In diffuse esophageal spasm (DES), repetitive, simultaneous, high-amplitude contractions of the esophagus lead to the classic symptoms of chest pain, dysphagia, or both. Patients with DES commonly have a history of irritable bowel syndrome, pylorospasm, spastic colon, and/or underlying psychiatric problems. DES is still a poorly understood esophageal hypermotility disorder and is often triggered by emotional factors, ingestion of cold substance, GE reflux, peptic ulcer disease, cholelithiasis, and pancreatitis.

Diagnostic Tests

Because of the clinical presentations, obtaining an accurate medical history is vital in making the diagnosis of DES. Since the classic symptoms of DES are similar to angina pectoralis from coronary artery disease, a cardiac workup is necessary. On barium esophagogram, *curling* or *corkscrew* esophagus, due to segmental and uncoordinated contractions of the circular muscle layer, is the hallmark of DES,[9] although this radiographic finding is quite variable.[9,14] Manometric findings include simultaneous, nonperistaltic, and spontaneous contractions that may be of increased amplitude. However, both barium esophagogram and manometry may be normal, since the episodes of esophageal spasm typically occur intermittently. Esophageal endoscopy should also be performed to rule out esophagitis, fibrosis, and an infiltrating tumor or other obstructing lesions distally.

Treatment

Since there is a psychiatric component in most cases of DES (documented psychiatric disorders are reported in more than 80 percent of patients with manometrically determined esophageal contraction abnormalities),[14] many patients may respond therapeutically with psychiatric counseling or with simple reassurance that their chest pain is not due to a life-threatening problem such as myocardial infarction. The patient should be advised to avoid emotional stress or physiologic stressor such as food that might have a history of triggering DES symptoms in that individual. If present, associated problems such as GE reflux disease or cholelithiasis should be treated. Medications such as sublingual nitroglycerin, longer-acting nitrates, and calcium channel blockers may be effective in curtailing the symptoms of DES. Repeated esophageal dilation with smooth, tapered bougies may provide relief weeks to months at a time. Pneumatic dilatation is to be avoided due to the risk of creating a major tear with forceful expansion of a hypertonic and spastic esophagus. Although a long, thoracic esophagomyotomy (from the level of the aortic arch to the LES) is an option, it is not uniformly recommended as in severe achalasia, since long-term improvement is not frequently achieved with this operation in DES. In rare instances in which esophagomyotomy is performed for DES, antireflux procedures should be cautiously applied, and fundoplication involving 360° wraps should not be used because of the already abnormal tone and contractions in the body of the esophagus.

OTHER ESOPHAGEAL MOTILITY DISORDERS

Related to DES is the *nutcracker (super-squeeze) esophagus*, in which the mean peristaltic amplitude exceeds 180 mmHg and at times reaches 225–430 mmHg.[14] The duration of these progressive contractions are also frequently increased, but there are normal peristaltic sequences. The clinical presentations, the methods of diagnosis, and the treatment options are similar to DES. Patients who manifest clinical and manometric evidence of both DES (i.e., repetitive and simultaneous contractions of the esophageal body) and achalasia (i.e., partial or absent reflex LES relaxation) are categorized as having *vigorous achalasia*. Other primary esophageal motility disorders include *hypertensive LES*, *hypotensive LES*, and *nonspecific esophageal motility disorders*.

Esophageal motility problems also occur secondary to various systemic illnesses such as diabetes, dermatomyositis, polymyositis, lupus erythematosus, and scleroderma. Esophageal dysmotility is especially prominent in *scleroderma*, and it results from the weakening of distal esophageal tone and contraction due to progressive fibrosis and atrophy of the esophageal smooth muscle layers. Patients complain mostly of heartburn from GE reflux and regurgitation, and bleeding and dysphagia are occasionally seen. Treatment modalities are predominantly targeted to control the underlying systemic disease, although there is no known effective therapy for patients with scleroderma. Symptomatic palliation can sometimes be achieved using antacids, standard antireflux medications, and head elevation during sleep. If there is stricture causing regurgitation, dysphagia, or odynophagia, esophageal dilatation procedures may provide symptomatic relief. Antireflux operations, specifically using the Collis gastroplasty-fundoplication technique, should be considered in patients who fail medical management. In advanced esophageal disease from scleroderma with intractable symptoms, transhiatal esophagectomy may offer significant relief from various complications of reflux.

Vascular Rings

Vascular rings are congenital anomalies that affect the esophagus and typically cause symptoms of dysphagia in young adulthood. Barium esophagogram or endoscopy demonstrates a more than usual narrowing of the esophagus at the level of the aortic arch and the great vessels. Because these vascular rings are frequently derived from aberrant vessels, angiography or magnetic reso-nance imaging (MRI) should be performed to demonstrate which vessels are involved. If the symptoms are severe enough, the treatment is surgical divi-sion of the vascular ring through a transthoracic approach.

Esophageal Webs

UPPER ESOPHAGEAL WEBS

The presence of upper or cervical esophageal webs is one of the manifestations of Plummer-Vinson syndrome, also known as Kelly-Patterson syndrome and sideropenic dysphagia. Plummer-Vinson syndrome typically afflicts White women older than 40 years of age, and the upper esophageal web is the pre-sumed cause of the dysphagia. Other manifestations of the syndrome include iron-deficiency anemia, atrophic oral mucosa, glossitis, weight loss, and koilony-chias. The diagnosis of upper esophageal web is suspected in patients who fit this profile and is made when barium esophagogram demonstrates one or more webs above the level of the aortic arch. Upper endoscopy will confirm this diagnosis and usually is adequate to treat these characteristically thin, flimsy webs by rupturing them with or without esophageal dilatation. It is also impor-tant to improve the nutritional status and correct the iron-deficiency anemia as soon as the diagnosis is made, since early treatment decreases the risk of devel-oping carcinoma of the hypopharynx, oral cavity, or esophagus, which has been known to occur in about 10 percent of these patients.

LOWER ESOPHAGEAL WEBS

Most of the lower esophageal webs, or Schatzki rings, are discovered inci-dentally on barium esophagograms performed for unrelated reasons. Some patients have symptoms of dysphagia to solid foods if there is significant nar-rowing from the ring. These rings are focal, annular strictures that project per-pendicular to the long axis of the esophagus at the esophagogastric junction; it is made up of mucosa and submucosa and not the muscles of the esophageal wall and histologically occurs at the squamocolumnar epithelial junction. The diagnosis of Schatzki ring indicates the presence of a hiatal hernia of the sliding type (see Hiatal Hernias and Gastroesophageal Reflux), but it does not nec-essarily mean that GE reflux or esophagitis exists. Besides the barium esoph-agogram, these rings can be diagnosed by endoscopy from their characteristic white, membranous narrowing in the lumen of the distal esophagus. Much like the upper esophageal web, Schatzki ring can easily be treated endoscop-ically or by balloon dilatation. Surgical resection of Schatzki ring is rarely necessary; however, when it is performed, the sliding hiatal hernia that is typ-ically associated with this ring should also be repaired.

Diverticula

An esophageal diverticulum is an acquired condition in which all or a portion of the normal esophageal wall (mucosa, submucosa, and muscle) protrudes away from the lumen. Three specific types of esophageal diverticulum are discussed here, based on the location of the occurrence—*pharyngoesophageal,* *midesophageal,* and *epiphrenic* diverticula. Esophageal diverticula can also be classified according to the mechanism of development—*pulsion-type* diverticulum, created by a protrusion of only the mucosal and submucosal layers as a result of high-intraluminal pressure forcing these layers through a defect in the musculature of the esophageal wall, and *traction-type* diverticulum, formed by an outward traction or pulling of all three layers of the esophageal wall from inflammation and scarring at a site adjacent to the esophagus, such as a peribronchial lymph node.

PHARYNGOESOPHAGEAL DIVERTICULUM

Definition and Clinical Presentations

Pharyngoesophageal or Zenker diverticulum is the most common type of esophageal diverticulum and presents predominantly in patients over 60 years of age. It occurs at the junction of the pharynx and esophagus and specifically arises within the Killian triangle of the inferior pharyngeal constrictor, which is a point of weakness between the oblique fibers of the thyropharyngeus muscle and the horizontal fibers of the cricopharyngeus muscle (Fig. 8-3). *Zenker diverticulum is a pulsion-type diverticulum,* and its development is partly due to cricopharyngeal achalasia (UES dysfunction), a condition in which there is incomplete relaxation of the UES leading to elevated intraluminal pressure. As this diverticulum enlarges, it hangs over to the *left side* of the cricopharyngeus muscle inferiorly in the prevertebral space, an important point to understand when it comes to the surgical management of this problem.

Early in the development of Zenker diverticulum, patients are usually asymptomatic. When symptoms do surface, they complain of a sticking sensation in the throat, excessive salivation, intermittent cough, as well as intermittent dysphagia, typically with solids. As the diverticulum enlarges, more severe symptoms and signs may develop, such as regurgitation of undigested food, unusual gurgling sounds during swallowing, halitosis, voice change, retrosternal pain, and respiratory compromise from aspiration. Some patients develop various maneuvers, such as throat clearing, coughing, or massaging the neck, to help get the food past the upper esophagus.

Diagnostic Tests

Although clinical presentations may suggest the presence of the diverticulum, the diagnosis is made with barium esophagogram. Lateral view is important in demonstrating the diverticulum because the protrusion is initially directed posteriorly; anterior view will show that the diverticulum is, as discussed earlier, usually draped to the left side. Plain radiographic studies will sometimes reveal air-fluid level within the diverticulum. Manometric studies are typically unrevealing and are therefore not necessary when Zenker diverticulum is the only diagnosis being considered. In fact, the probe used for manometry may pose a risk of perforating the diverticulum. Computed

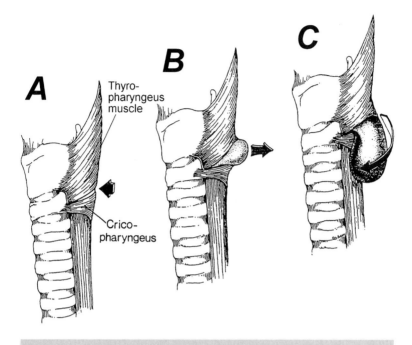

Figure 8-3 ***(A) Zenker (pharyngoesophageal) diverticulum occurs at the point of weakness between the oblique fibers of the thyropharyngeus muscle and the horizontal fibers of the cricopharyngeus muscle (short arrow). (B) The pharyngeal mucosa and (C) submucosa herniate through this area and typically expand caudally toward the left side into the superior mediastinum.*** (*Source: Modified with permission from Zwischenberger JB, Alpard SK, Orringer MB. Esophagus. In Townsend CM, Beauchamp RD, Evers BM, et al., eds., Sabiston Textbook of Surgery: The Biological Basis of Modern Surgical Practice, 16th ed. Philadelphia, PA: W.B. Saunders, 2001: 715.*)

tomography (CT), MRI, and other radiographic studies also do not add much to the diagnosis or the management of Zenker diverticulum. Endoscopy should be performed only when filling defects or ulcers are seen on barium esophagogram, but the procedure must be performed with extra caution since there is a real risk in entering and perforating the diverticulum. It would not be inappropriate to delay the manometric and endoscopic studies after successful surgical treatment of the diverticulum.

Treatment

All symptomatic patients should undergo surgical treatment, regardless of the size of the diverticulum. The standard treatment of Zenker diverticulum is esophagomyotomy with concomitant resection of the diverticulum through a left cervical incision. Instead of resecting the diverticulum, an alternative approach is to perform diverticulopexy, a procedure in which the pouch is suspended with the mouth or neck in the most dependent position so that any food particle entering the diverticulum would easily drain out on its own. Another method of treating Zenker diverticulum is called pharyngoesophagotomy, or the Dohlman procedure, which entails *endoscopically* dividing the common wall between the diverticulum and esophageal wall. All of these approaches have excellent results with low rates of recurrence.

MIDESOPHAGEAL DIVERTICULUM

Midesophageal or parabronchial diverticula are typically found near the tracheal bifurcation, are more commonly found on the right side, and usually have a wide neck. These diverticula are true diverticula, containing all three layers of the esophageal wall. Midesophageal diverticula have historically been attributed to mediastinal lymphadenitis and fibrosis from tuberculosis and histoplasmosis and are therefore traction-type diverticula. With a decline in the incidence of tuberculosis in recent decades, these postinflammatory diverticula have decreased in number, and more midesophageal diverticula are considered to be that of the pulsion type today. For that reason, esophageal manometry is an important tool in evaluating patients with midesophageal diverticulum. However, just as in Zenker diverticulum, barium esophagogram establishes the diagnosis, and this study should be performed first. Endoscopy is important in ruling out other structural abnormalities and sometimes needed to pass the manometry probe safely into the stomach.

EPIPHRENIC DIVERTICULUM

Definition and Clinical Presentations

Epiphrenic or supradiaphragmatic diverticula appear in the distal third of the esophagus. They are pulsion-type diverticula and, like midesophageal diverticula, occur more frequently on the right side. The size of the diverticulum usually does not dictate the severity or the type of symptoms, and patients who have symptoms such as dysphagia regurgitation, vomiting, chest and epigastric pain, and halitosis typically have associated motility disorders.

Diagnostic Tests

As in other types of esophageal diverticulum, epiphrenic diverticulum is diagnosed by barium esophagogram. Because underlying motor disorders are common in symptomatic patients, manometric studies are needed. Also, because a distal esophageal stricture or tumor can cause this type of diverticulum, endoscopic evaluation needs to be carried out.

Treatment

Patients with a small (less than 3 cm) epiphrenic diverticulum and with only mild symptoms do not require treatment. For those with severe symptoms or with anatomically dependent pouches that are enlarging, surgical treatment consisting of resection of the diverticulum and a long thoracic esophagomyotomy extending from the aortic arch to the GE junction is appropriate. Controversy exists due to the distal extent of the myotomy as well as due to the need for a concomitant antireflux procedure. If an antireflux procedure is performed, a partial fundoplication, as opposed to a 360° fundoplication, is recommended to reduce the risk of functional obstruction in the future. With proper esophagomyotomy, the recurrence of the diverticulum and the disruption of the suture line are rare.

Tears and Perforations[2]

MALLORY-WEISS SYNDROME

Bleeding from stomach or esophageal laceration as a result of forceful vomiting is known as Mallory-Weiss syndrome. This problem typically occurs after consuming large quantities of food and alcohol. Endoscopy will establish the diagnosis and the site of bleeding. Conservative management is usually adequate in most cases. Nasogastric lavage with ice water may slow down the hemorrhage. Intravenous vasopressin infusion may also be used to constrict the culprit vessels and control the bleeding. In cases in which surgical measure is required, an upper midline laparotomy or a left thoracotomy approach may be used to create a high gastrostomy in order to oversee the bleeding vessel under direct vision.

BOERHAAVE SYNDROME

Boerhaave syndrome refers to spontaneous perforation of all layers of the esophageal wall, classically as a result of severe vomiting from heavy alcohol and food intake, but it can also occur with any event that rapidly raises the intraesophageal pressure while the UES is closed. After vomiting, patients present with epigastric and lower thoracic pain, which may radiate to the left shoulder due to diaphragmatic irritation. Dyspnea may develop because of the fluid in the pleural cavity. Most commonly, the perforation is located in the left, posterior aspect of the lower esophageal wall, approximately 3–5 cm above the GE junction. The next most common location of the perforation is on the right side of the midthoracic esophagus at the level of the azygos vein. Radiographic studies will demonstrate mediastinal air or hydropneumothorax. Water-soluble esophagogram or CT scan with oral contrast will confirm the diagnosis. Once the diagnosis is made, the initial line of therapy includes fluid resuscitation and broad-spectrum intravenous antibiotics. The mediastinal and pleural cavities are drained. If the perforation is significant (i.e., not microperforation), then operative management with primary closure, reenforced with a tissue flap, is preferred. The choices of tissue used for buttressing the primary repair include intercostal muscle bundle flap, pleural flap, pedicled pericardial fat, and omental flap. However, if the opening cannot be primarily closed due to friable and inflamed tissue, typically from a delay in diagnosis (traditionally defined as greater than 24 h), then the fundus of the stomach can be mobilized and be used as a Thal patch. Another option would be to perform esophageal exclusion proximal and distal to the perforation, drain the perforated area, create a cervical esophagostomy through the left side, and place a gastrostomy tube for nutritional support. A more extreme alternative would be to perform esophagectomy, especially if underlying esophageal cancer is suspected.

IATROGENIC PERFORATIONS

Any diagnostic or therapeutic procedures or operations that involve the upper gastrointestinal tract have a chance of causing injuries to the esophagus. By sheer number of cases, *the most common cause of iatrogenic perforation is diagnostic flexible esophagoscopy*. The most frequent site of injury is in the cervical esophagus at the level of cricopharyngeus muscle near the upper sphincter, not uncommonly against a vertebral spur that is present posteriorly. Other frequent sites of iatrogenic perforation are the midthoracic esophagus at the level of the left mainstem bronchus and the lower esophagus at the diaphragmatic hiatus. The risk of iatrogenic perforation with diagnostic esophagoscopy is about 0.1 percent (0.09 percent for flexible fiber-optic esophagoscopy and 0.07 percent for rigid esophagoscopy).

On the other hand, the risks of perforation with *therapeutic* procedures vary with the types of procedures. For example, in treating achalasia, surgical esophagomyotomy carries a risk of only 1 percent, whereas pneumatic dilatation has a risk of 4 percent. That risk is significantly lower (0.5 percent) when using semiflexible bougies that are guided by an endoscopically placed wire.

Hiatal Hernias and Gastroesophageal Reflux[3,4]

Definition and Clinical Presentations

Hiatal hernia is a condition in which a variable portion of an abdominal organ, typically the stomach, becomes displaced above the diaphragm through the esophageal hiatus. When only the stomach is considered, there are essentially two types of hiatal hernias (Fig. 8-4). However, in a more elaborate classification system that includes the involvement of other abdominal organs, four have been described. In *type I hiatal hernia* (sliding or axial type), the GE junction is displaced above the level of the diaphragm through the esophageal hiatus. The LES, or the HPZ in the distal esophagus, is exposed to the negative pressure of the thoracic cavity, and this is presumed to predispose patients with type I hiatal hernia to problems with GE reflux. In *type II hiatal hernia* (paraesophageal or rolling type), a portion of the stomach herniates into the mediastinum, but the GE junction remains below the level of the diaphragm, thereby keeping the LES within the positive pressure environment of the peritoneal cavity. In *type III hiatal hernia*, features from both

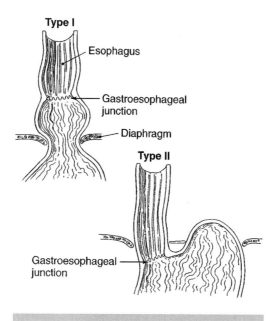

Figure 8-4 **Involvement of the stomach in hiatal hernia can essentially be divided into two general types, based on the relative position of the GE junction. In type I hiatal hernia (sliding or axial type), the GE junction passes through the esophageal hiatus and is above the diaphragm. In type II hiatal hernia (paraesophageal or rolling type), a portion of the stomach herniates through the esophageal hiatus but the GE junction remains within the abdominal cavity.** (*Source: Reprinted with permission from Jacobs DO. The esophagus. In Niederhuber JE, ed., Fundamentals of Surgery. Stamford, CT: Appleton and Lange, 1998: 279.*)

type I and type II are present; that is, both the GE junction and a part of the gastric fundus are above the esophageal hiatus. In *type IV hiatal hernia*, there is a large paraesophageal hernia that includes other organs such as the large or small intestine. Clinically, types II, III, and IV hiatal hernias should initially be considered together because of the mechanical problems that each one of these can create (e.g., incarceration and strangulation). However, because the GE junction is also displaced into the mediastinum in types III and IV, the GE reflux issues related to type I hiatal hernia should also be kept in mind.

Type I hiatal hernia is common and is usually discovered incidentally on chest radiograph. It is considered by many not to be a true pathologic condition since the GE junction has been demonstrated to move above the level of the diaphragm in normal individual during a Valsalva maneuver. However, type I hiatal hernia is associated with GE reflux and subsequent reflux esophagitis; type I hiatal hernia is present in about 80 percent of patients with pathologic reflux. Only when the hiatal hernia is associated with GE reflux do patients become symptomatic. The typical symptoms include heartburn (80 percent) and regurgitation (54 percent). Other symptoms reported by a significant proportion (~30 percent) of patients with type I hiatal hernia are abdominal pain and cough. Types II, III, and IV hiatal hernias are not as frequently seen as type I, and they are rarely associated with GE reflux, but the herniated portion of the stomach is more likely to strangulate and infarct. They can be asymptomatic, even when a large portion of the stomach is involved; when present, predominant symptoms include epigastric, subcostal, and chest pain, dysphagia, and heartburn. Regurgitation, upper gastrointestinal bleeding, and hoarseness may occasionally occur if there are complications of the hernia. To avoid potentially catastrophic consequences, asymptomatic type II hiatal hernia should be surgically managed on an elective basis in patients with no contraindications; if symptoms do develop, they should be repaired emergently.

Diagnostic Tests

Radiographic studies such as barium esophagogram will help define the type of hiatal hernia present, but in GE reflux disease, other studies are needed to evaluate the presence of pathologic reflux. These include endoscopy to visualize the mucosa, endoscopic biopsy to document the mucosal and submucosal pathology, 24-h pH study to assess the extent of esophageal exposure to acid, and manometric recordings to evaluate any physiologic abnormalities in motor function.

Treatment

For GE reflux disease, the least aggressive and invasive treatment modalities should be attempted first. Initial recommendations might be to practice lifestyle changes such as cessation of smoking and avoidance of caffeine, fatty meals, or large meals before bedtime. The next level of treatment is medical management, which includes antacids, prokinetic agents, H_2-blockers, and proton pump inhibitors. A 6-week trial of acid suppression therapy with a double dose of a proton pump inhibitor not only might relieve the symptoms but also helps confirm the diagnosis if the patient responds favorably.

Because of the tremendous success in the minimally invasive surgical techniques, operative management of GE reflux disease should be considered an alternative to medical therapy rather than the last resort. The underlying principle of any of the operative approaches is to reenforce the tone of the distal esophagus by partially or completely wrapping it with the fundus of the

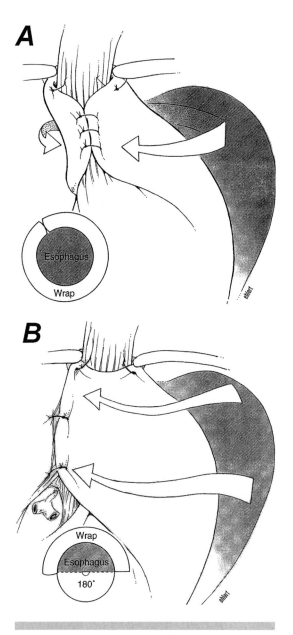

Figure 8-5 **There are three basic types of fundopli-cations: (A) Nissen fundoplication (360° wrap); (B) Thal and Dor fundoplications (partial anterior wrap); (C) Toupet fundoplication (partial posterior wrap).** (*Source: Reprinted with permission from Zwischenberger JB, Alpard SK, Orringer MB. Esophagus. In Townsend CM, Beauchamp RD, Evers BM, et al., eds., Sabiston Textbook of Surgery: The Biological Basis of Modern Surgical Practice, 16th ed. Philadelphia, PA: W.B. Saunders, 2001: 763.*)

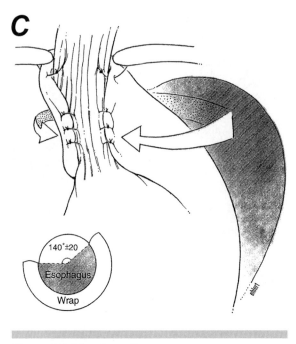

Figure 8-5 **(Continued)**

stomach (fundoplication). The three basic types of fundoplications are: *360° wrap* (Nissen fundoplication), *partial anterior wrap* (Thal and Dor fundoplications), and *partial posterior wrap* (Toupet fundoplication) (Fig. 8-5). In all of these approaches, the wrap is formed over a 2.5- to 3-cm distance. In general, the 360° wrap, Nissen fundoplication is used for patients with normal esophageal motility, and the partial fundoplications (the 180° anterior wrap or the 220–250° posterior wrap) are reserved for patients with abnormal esophageal manometric measurement, such as a distal esophageal pressure amplitude of less than 30 mmHg.

BENIGN TUMORS[11,14]

The great majority of esophageal tumors are malignant. Benign tumors constitute only 0.5–0.8 percent of all esophageal neoplasms. Benign esophageal tumors can be classified into *epithelial* (such as papillomas, polyps, adenomas, and cysts), *nonepithelial* (such as myomas, vascular tumors, and mesenchymal tumors), and *heterotopic* tumors. Since leiomyomas represent the most common type of the benign esophageal tumors (60 percent), the discussion here will focus mainly on this tumor. Cysts (20 percent) and polyps (5 percent) make up the second and third most common benign neoplasms of the esophagus.

Leiomyomas

Definition and Clinical Presentations

Leiomyomas are the most common benign tumor of the esophagus. More than 80 percent of them are found in the distal two-thirds of the esophagus. Leiomyomas are smooth muscle tumors that are well encapsulated and typically solitary. They occur in patients 20 and 50 years of age (slightly older in females). In 3–10 percent of the patients, esophageal leiomyomas are multiple. Most esophageal leiomyomas are asymptomatic, but larger (greater than 5 cm) ones may cause dysphagia, odynophagia, bleeding, or even obstruction.

Diagnostic Tests

The characteristic radiographic finding of esophageal leiomyomas on barium esophagogram is a smooth concave filling defect with sharp, intact mucosal shadow with abrupt angle where the tumor meets the normal esophageal wall (Fig. 8-6). Endoscopic evaluation should be performed to rule out malignancy, but if the appearance is characteristic of a leiomyoma, some experts recommend that a biopsy should be avoided to prevent scarring at the biopsy site, which might make the standard surgical treatment of enucleation more difficult in the future. Although esophageal ultrasound may provide further evidence in diagnosing leiomyomas, it is not necessary. Other studies are certainly not necessary prior to instituting appropriate treatment if leiomyoma is the only diagnosis being considered.

Treatment

Leiomyomas that are larger than 5 cm or cause symptoms should be surgically removed. After the outer longitudinal muscle is divided along the direction of its fiber, the tumor is gently enucleated from its underlying submucosa, and the opening through the longitudinal muscle layer is then reapproximated. There has been no report of recurrence after this procedure.

ESOPHAGEAL CANCER[5,11,12,14]

Epidemiology

More than 99 percent of esophageal tumors are of the malignant variety. However, esophageal cancer is relatively uncommon in the United States, with an annual rate of less than 10 per 100,000. Most are diagnosed between the sixth and the eighth decade of life, and, in general, men are two to four times more likely to be afflicted than females. Nevertheless, it is a lethal problem— once diagnosed, the overall 5-year survival rate is typically less than 10 percent,

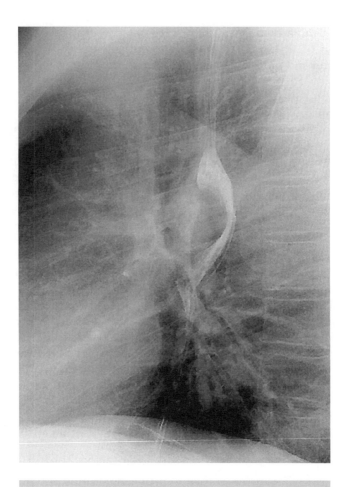

Figure 8-6 **The characteristic radiographic finding of an esophageal leiomyoma on barium esophagogram, showing a smooth concave filling defect, created by a well-defined lesion, with sharp, intact mucosal shadow with abrupt angle where the tumor meets the normal esophageal wall.** (*Source: Courtesy of William Thompson, M.D., and Anamaria Gaca, M.D., Department of Radiology, Duke University Medical Center.*)

and it is responsible for approximately 10,000–12,000 deaths per year in the United States. Internationally, esophageal cancer is much more prevalent, accounting for greater than 300,000 new cases per year. It is endemic in certain parts of the world. For example, in northeast Iran and in parts of northern

China, there are well over 100 new cases per 100,000 population each year. Furthermore, esophageal cancer has also been consistently one of the top 10 leading causes of cancer deaths worldwide.

Etiologic and Risk Factors

Based on epidemiologic studies, alcohol and tobacco use are strongly associated with esophageal cancer; individuals having a strong history of using both of these substances are 25–100 times more likely to develop esophageal cancer. Also implicated as causative factors are nitrosamines, foods contaminated by fungi and yeast that produce mutagens, ingestion of hot beverages causing chronic irritation of the esophageal mucosa, betel leaf, slaked lime, and resin from the acacia. Premalignant esophageal conditions include achalasia, reflux and radiation esophagitis, Barrett esophagus, caustic burns, Plummer-Vinson syndrome, leukoplakia, esophageal diverticula, and familial keratosis palmaris et plantaris (tylosis).

Histologic Cell Types

Although malignant esophageal tumors can be any one of several histologic cell types, including anaplastic small cell or oat cell carcinoma, adenoid cystic carcinoma, malignant melanoma, and carcinosarcoma, the most common cell types are squamous cell carcinoma and adenocarcinoma.

SQUAMOUS CELL CARCINOMA

Worldwide, squamous cell carcinoma represents approximately 95 percent of all esophageal cancers. Squamous cell carcinoma is a malignant tumor of the epithelial type, and it originates from the mucosa of the esophagus. Most cases of squamous cell esophageal cancer are in stage III or IV at the time of diagnosis. Squamous cell carcinomas typically occur in the upper and middle third of the esophagus, although in about 30 percent of patients, they are found in the distal third. There are four gross pathologic growth patterns: fungating, ulcerating, infiltrating, and polypoid. The fungating squamous cell carcinoma is the most common, representing about 60 percent of esophageal cancer of the squamous cell type; the polypoid variety is the least common (less than 5 percent of the cases), but it is associated with the best 5-year survival rate (about 70 percent).

ADENOCARCINOMA

The incidence of adenocarcinoma has dramatically increased recently, especially in industrialized countries. In fact, adenocarcinoma has now surpassed squamous cell carcinoma as the most common type of esophageal cancer in the United States. Unlike squamous cell carcinoma, adenocarcinoma afflicts Whites 4 times more frequently than Blacks; male are affected more than female. Adenocarcinoma typically occurs in the distal third of the esophagus, and it originates from submucosal glands or from columnar epithelium that is heterotopically located or has formed from metaplastic degeneration. Esophagus with columnar-type epithelium that has replaced the normally present squamous cell epithelium is called Barrett esophagus. Three different types of columnar epithelium can be found in Barrett esophagus—specialized intestinal metaplasia, gastric fundic type, and junctional type—of which specialized intestinal metaplasia is the most frequently seen as well as the most strongly associated with dysplasia and carcinoma in Barrett esophagus. The malignant cells of adenocarcinoma, as compared to normal cells from which they originated, have a characteristic reduced cytoplasmic-to-nuclear ratio. Individuals with Barrett esophagus are 40 times more at risk for developing esophageal adenocarcinoma than the general population; it is estimated that adenocarcinoma arises from 8 to 15 percent of patients with Barrett esophagus. The finding of dysplasia in Barrett mucosa is essentially synonymous with carcinoma in situ and is an indication for surgical resection.

Definition and Clinical Presentations

Patients with esophageal cancer may initially present with nonspecific retrosternal discomfort and indigestion. With time, progressive dysphagia is the chief complaint, occurring in 80–95 percent of patients who eventually are diagnosed with esophageal cancer. Weight loss ensues as a result of poor nutritional intake due to dysphagia or odynophagia, or as a consequence of metastatic spread of the malignancy. Other symptoms and signs include hematemesis, when the mucosal surface of the tumor becomes ulcerated, and coughing or hoarseness, especially when the tumor involves the cervical esophagus.

Diagnostic Tests

Plain radiographs will sometimes provide nonspecific clues, such as abnormal azygoesophageal recess, mediastinal widening, posterior tracheal indentation, that might suggest the presence of esophageal tumor. Barium esophagogram, which should be ordered in anyone with the complaint of dysphagia, is helpful in determining the size, the extent, and the location of the tumor and in demonstrating the presence of any obstruction or fistulas. Today, endoscopy with biopsy is the gold standard in confirming the presence of the malignancy and establishing a tissue diagnosis; often, it is the method by which carcinoma in situ or early stage cancer is detected through routine surveillance in patients with high-risk factors. A CT scan is done to evaluate any possible involvement of regional lymph nodes and any distant metastases. Positron emission tomography (PET) imaging, using fluorodeoxyglucose (FDG) that is preferentially taken up by malignant cells, can be used in supplementing the information obtained from CT scan and other studies; the advantage of PET imaging is the superior sensitivity for detecting distant metastases. Endoscopic ultrasound (EUS) is a technology that has been popularized recently because of its ability to more accurately assess both the depth of tumor invasion (T status) and the status of periesophageal lymph nodes. The accuracy of T stage determination by EUS has been shown to be between 60 and 90 percent.

Staging

Once the diagnosis of esophageal cancer is made by barium esophagogram and esophagoscopy, establishing the stage of the cancer is important in deciding the appropriate therapeutic options. Clinical staging can be accomplished based on many of the diagnostic studies (e.g., CT scan, PET imaging, and/or EUS) mentioned earlier; determining the pathologic staging will have to wait until a surgical specimen is available. The staging system most commonly used worldwide is the TNM format devised by the American Joint Committee on Cancer (AJCC) (Table 8-2).[5] T indicates the level of primary tumor invasion into the esophageal wall; N denotes the absence or presence of regional lymph node involvement; and M indicates whether there is distant metastasis or not. The overall 5-year survival rate is approximately 5 percent for esophageal cancer; based on the staging system, the 5-year survival rate is 50–55 percent for stage I, 15–38 percent for stage II, 6–17 percent for stage III, and less than 5 percent for stage IV.

Treatment

Despite the advances in surgery, chemotherapy, and radiation therapy, there has been little success in consistently achieving long-term survival for patients with esophageal cancer. Much of this might be due to the limitation of early detection of esophageal cancer. This is evidenced by the fact that more than three quarters of the patients who underwent surgical resection already have stage III or IV cancer. Furthermore, when a *curative* resection is documented, the 5-year survival rate is still only 30 percent. Therefore, the primary goal of any treatment is to provide symptomatic relief, most frequently from dysphagia, and at least to restore the patient's ability to comfortably swallow liquids.

The methods of palliative treatment include dilatation, stenting, photodynamic therapy, external-beam and intracavitary radiation therapy, and endoscopic laser therapy. The average length of survival with any of these palliative measures is less than 6 months. Palliative surgery using colon interposition or reversed gastric tube to bypass unresected esophagus have been used and are associated with at least a 25 percent operative mortality and a survival that averages only 6 months.

In patients with localized esophageal cancer, a more definitive operation provides the best chance of long-term survival. Three general approaches are available. First, a left thoracoabdominal approach (*Sweet operation*) can be used for distal esophageal tumors (Fig. 8-7). This operation allows the best

Table 8-2 **The TNM Staging System Devised by the AJCC**

Definition of TNM

Primary tumor (T)

TX	Primary tumor cannot be assessed
T0	No evidence of primary tumor
Tis	Carcinoma-in-situ
T1	Tumor invades lamina propria or submucosa
T2	Tumor invades muscularis propria
T3	Tumor invades adventitia
T4	Tumor invades adjacent structures

Regional lymph nodes (N)

NX	Regional lymph nodes cannot be assessed
N0	No regional lymph node metastasis
N1	Regional lymph node metastasis

Distant metastasis (M)

MX	Distant metastasis cannot be assessed
M0	No distant metastasis
M1	Distant metastasis
	Tumors of the lower thoracic esophagus
M1a	Metastasis in celiac lymph nodes
M1b	Other distant metastasis
	Tumors of the midthoracic esophagus
M1a	Not applicable
M1b	Nonregional lymph nodes and/or other distant metastasis
	Tumors of the upper thoracic esophagus
M1a	Metastasis in cervical nodes
M1b	Other distant metastasis

Stage grouping

Stage 0	Tis	N0	M0
Stage 1	T1	N0	M0
Stage IIA	T2	N0	M0
	T3	N0	M0
Stage IIB	T1	N1	M0
	T2	N1	M0
Stage III	T3	N1	M0
	T4	Any N	M0
Stage IV	Any T	Any N	M1
Stage IVA	Any T	Any N	M1a
Stage IVB	Any T	Any N	M1b

Source: Reprinted with permission from Table 1 of Patel M, Ferry K, Franceschi D, et al. Esophageal carcinoma: current controversial topics. *Cancer Invest* 22:898, 2004.

exposure of the lower third of the esophagus as well as the GE junction and the diaphragmatic hiatus, and it facilitates a more complete abdominal lymphadenectomy, which can be vital in staging cancer of the lower esophagus. Second, a combined right thoracotomy and upper midline laparotomy (*Ivor-Lewis operation*) can be used either for a lower esophageal tumor or a higher thoracic esophageal tumor (Fig. 8-8). Because the incision does not limit the exposure of the proximal extent of the thoracic esophagus, a wider margin on the tumor can be obtained and the anastomosis between the reconstructed stomach and the proximal esophagus can be performed more easily than the Sweet operation; the recurrence rate at the anastomotic margin is therefore thought to be lower with the Ivor-Lewis esophagectomy. Finally, the transhiatal approach (*Orringer esophagectomy*) uses an upper midline laparotomy and a left cervical incision (Fig. 8-9). Through the upper

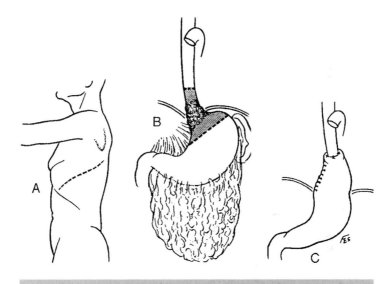

Figure 8-7 **An overview of Sweet operation, which can be performed for distal esophageal tumors. (A) A left thoracotomy or thoracoabdominal approach is used. (B) Tumor is removed by resecting a portion of the distal esophagus and the stomach. (C) The stomach is mobilized for intrathoracic esophagogastric anastomosis.** (*Source: Reprinted with permission from Zwischenberger JB, Alpard SK, Orringer MB. Esophagus. In Townsend CM, Beauchamp RD, Evers BM, eds., Sabiston Textbook of Surgery: The Biological Basis of Modern Surgical Practice, 16th ed. Philadelphia, PA: W.B. Saunders, 2001: 739, which was adapted from Ellis FH Jr, Shahian DM. Tumors of the esophagus. In Glenn WWL, Baue AE, Geha AS, et al., eds., Thoracic and Cardiovascular Surgery, 4th ed. Norwalk, CT: Appleton and Lange, 1983: 566.*)

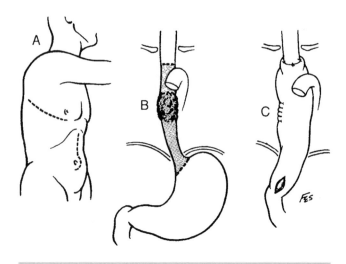

Figure 8-8   ***An overview of Ivor-Lewis operation.***
(A) Exposure is made through a combined right thoraco-
tomy and upper midline laparotomy. (B) This approach can
be used either for a lower esophageal tumor or a higher
thoracic esophageal tumor; the length of the esophagus
required to remove the tumor is resected. (C) The stomach
is mobilized for intrathoracic esophagogastric anastomosis.
(*Source: Reprinted with permission from Zwischenberger JB,*
Alpard SK, Orringer MB. Esophagus. In Townsend CM,
Beauchamp RD, Evers BM, et al., eds., Sabiston Textbook of
Surgery: The Biological Basis of Modern Surgical Practice,
16th ed. Philadelphia, PA: W.B. Saunders, 2001: 739, which
was adapted from Ellis FH Jr. Esophagogastrectomy for carci-
noma: technical considerations based on anatomic location of
lesion. Surg Clin North Am 60:273, 1980.)

midline abdominal incision, the esophagus is resected after being bluntly dissected from adjacent structures, and the stomach, fashioned into a tubular structure by stapling off a portion of the proximal lesser curvature, is pulled through the posterior mediastinal space out through the left neck incision, where it is anastomosed with the cervical esophagus proximally. The clear advantage of the Orringer technique is that a thoracotomy is avoided, thus minimizing some of the pulmonary complications. In addition, if there is a postoperative leak at the esophageal anastomosis, the contamination in the neck wound would be more manageable than that in the mediastinum. Because of the nature of the blunt dissection technique, the theoretical concern is that a more complete mediastinal lymphadenectomy

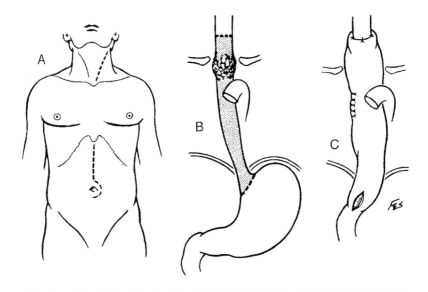

Figure 8-9 **An overview of Orringer (transhiatal) esophagectomy. (A) Exposure is made through an upper midline laparotomy and a left cervical incision. (B) The entire length of the esophagus is resected. (C) The stomach is mobilized for cervical-esophagogastric anastomosis.** (*Source: Reprinted with permission from Zwischenberger JB, Alpard SK, Orringer MB. Esophagus. In Townsend CM, Beauchamp RD, Evers BM, et al., eds., Sabiston Textbook of Surgery: The Biological Basis of Modern Surgical Practice, 16th ed. Philadelphia, PA: W.B. Saunders, 2001: 741, which was adapted from Ellis FH Jr. Esophagogastrectomy for carcinoma: technical considerations based on anatomic location of lesion. Surg Clin North Am 60:275, 1980.*)

cannot be performed and the patient survival rate would therefore be compromised; this concern has never been substantiated, as the current survival rates between any of these three operative approaches are indistinguishable. A variation of the Orringer esophagectomy is to make one additional incision on the right chest with a thoracoscopy or thoracotomy (*three-hole esophagectomy*); although the putative benefit is to obtain a more thorough mediastinal lymphadenectomy, the main advantage of this approach is to facilitate a visually more direct dissection of the midesophageal region if the primary tumor is especially large or appears to be adherent to adjacent structures through inflammation.

The effectiveness of *neoadjuvant* (preoperative) and *adjuvant* (postoperative) therapies with drugs and radiation has been a point of controversy. The literature is filled with studies that have led to mixed conclusions. However, by most accounts, there is no convincing evidence that either neoadjuvant or adjuvant therapy improves survival as compared to surgery alone.

REFERENCES

1. Duranceau A. The esophagus. In Sabiston DC, Lyerly HK, eds., *Essentials of Surgery*, 2nd ed. Philadelphia, PA: W.B. Saunders, 1994, Chap. 25.

2. Duranceau A. The esophagus: part VII, perforation of the esophagus. In Sabiston DC, Lyerly HK, eds., *Textbook of Surgery: The Biological Basis of Modern Surgical Practice*, 15th ed. Philadelphia, PA: W.B. Saunders, 1997, Chap. 26.

3. Duranceau A, Jamieson GG. The esophagus: part VIII, hiatal hernia and gastroesophageal reflux. In Sabiston DC, Lyerly HK, eds., *Textbook of Surgery: The Biological Basis of Modern Surgical Practice*, 15th ed. Philadelphia, PA: W.B. Saunders, 1997, Chap. 26.

4. Eubanks TR, Pellegrini CA. Hiatal hernia and gastroesophageal reflux disease. In Townsend CM, Beauchamp RD, Evers BM, et al., eds., *Sabiston Textbook of Surgery: The Biological Basis of Modern Surgical Practice*, 16th ed. Philadelphia, PA: W.B. Saunders, 2001, Chap. 38.

5. Fleming I, Cooper J, Henson D. *AJCC Cancer Staging Manual*, 5th ed. Philadelphia, PA: Lippincott-Raven, 1997.

6. Jacobs DO. The esophagus. In Niederhuber JE, ed., *Fundamentals of Surgery*. Stamford, CT: Appleton and Lange, 1998, Chap. 25.

7. Orringer MB. The esophagus. Part I. Historical aspects and anatomy. In Sabiston DC, Lyerly HK, eds., *Textbook of Surgery: The Biological Basis of Modern Surgical Practice*, 15th ed. Philadelphia, PA: W.B. Saunders, 1997, Chap. 26.

8. Orringer MB. The esophagus. Part II. Physiology. In Sabiston DC, Lyerly HK, eds., *Textbook of Surgery: The Biological Basis of Modern Surgical Practice*, 15th ed. Philadelphia, PA: W.B. Saunders, 1997, Chap. 26.

9. Orringer MB. The esophagus. Part III. Disorders of esophageal motility. In Sabiston DC, Lyerly HK, eds., *Textbook of Surgery: The Biological Basis of Modern Surgical Practice*, 15th ed. Philadelphia, PA: W.B. Saunders, 1997, Chap. 26.

10. Orringer MB. The esophagus. Part IV. Diverticula and miscellaneous conditions of the esophagus. In Sabiston DC, Lyerly HK, eds., *Textbook of Surgery: The Biological Basis of Modern Surgical Practice*, 15th ed. Philadelphia, PA: W.B. Saunders, 1997, Chap. 26.

11. Orringer MB. The esophagus. Part VI. Tumors of the esophagus. In Sabiston DC, Lyerly HK, eds., *Textbook of Surgery: The Biological Basis of Modern Surgical Practice*, 15th ed. Philadelphia, PA: W.B. Saunders, 1997, Chap. 26.

12. Patel M, Ferry K, Franceschi D, et al. Esophageal carcinoma: current controversial topics. *Cancer Invest* 22:897–912, 2004.

13. Smith CD. Esophagus. In Norton JA, Bollinger RR, Chang AE, et al., eds., *Surgery: Basic Science and Clinical Evidence*. New York: Springer-Verlag, 2001, Chap. 26.

14. Zwischenberger JB, Alpard SK, Orringer MB. Esophagus. In Townsend CM, Beauchamp RD, Evers BM, et al., eds., *Sabiston Textbook of Surgery: The Biological Basis of Modern Surgical Practice*, 16th ed. Philadelphia, PA: W.B. Saunders, 2001, Chap. 37.

STOMACH

Carlos E. Marroquin, MD

EMBRYOLOGY

The stomach originates in the tubular embryonic foregut during the fifth week of gestation.[1] It first appears as a fusiform dilatation of the caudal part of the foregut. The dorsal border enlarges faster than the ventral border, producing the greater curvature. By the seventh week, it assumes its normal anatomic shape and position by descent, clockwise rotation, and dilatation, with disproportionate elongation of the greater curvature.

ANATOMY

The stomach is the most proximal abdominal organ of the alimentary tract. The region of the stomach that attaches to the esophagus is called the *cardia*. The stomach is made up of the *fundus*, the *body*, and the *pyloric antrum* (Fig. 9-1). The pylorus forms a circular muscle or sphincter that guards the junction between the stomach and duodenum. The stomach has a greater and lesser curvature. The greater curvature is attached to the greater omentum. The stomach is a richly perfused organ. It derives blood supply from the left and right gastric arteries, the left and right gastroepiploic arteries, the short gastric arteries, and the inferior phrenic arteries. The left and right gastric arteries course along the lesser curvature while the left and right gastroepiploic arteries course along the greater curvature. The short gastric arteries travel in a veil of tissue constituting the gastrosplenic ligament.

PHYSIOLOGY

The stomach serves to mix food with gastric secretions performing both a mechanical and chemical reduction of food into *chyme*. Once chyme formation is complete, the pylorus sphincter relaxes allowing the stomach to propel chyme into the duodenum via muscular contractions. The mucosa of the

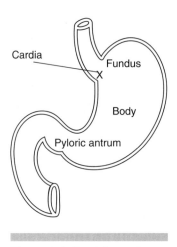

Figure 9-1 **Gastric anatomy.**

stomach is glandular and there are three distinct histologic zones.[2] The region of the cardia is a small area around the entrance of the esophagus where there is a preponderance of mucous-secreting glands. The fundus and body contain the bulk of gastric glands which synthesize and secrete gastric juice. Gastric juice is a watery secretion containing hydrochloric acid and pepsin. Pepsin is a digestive enzyme which hydrolyses protein into polypeptide fragments. The glands of the fundus and body contain three populations of cells. *Mucous neck cells* secrete mucous to protect the gastric mucosa from autodigestion by acid and pepsin. *Parietal cells* secrete hydrochloric acid and intrinsic factor which binds vitamin B_{12} facilitating its absorption in the ileum, and pepsin-secreting chief cells. Finally, the *glands* of the pyloric region secrete mucous and associated endocrine cells, G cells, and the hormone gastrin.

Parietal cells have receptors for acetylcholine, gastrin, and histamine. As a result, gastric secretion is regulated by acetylcholine, gastrin, and histamine which bind their receptor leading to stimulation of acid secretion. Stimulation of gastric secretion has been divided into three separate phases: the cephalic phase, gastric phase, and intestinal phase.[3] The *cephalic phase* originates with sight, smell, thought, and taste of food and is initiated in the cerebral cortex. The afferent impulse is delivered through the vagal nerve fibers innervating the stomach. The vagus acts directly on the parietal cells through acetylcholine and indirectly through the release of gastrin-releasing peptide to stimulate gastrin release. The *gastric phase* originates with food entering the stomach and subsequently stimulating the release of acetylcholine from vagal and local nerves, gastrin from G cells, and histamine from enterochromaffin-like cells. Finally, the *intestinal phase* of gastric secretion is stimulated by food entering the duodenum and contributes only a small portion of the stimulation to gastric secretion. Paradoxically, the intestinal phase of gastric secretion is predominantly an inhibitory signal which inhibits ongoing gastric secretion. During this phase, several intestinal hormones (e.g., secretin, cholecystokinin [CCK], somatostatin, and gastric inhibitory peptide [GIP]) are released which serve to inhibit gastric secretion.

GASTRIC ULCERS

Symptoms of burning or pain in the upper abdomen, usually occurring about an hour or so after meals or even during the night, are classic in patients with gastric ulcers. These symptoms are relieved temporarily by antacids, milk, or medications that reduce stomach acid production. Gastric ulcers[4,5] are classified by location (Fig. 9-2) and whether acid hypersecretion is involved in their pathogenesis (Table 9-1). *Type I ulcers* are the most common representing approximately 60 percent of all ulcers. Type I ulcers are commonly found along the lesser curvature, where the lesser curvature acutely angles to the right marking the end of the body and the beginning of the antrum, near the incisura angularis. Ulcers that arise coincident with duodenal ulcers and are associated with high acid production are classified as *type II ulcers* and represent about 20 percent of ulcers. Ulcers in the prepyloric and pyloric region are classified as *type III gastric ulcers* and constitute about 20 percent of all ulcers, and because of their common association with

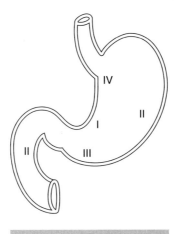

Figure 9-2 **Location of gastric ulcers.**

Table 9-1 **Classification of Gastric Ulcers**

Ulcer Type	Location	Acid Hypersecretion	Surgical Therapy	Recurrence Rate (%)
I	Incisura or lesser curvature (most common)	No	Distal gastrectomy with Billroth I	2
			Truncal vagotomy and pyloroplasty	10–20
			Highly selective vagotomy	15
II	Body of stomach and duodenum	Yes	Bilateral truncal vagotomy and antrectomy with Billroth I or II	<5
			Truncal vagotomy and pyloroplasty	10–20
			Highly selective vagotomy	15
III	Prepyloric	Yes	Bilateral truncal vagotomy and antrectomy with Billroth I or Billroth II	<5
			Truncal vagotomy and pyloroplasty	10–20
			Highly selective vagotomy	12–44
IV	Gastroesophageal junction (uncommon)	No	Pauchet procedure Csendes procedure Kelling-Madlener procedure	
V	Any anatomic location (medically induced)	No	Vagotomy and pyloroplasty	

high acid production are believed to have a similar origin as their duodenal counterparts. *Type IV ulcers* are found high on the lesser curvature near the gastroesophageal junction, and likely represent high type I ulcers. Finally, ulcers that result secondary to nonsteroidal anti-inflammatory drugs (NSAIDs) or steroid use do not conform to this classification. These ulcers typically occur in the antrum but may be located anywhere in the stomach and may be multiple as opposed to the single ulcer seen in gastric ulcer disease. As a result, iatrogenic ulcers related to NSAIDs and steroid use are referred to as *type V ulcers*.

It is now known that approximately 80 percent of ulcers are caused by a bacterium, *Helicobacter pylori*.[4,5] Although the majority of gastric ulcers are now known to be associated with *H. pylori* infection, there is a subset of patients who develop ulcers in association with NSAID use. This subgroup of patients may account for 10–30 percent of ulcers. One other less frequently seen cause of ulcers in patients who are *H. pylori* negative is the Zollinger-Ellison syndrome (ZES).

There are several ways to diagnose *H. pylori* infection.[6] Biopsies are obtained during endoscopy and the tissue is assessed histologically for the bacteria. This histologic evaluation is the gold standard for diagnosing *H. pylori*. Alternatively, the tissue can be placed in a capsule containing urea. This is known as the *biopsy urease test*—a colorimetric test based on the ability of *H. pylori* to produce urease; it provides rapid testing at the time of biopsy. If *H. pylori* is present, urea is broken down producing a change in the color of the gel in the capsule. A *breath test* is also available in which the patient is given 13C- or 14C-labeled urea to drink. A strong enzyme in the bacteria breaks down the urea into carbon dioxide. The labeled carbon can then be measured as CO_2 in the patient's expired breath to determine whether *H. pylori* is present. Antibodies (IgG) against *H. pylori* can also be detected in the patient's serum. However, antibodies are detectable even if the infection has been cleared. Therefore, a person can have a positive blood test in the absence of infection. Finally, cultures of biopsy specimens can be grown in a microbiology laboratory as a means of detecting the presence of the bacteria.

MEDICAL THERAPY

Physicians are treating the acute ulcer with acid-reducing medicines and treating the infection with antibiotics. *Pepto-Bismol* has been one of the mainstays of therapy. The bismuth component is bactericidal. *H. pylori* is buried deep in the stomach mucosa, so it is difficult to eradicate. Several antibiotic drugs are always used together to prevent the bacteria from developing resistance to any one of them (Table 9-2). The two main antibiotics used are metronidazole and clarithromycin.[7] Good clinical evidence of efficacy has been provided for several triple or quadruple antibiotic therapies. These therapies are associated with cure rates of 80–90 percent. Therapies combining only a proton pump inhibitor and amoxicillin or clarithromycin are no longer regarded as effective. Several treatment regimens have been shown to be effective, but no single treatment regimen is considered the final treatment of choice.

Table 9-2 **Medical Therapy of H. pylori**

Component Drugs			Length of Treatment (Days)
Regimens Based on Clarithromycin			
Ranitidine, 400 mg twice daily	Clarithromycin, 500 mg twice daily		14
Ranitidine, 400 mg twice daily	Clarithromycin, 500 mg twice daily	Amoxicillin, 1000 mg twice daily	7–10
Proton pump inhibitor twice daily	Clarithromycin, 500 mg twice daily	Amoxicillin, 1000 mg twice daily	7–10
Regimens Based on Metronidazole			
Bismuth compound four times daily	Tetracycline, 500 mg four times daily	Metronidazole, 400–500 mg three to four times daily	14
Proton pump inhibitor twice daily	Amoxicillin, 500 mg two to three times daily	Metronidazole, 400–500 mg two to three times daily	7–10
Proton pump inhibitor twice daily	Colloidal bismuth four times daily	Tetracycline, 500 mg four times daily	4–7
Regimens Based on Clarithromycin Plus Metronidazole			
Ranitidine, 400 mg twice daily	Clarithromycin, 500 mg twice daily	Metronidazole, 400–500 mg twice daily	7
Proton pump inhibitor twice daily	Clarithromycin, 500 mg twice daily	Metronidazole, 400–500 mg twice daily	7

SURGICAL THERAPY

The only time surgery should serve as the first-line therapy is in patients with giant (greater than 3 cm) gastric ulcers.[4,5] Elective surgery is the first-line therapy in these patients because of the high rate of complications associated with these lesions and the high rate of medical failure. Otherwise, surgical therapy is reserved for complications resulting from ulcers or for the management of ulcers refractory to medical therapy. Ulcers are considered refractory to medical therapy if the ulcer fails to heal with optimal medical management, or if the patient is noncompliant or does not tolerate medical treatment. By and large, surgery is reserved for dealing with complications that result from gastric ulcers such as bleeding, perforation, and obstruction.

Elective surgery for refractory gastric ulcers is rarely performed. Type I gastric ulcers are treated with distal gastrectomy, including the ulcer, and a gastroduodenal anastomosis, or Billroth I (Fig. 9-3). Type II ulcers can be located anywhere in the distal body of the stomach and are associated with duodenal ulcers. These ulcers are also known to be associated with acid secretion. Therefore, a truncal vagotomy and antrectomy removes the mucosa at risk and eliminates the acid secretory state associated with the

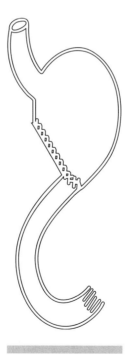

Figure 9-3 **Billroth I/ gastroduodenostomy.**

ulcer formation. If a Billroth I anastomosis cannot be performed due to extensive duodenal inflammation, a gastrojejunostomy, or Billroth II is performed (Fig. 9-4). Type III ulcers are located in the pyloric region. The procedure of choice is a vagotomy and antrectomy with Billroth I unless extensive scarring and inflammation necessitates a gastrojejunostomy. The greatest disadvantage associated with these procedures is the high incidence of postgastrectomy syndromes[8,9] (Table 9-3). Fortunately, these can be managed with mild-to-moderate dietary alterations. Despite greater recurrence rates, some surgeons prefer lesser procedures which do not require gastric resection such as a truncal vagotomy and pyloroplasty or a highly selective vagotomy to treat type I, II, and III ulcers. In addition to a procedure to reduce acid production (vagotomy), the ulcer is generally excised in order to rule out the presence of malignancy. In the rare instance when the ulcer cannot be incorporated into the surgical specimen or excised, multiple biopsies should be taken of both the center and the edge of the ulcer to rule out an underlying malignancy.

Type IV or ulcers at the gastroesophageal junction present a surgical challenge. The procedure of choice is known as a *Pauchet procedure*[4,5] and involves a distal gastrectomy combined with a Billroth I. The gastrectomy involves an extensive resection extending onto the proximal portion of the lesser curvature in order to incorporate the ulcer. Another alternative is

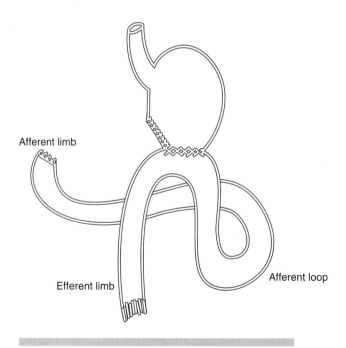

Afferent limb

Efferent limb

Afferent loop

Figure 9-4 **Billroth II/gastrojejunostomy.**

Table 9-3 *Postgastrectomy Syndromes*

Syndrome	Etiology	Signs and Symptoms	Treatment
Recurrent ulcer	Incomplete vagotomy Retained antrum Zollinger-Ellison syndrome Recurrent *H. pylori* Surreptitious NSAIDs Gastric cancer Marginal ulcer	Recurrent abdominal pain and dyspepsia	Completion vagotomy Completion antrectomy Resect gastrinoma Triple or quadruple antimicrobial therapy Discontinue NSAID use Gastrectomy Reresection and completion vagotomy
Early dumping syndrome	Destruction or bypass of the pyloric sphincter	Weakness, light head, diaphoresis, and tachycardia 15–30 min after hypertonic liquid meal. Associated with abdominal cramping/discomfort and diarrhea	Change meals to low carbohydrate with high fiber content and restrict fluids with meals Octreotide convert to Roux-en-Y
Late dumping syndrome	Destruction or bypass of the pyloric sphincter	Hypoglycemia about 2–3 h after meals due to extreme fluctuations in glucose and insulin	Administer glucose Acarbose, an α-glucosidase inhibitor may ameliorate symptoms of late dumping syndrome Convert to Roux-en-Y
Postvagotomy diarrhea	Intestinal dysmotility Accelerated transit Bile acid malabsorption	Diarrhea with associated electrolyte abnormality and dehydration with no other postgastrectomy symptoms	Cholestyramine, Lomotil, and/or tincture of opium Interposition of reversed jejunal segment

(Continued)

Table 9-3 *Postgastrectomy Syndromes (Continued)*

Syndrome	Etiology	Signs and Symptoms	Treatment
Gastroparesis	Loss of motor function	Nausea, vomiting, and bloating	Reglan, erythromycin, or Zelnorm
Alkaline reflux gastritis	Reflux of pancreatic, duodenal, and biliary contents into denervated stomach	Pain with associated nausea and bilious vomiting	Convert to Roux-en-Y with a 50– cm efferent jejunal limb
Afferent loop syndrome usually after a Billroth II	Long afferent limb associated with trapped biliary and pancreatic secretions which produce distention of the proximal limb	Pain with bilious vomiting	Convert to Roux-en-Y
Blind loop syndrome usually after a Billroth II	Long afferent limb with bacterial overgrowth	Weakness associated with anemia and positive Schilling test	Supplement fat-soluble vitamins and vitamin B_{12} Broad-spectrum antibiotics
Anemia	Decreased intrinsic factor that results in decreased vitamin B_{12}	Weakness that evolves with associated anemia	Vitamin B_{12} injections
Gastrojejunocolic fistula	Marginal ulcer in jejunum	Diarrhea, malnutrition, and feculent vomiting	Excise the gastrojejunal segment and reconstruct Avoid contact of new suture line with colon with omental interposition

known as the *Csendes procedure*[4,5] which includes resection of the lesser curvature with Roux-en-Y esophagogastrojejunostomy. Finally, if the ulcer cannot be excised because its size or location makes it technically impossible, a Kelling-Madlener procedure provides a less aggressive approach and incorporates an antrectomy with a Billroth I reconstruction with bilateral truncal vagotomy. Multiple biopsies of the ulcer are obtained to rule out malignancy. Finally, patients who develop ulcers in association with NSAID or steroid use can have ulcers located anywhere in the stomach and can be associated with high and low acid production. These patients are best treated with vagotomy and pyloroplasty.

It is more common to operate on patients who experience complications from their ulcers. A common reason for surgical exploration is upper gastrointestinal (UGI) bleeding. However, before these patients are explored, they must be resuscitated and properly evaluated and treated. Medical and endoscopic management are often successful as first-line therapy for ulcerogenic bleeding.[4] Patients with suspected upper GI bleeding must first be resuscitated with two large bore IVs, and appropriate laboratory interrogation and medical management should be initiated. Serial hematocrit and coagulation assays should be followed and corrected if abnormal, and acid suppression therapy should be initiated with proton pump inhibitors or H_2-blocker infusion. The diagnosis needs to be confirmed with a large volume gastric lavage. A nasogastric (NG) tube is placed and irrigated with a minimum of 500 cc of normal saline. The intent is to lavage until the effluent is clear or bilious. If the aspirate that follows the large volume lavage is bloody, one can assume active bleeding is present. Once an upper GI source of bleeding is documented, a GI consult should be obtained for endoscopy. Upper endoscopy serves as both a diagnostic maneuver to establish the location of bleeding and is also therapeutic. In fact, the risk of bleeding from a gastric ulcer decreases significantly after endoscopic therapy.[4] This is critical given that patients who experience bleeding from an upper GI source are often older individuals who are poor operative candidates. In fact, emergent surgery for bleeding gastric ulcers is associated with a high mortality rate; on the order of 10–30 percent.

Patients who develop a transfusion requirement (4 U) or who are found to have active bleeding or a visible vessel at endoscopy will require an operative intervention. Surgical options depend on the patient's condition. When an unstable patient is taken to the operating room for ongoing hemorrhage, simple excision or oversewing of the ulcer with vagotomy and pyloroplasty is acceptable with prompt return to the intensive care unit for continued resuscitation. Both excision and oversewing are performed through an anterior gastrotomy. Hemodynamically stable patients should undergo a definitive procedure usually consisting of a distal gastrectomy incorporating the ulcer with a Billroth I reconstruction. Patients whose ulcers are associated with NSAID use and acid secretion (types II and III) should also undergo a bilateral truncal vagotomy to control acid production.

Perforation is also a complication of gastric ulcers.[4,5] Patients with evidence of perforation require a laparotomy. The procedure of choice is a distal gastrectomy including the ulcer with gastroduodenal anastomosis. As in cases of bleeding, a vagotomy should be preformed for patients whose ulcers are associated with hypersecretion or NSAIDs. Rarely, hemodynamically stable patients with prohibitive comorbidities and evidence of a sealed perforation can be managed expectantly. These patients require NG-tube decompression and supportive care in a monitored setting. Patients with no prior history of ulcers whose initial presentation is perforation can be treated with ulcer biopsy or excision and primary repair with omentum. These patients need to be worked up and treated for *H. pylori*. Omental patch closure in this population is considered reasonable by some, as this patient population is considered at low risk for recurrence once *H. pylori* is eradicated. Patients with known history of ulcer disease should undergo resection of the ulcer with a vagotomy and antrectomy. However, if the patient is a poor surgical candidate because of hemodynamic instability, the procedure can be limited to simple excision or oversewing with vagotomy and pyloroplasty. A vagotomy and pyloroplasty reduces the risk of recurrence to approximately 10 percent with lower operative risks. Although a vagotomy and antrectomy is associated with the lowest risk of recurrence, it is associated with a greater incidence of postgastrectomy syndromes (Table 9-3).

Obstruction is a rare complication of gastric ulcers. In the majority of patients with gastric outlet obstruction due to gastric ulcer disease, the ulcer has been present for a long period of time. Long enough to allow inflammation and scarring to develop into an obstruction. These patients are commonly dehydrated and have significant electrolyte abnormalities. Therefore, initial management is conservative with NG decompression and IV hydration. Rarely will nonoperative management resolve the obstruction. Once the patient is resuscitated and electrolyte abnormalities corrected, the procedure of choice involves an antrectomy with a Billroth I anastomosis. Since obstructive lesions are associated with type II and III ulcers, a vagotomy is added to the procedure. Some surgeons prefer a bypass procedure using a gastrojejunostomy to bypass the obstructed segment. This is particularly useful if one finds the inflammatory process involves the duodenal stump.

POSTGASTRECTOMY SYNDROMES

Although not commonly thought of as a part of the postgastrectomy constellation,[8,9] ulcer recurrence is a postgastrectomy complication. Patients with recurrence of their gastric ulcers were either not worked up adequately or underwent an inadequate operation. In the former scenario, an inadequate workup missed a gastrinoma, a gastric malignancy, *H. pylori* infection, or history of NSAID abuse. In the latter scenario, an incomplete vagotomy or incomplete gastric resection was performed leaving behind a portion of the antrum. G cells in the antrum secrete gastrin that stimulates parietal cells to make acid.

Hypergastrinemia can result from the presence of a gastrinoma (ZES), retained antrum, or G-cell hyperplasia from a postvagotomy state. A gastrinoma can be distinguished from G-cell hyperplasia with either a secretin stimulation test or a meal stimulation test. Secretin causes paradoxical release of gastrin from a gastrinoma, but has little effect on gastrin release from normal antrum or antrum with G-cell hyperplasia. A meal will have little to no effect on gastrin release from a patient with ZES. Yet, a meal results in significant gastrin release in patients with G-cell hyperplasia. Regardless of the etiology, patients should have a thorough workup prior to committing them to additional surgical procedures. In addition to a medical workup with fasting serum gastrin and basal acid output measurements, an endoscopic gastroduodenoscopy should be obtained with biopsies for *H. pylori*, gastric cancer, and formation of marginal ulcerations. If both the serum gastrin and basal acid output are elevated, a workup for ZES should be undertaken. Patients should also receive a meal followed by measurement of acid output. A significant increase in acid production is suggestive of an incomplete vagotomy.

Management should be tailored to the results of the workup. Patients who are found to be infected with *H. pylori* should be treated with triple or quadruple therapy, and patients who are found to have elevated salicylate levels should be encouraged, emphatically, to discontinue the use of NSAIDs. Otherwise, patients who underwent an inadequate operation should be followed with a complete vagotomy and/or complete antrectomy if a patient was left with a retained antrum in the duodenal margin. If a gastrinoma is found, it should be localized and resected. The presence of a marginal ulcer requires gastric resection and completion vagotomy. Finally, if an elusive gastric cancer turns out to be the cause of a recurrent ulcer, this will commonly be managed with a subtotal gastrectomy.

There are two types of dumping syndromes that are described in patients who have undergone a gastrectomy or pyloroplasty. Dumping syndromes occur due to the iatrogenic loss of the pyloric sphincter. *Early dumping syndrome* occurs 15–30 min after a meal and is manifested by the onset of weakness, dizziness or lightheadedness, diaphoresis, and tachycardia. Abdominal cramping/discomfort and diarrhea often follow. Dietary manipulations are often effective in the management of early dumping syndrome, and the addition of octreotide before meals may help the extreme hormonal fluctuations often seen in patients with dumping syndrome. *Late dumping syndrome* or *postprandial hypoglycemia* is experienced approximately 2–3 h after meals due to extreme fluctuations in serum glucose levels and subsequent insulin secretion. Late dumping syndrome can be managed by simply administering glucose in the form of snacks or juices with symptomatic relief. In the rare instance in which surgical intervention is necessary in patients who have exhausted all nonoperative options, conversion to a Roux-en-Y gastroje-junostomy provides the best option. Several other procedures have been attempted with limited success.

Diarrhea can also plague a patient following gastrectomy. Unremitting diarrhea following a vagotomy and antrectomy that is not associated with any other symptoms of dumping or malabsorption is most likely related to the vagotomy. Postvagotomy diarrhea usually responds to medical therapy with cholestyramine, Lomotil, or tincture of opium and commonly improves over time. It is uncommon for one to require surgical therapy of postvagotomy diarrhea. However, in the extreme, interposition of a reversed jejunal segment approximately 100 cm beyond the ligament of Treitz has been found to be useful in the management of refractory postvagotomy diarrhea.

Vomiting and epigastric pain with associated bloating following gastrec-tomy can result from gastroparesis. Delayed gastric emptying in the absence of a mechanical obstruction following a gastrectomy is usually due to loss of motor function. Peristaltic waves are normally triggered in the stomach by a food bolus and these waves progress distally to the antrum as the stomach converts the food bolus into chyme prior to ejecting it into the duodenum. Gastric motility is dependent on the fundus, body, antrum, and pylorus working as a unit and is measured by the rate at which foodstuff is emptied from the stomach. Contractions in the body and antrum occur in response to an organized electrical rhythm, referred as the *gastric pacemaker*. Vagal nerve input as well as GI hormones and peptides stimulate activity of the gastric pacemaker and smooth muscle contractility of the stomach. This loss of motor function can occur as a direct result of the vagotomy, one reason sur-geons commonly perform a drainage procedure with a vagotomy, or from physical resection which disrupts the coordinated contractions of the stom-ach smooth muscle.

Once a mechanical obstruction has been ruled out, patients suspected of developing postoperative gastroparesis should be worked up with a nuclear medicine gastric emptying study or an upper GI series. The nuclear medicine scan will be able to quantify both liquid and solid phase emptying time. Postoperative gastroparesis usually resolves with medical therapy and or dietary modification. Commonly used agents include metoclopramide, domperidone, erythromycin, and Zelnorm. Surgical intervention is required infrequently for the management of gastroparesis. However, conversion to a subtotal gastric resection with Billroth II anastomosis with distal enteroen-terostomy or a near total gastric resection with Roux-en-Y gastrojejunostomy should be employed when refractory gastroparesis results.

The reflux of intestinal contents into the stomach can cause severe pain with associated nausea and vomiting and is referred to as bile reflux gastritis or alkaline reflux gastritis. Bilious vomiting and excessive reflux of intestinal juices into the stomach can produce significant debility. This is usually a late manifestation following gastrectomy and is a diagnosis of exclusion. Bile reflux may be quantified with a *hepatoiminodiacetic acid* (HIDA) scan. Alkaline efflux gastritis is more commonly seen following a Billroth II anastomosis, but can be seen with a Billroth I reconstruction or a vagotomy and pyloroplasty. Conservative management including dietary modifications with high fat and amino acid regimens to augment pyloric tone, acid suppression therapy, gastric mucosal protection with Carafate and prostaglandins, prokinetic agents to improve gastric emptying, and Actigall and aluminum hydroxide containing antacids and cholestyramine to bind bile acids have all produced varying but disappointing success. Patients who experience no relief from medical therapy may benefit from elimination of the bile from the vomitus. This can be achieved with a Roux-en-Y gastrojejunostomy where the Roux limb is at least 45 cm long.

Unfortunately, the management of one postgastrectomy syndrome, alkaline/biliary reflux, has created another. The Roux syndrome is a late complication characterized by nausea, vomiting, bloating, and abdominal pain. This constellation of symptoms can be difficult to distinguish from gastroparesis, and like gastroparesis, it is important to perform a thorough workup looking for other causes. Upper GI studies are normal with evidence of delayed gastric emptying on nuclear scintigraphy. Patients with Roux syndrome do not resolve with medical management. These patients invariably require operative intervention, and the procedure of choice involves gastric resection and construction of a new Roux limb. Patients who undergo Roux-en-Y gastrojejunostomy for alkaline/biliary reflux gastritis can be managed with conversion to a Billroth II with Braun jejunojejunostomy.

Afferent loop syndrome is a complication observed after a gastrectomy with Billroth II reconstruction. The signs and symptoms include right upper quadrant or epigastric pain that is relieved by bilious (dark brown material) vomiting. This is due to an afferent limb that is too long and results in trapped biliary and pancreatic secretions which produce distention and obstruction of the afferent limb. There are two forms of afferent loop syndrome: acute and chronic. In the *acute form*, the afferent limb is obstructed and is manifested in the immediate postoperative period. Early diagnosis is crucial as a delay in diagnosis translates into a delay in therapy which can be catastrophic resulting in perforation. The therapy is always surgical with the goal to relieve the obstruction and revise the Roux limb.

Chronic afferent loop syndrome has multiple etiologies: adhesions, internal hernia, volvulus, anastomotic stricture, and intussusception. The common denominator in all of these is the formation of a partial afferent limb obstruction. The clinical presentation is pathognomonic of afferent loop and the severity of symptoms is directly proportional to the degree of obstruction. These patients need to be evaluated with an upper GI series looking for a dilated afferent limb. A nuclear gastric emptying scan is useful in distinguishing this afferent limb syndrome from alkaline reflux gastritis. Treatment is always surgical and usually involves conversion to a Billroth I anastomosis or simply fashioning a Braun anastomosis (enteroenterostomy) approximately 30 cm below the gastrojejunostomy. Blind loop syndrome is a direct consequence of afferent loop syndrome. Bacterial overgrowth occurs in the chronically obstructed afferent loop resulting in megaloblastic anemia due to vitamin B_{12} deficiency. These patients are weak and have an associated anemia. The treatment involves parenteral vitamin B_{12} and supplement fat-soluble vitamins. These patients also receive an empiric course of broad-spectrum antibiotics to decrease the bacterial burden in the afferent limb.

Efferent loop syndrome is far less common than its more common counterpart. Patients with efferent loop syndrome present with crampy left upper quadrant and epigastric pain that is associated with bilious vomiting. The differential diagnosis includes afferent loop obstruction and alkaline reflux gastritis. Anything that can lead to obstruction of the efferent loop such as adhesions, internal hernia, volvulus, anastomotic stricture, or intussusception can produce an efferent loop syndrome. An upper GI series with small bowel follow through is the most useful means of making the diagnosis. Since this is the result of a mechanical obstruction, the treatment is always operative once the diagnosis is made and the exact procedure is dictated by the findings.

Anemia and metabolic disorders are a common sequela of gastrectomy. Anemia is commonly seen and results from vitamin B_{12} deficiency (macrocytic), intrinsic factor deficiency (megaloblastic), folate deficiency (macrocytic), or iron deficiency (microcytic). Iron-deficiency anemia is the most common form of anemia seen following gastrectomy as iron absorption takes place in the proximal GI tract and is facilitated by an acidic environment. Since vitamin B_{12} absorption is dependent on intrinsic factor, produced by parietal cells in the gastric body and fundus, vitamin B_{12} deficiency results from a decreased production of intrinsic factor with a resultant macrocytic anemia. Anemia is relatively easy to resolve with supplementation. Fat malabsorption with associated steatorrhea and deficiency of fat-soluble vitamins is the result of bacterial overgrowth in the afferent limb following a Billroth II reconstruction. Calcium absorption takes place in the duodenum which is bypassed with gastrojejunostomy. Therefore, deficiencies of vitamin D (a fat-soluble vitamin) and calcium malabsorption result in osteoporosis and osteomalacia. Again, supplementation will resolve these metabolic derangements once the diagnosis is made. Finally, weight loss can be seen following gastric resection and is usually due to malabsorption or reduced caloric intake. Malabsorption occurs as a result of surgery when the loop gastroenterostomy is created distally in the small intestine, ileum, reducing the overall surface area involved in the absorptive process. Additionally, food enters the small bowel far away from the site of bile and pancreatic secretions which aid digestion and absorption. Weight loss also occurs because caloric intake is reduced as a means of coping with other side effects of the surgical procedure (e.g., diarrhea and pain).

Gastrocolic fistulae can occur in the postgastrectomy setting following the formation of a marginal ulceration in the jejunum. Once the marginal ulceration forms in the jejunal segment of the gastrojejunostomy, the rare occurrence of a gastrojejunocolic fistula can be observed. Patients subsequently develop diarrhea, malnutrition, and feculent vomiting. Stool migrates into the proximal small bowel and diarrhea and malnutrition result from bacterial overgrowth in the stomach and small bowel. Complete en bloc excision is the procedure of choice. Lastly, patients who underwent a gastric resection for benign ulcer disease are at increased risk of developing adenocarcinoma of the gastric remnant. Although this postgastrectomy complication (stump carcinoma) is more commonly seen following a Billroth II, all patients who have undergone a gastric resection over 10 years ago should have surveillance with periodic esophagogastroduodenoscopy (EGD) and biopsies.

STRESS GASTRITIS

Stress gastritis develops in critically ill patients.[4,5] They are characterized by their diffuse and superficial nature and occurrence in the presence of trauma, burns, shock, and sepsis; specifically, in the setting of prolonged ventilation and coagulopathy. They manifest with bleeding which in the extreme can compromise the hemodynamic status of an already critically ill patient. There are three types of stress ulcers that are associated with specific settings. *Stress ulcers* or *erosive gastritis* is the prototypical diffuse lesions seen in the stomach of critically ill patients. *Curling ulcers* are diffuse ulcers which can be seen in the stomach, duodenum, and occasionally throughout the GI tract and are associated with burns. *Cushing ulcers* are usually confined to the stomach and duodenum and are seen in the setting of head injury. Because of the association with critical illness, all patients who remain on a ventilator for over 48 h and/or have an underlying coagulopathy should receive ulcer prophylaxis. Moreover, any patient with a recent history of upper GI bleeding secondary to a history of a gastric ulcer in the past year should receive ulcer prophylaxis. Finally, all patients with two or more risk factors should also receive prophylaxis (Table 9-4). Medical prophylaxis reduces the incidence of clinically significant bleeding. Prophylaxis should consist of an H_2-blocker or proton pump inhibitor delivered in the form of a continuous infusion, and sucralfate to protect the gastric mucosa. The main side effect of prophylaxis is the development of pneumonia as a result of permissive bacterial overgrowth secondary to acid suppression. Sucralfate has the advantage of decreasing gram-negative bacteria in the stomach, which helps prevent aspiration pneumonia. In the extreme, patients who develop hemodynamic instability secondary to diffuse stress gastritis may require surgery. Gastric devascularization with truncal vagotomy is the procedure of choice. Gastric resections in this setting are associated with a prohibitive mortality.

Table 9-4 **Risk Factors for Stress Gastritis**

Prophylaxis for any patient with one factor
1.   Prolonged (>48 h) ventilator requirement
2.   Coagulopathy
3.   UGI bleeding within last year
4.   Known ulcer within last year
5.   Head trauma patients with Glasgow Coma Score <10
6.   Thermal injury to >35% body surface area
7.   Following partial hepatectomy
8.   Patients with liver failure
9.   Multiple trauma patients
10.   Following spinal cord injuries
11.   Following solid organ transplantation

Prophylaxis for any patient with two factors
1.   Sepsis
2.   Prolonged ICU admission (>1 week)
3.   Occult bleeding for more than 6 days
4.   High-dose steroid use

ZOLLINGER-ELLISON SYNDROME

Zollinger-Ellison syndrome was first described by Zollinger and Ellison as a condition caused by non-insulin-secreting tumors of the pancreas which lead to the development of an ulcerogenic state.[10] These tumors were eventually found to elaborate gastrin. Gastrinomas are rare tumors that arise from neuroendocrine cells which produce a unique clinical picture (Table 9-5). The majority of gastrinomas are sporadic. Approximately 25 percent of gastrinomas are associated with the multiple endocrine neoplasia type I (MEN I) syndrome. The presence of hypercalcemia associated with peptic ulcer disease should prompt a workup for ZES. The diagnosis is made by measuring a serum gastrin level. Patients with a gastrinoma generally have levels greater than 1000 pg/mL. In cases where the gastrin is not clearly elevated, but suspicion is high, one can use a secretin stimulation test. Secretin is administered intravenously (2 U/kg) after obtaining a baseline gastrin level. Gastrin levels are subsequently measured at 15- and 30-min intervals following infusion. If gastrinoma is present, one will see a rise of more than 200 pg/mL.

Once a diagnosis of gastrinoma is made, it becomes imperative to localize the lesion and to rule out disseminated disease with a staging computed tomography (CT) scan. Gastrinomas have somatostatin receptors. As a result, the best localizing study for gastrinomas is a somatostatin receptor

Table 9-5 **Characteristics of ZES**

1. Recurrent ulcer disease despite medical therapy
2. Ulcers in atypical locations (distal duodenum or jejunum)
3. Presence of multiple ulcers
4. Peptic ulcer disease in association with diarrhea
5. Presence of ulcers in association with hypercalcemia
6. Pancreatic neuroendocrine tumors
7. Predominantly (75%) sporadic
8. Associated with MEN I syndrome (25%)
9. Approximately half of patients have solitary lesions
10. Approximately half of patients have multiple lesions
11. Multiple lesions are seen in association with MEN I syndrome
12. Approximately 50% of lesions metastasize to lymph nodes and liver

scintigraphy. The sensitivity of this test is better than 85 percent and has the ability to detect lesions smaller than 1 cm. Although acid suppression therapy has effectively eliminated the need to perform total gastrectomies in these patients, approximately 50 percent of lesions are malignant demonstrated by their capacity to metastasize to local lymph nodes and liver. Therefore, patients should undergo resection of the tumor whenever deemed feasible and no distant metastatic disease can be identified. Surgery for ZES requires a methodic approach with a systematic abdominal exploration using intraoperative ultrasound to assess the neck, body, and tail of the pancreas and intraoperative endoscopy to assess the duodenal wall with transillumination. If the tumor is still not localized at this point, a duodenotomy is made to allow thorough palpation of the duodenal wall. If the gastrinoma is found in the pancreas, it can often be enucleated as long as it does not involve the pancreatic duct. If a lesion is found in the head of the gland involving the duct, one can perform a Whipple surgery, and if it is found in the body or tail, one can perform a distal pancreatectomy. Suspicious portal, perigastric, and celiac nodes are all biopsied. If the lesion cannot be localized, patients can be treated indefinitely with acid suppression or they can undergo a highly selective vagotomy. Patients who are managed conservatively with acid suppression therapy should still have periodic surveillance with a somatostatin scan as lesions may declare themselves over time.

Patients with metastatic disease of the liver should be managed with principles of surgical oncology. The primary tumor must be controlled and the patient should be medically capable of tolerating a liver resection. There must be no extrahepatic disease and the resection must be one that can be performed safely without compromising hepatic function with no residual disease. Patients who are unresectable are treated with systemic therapy and/or local regional therapies. Systemic therapy consists of chemotherapy in the form of streptozocin, doxorubicin, and 5-fluorouracil or immune and hormone modulating agents like interferon and somatostatin analogues have been used. Regional therapies for patients with unresectable hepatic disease or patients who may not tolerate resection include chemoembolization or radiofrequency ablation. Overall, patients who undergo complete resection of their primary gastrinoma with no evidence of metastatic disease have an excellent prognosis. This prognosis is reduced significantly for patients who are found to have hepatic disease.

MALLORY-WEISS SYNDROME

When patients, generally male, present with a history of upper GI bleeding which developed after an episode of vomiting, one must suspect a Mallory-Weiss tear. The process of vomiting can generate significant intragastric pressures and a large gradient between intragastric and intrathoracic pressures. When vomiting occurs, large fluxes in pressure gradients take place and these increases in pressures are transmitted to the gastric wall and mucosa and can result in mucosal lacerations at the gastroesophageal junction and bleeding. Clinical scenarios in which Mallory-Weiss tears are seen include vomiting in the presence of a paraesophageal hernia, pregnancy with hyperemesis gravidarum, blunt abdominal trauma, GI-associated refractory nausea and vomiting, medical-therapy-associated nausea and vomiting, activities which involve straining (childbirth, weight lifting, and bowel movements), and endoscopy. The common denominator in these scenarios involves an acute increase in the intra-abdominal pressures and sudden large pressure gradients can produce linear mucosal lacerations. EGD is diagnostic and is critical in terms of ruling out esophageal varices and gastric or duodenal ulcers as the source of the upper GI bleeding. Once the diagnosis is made, supportive care results in virtual resolution with little to no sequelae. In cases where hemodynamic instability results with ongoing blood losses, an exploratory laparotomy with gastrotomy and oversewing the tears should suffice.

GASTRIC CANCER

Gastric cancer, or cancer of the stomach, is the second leading cause of cancer deaths worldwide. However, there are considerable differences in the geographic distributions of gastric cancer.[11,12] In fact, in Japan where gastric cancer is a relatively common malignancy, screening for gastric cancer rivals the western practice of screening for colon cancer. The overwhelming majority (90–95 percent) of gastric cancers are adenocarcinomas arising from mucous producing cells of the gastric mucosa and have a characteristic signet ring appearance.[12] Stomach cancer is extremely virulent with aggressive metastatic behavior. The natural history of gastric adenocarcinoma is one of early metastasis spreading through lymphatic, hematogenous, and local extension. It is more common to find a gastric cancer along the lesser curve of the stomach than the greater curve of the stomach. There are many classifications of gastric cancer. One commonly referred to is the *Lauren classification* which divides gastric cancers into two types: intestinal and diffuse. The *intestinal* type is glandular and arises from the gastric mucosa and is seen in an older population of patients. The *diffuse* type is associated with an invasive pattern and appears to arise from the lamina propria and is seen in a younger population. The diffuse type is associated with a more aggressive natural history. Although we have noted a decline in the incidence and mortality of gastric cancer in the United States and other countries, it appears that this decline is due to a decline in the intestinal type. Results of one study indicates a progressive decrease in the incidence of the intestinal type of gastric cancer and an increase in the diffuse type of gastric carcinoma, especially the signet ring cell type.[13] In one form of gastric cancer, the tumor can involve the entire stomach with sheets of malignant cells infiltrating the gastric wall. This condition is referred to as *linitis plastica* and is associated with a poor prognosis with rare 5-year survival.

Although diet appears to play a central role in the development of gastric cancer, many factors appear to contribute to the risk of developing stomach cancer (Table 9-6). Diets that consist of smoked or cured meats and high-salt

Table 9-6 **Risk Factors Associated with Gastric Cancer**

1. Diet
2. Smoking
3. Excessive alcohol consumption
4. Male gender
5. African American race
6. Low socioeconomic status
7. Miners, metal workers, and rubber workers
8. H. pylori infection
9. Epstein-Barr virus
10. Pernicious anemia
11. Atrophic gastritis
12. Intestinal metaplasia
13. Gastric villous adenoma
14. History of surgery for benign ulcer disease
15. Familial predisposition

content are associated with an increased risk and diets that are full of fresh fruit and vegetables with antioxidants are associated with a decreased risk. In addition to environmental factors, familial predisposition also places patients at increased risk. Families with hereditary nonpolyposis colon cancer[14] are at increased risk of developing gastric cancer as are patients with E-cadherin mutations. Another factor that has been proposed to be associated with the development of gastric cancer is infection with *H. pylori*.[15] Chinese researchers have demonstrated that eradication of *H. pylori* does not appear to reduce the risk of developing gastric cancer in patients with preexisting precancerous areas of the stomach. However, in patients who do not have precancerous areas of the stomach at the time of treatment against *H. pylori*, eradication of the bacteria appears to reduce the risk of developing gastric cancer.[16]

The symptoms of gastric cancer are often misleading and in an era of over-the-counter medications for dyspepsia, it is not uncommon for a patient to report treating early symptoms with antacids. Once the signs and symptoms become prominent, disease is usually advanced. Abdominal pain, weight loss, and anemia are common. When the lesion is located proximally, as occurs with the diffuse type, patients may present with dysphagia. However, if the lesion is located distally, as occurs with the intestinal type, patients may present with nausea, vomiting, and symptoms consistent with gastric outlet obstruction. On physical examination, one may find evidence of advanced disease. It was noted by Sister Joseph in the early days of the Mayo Clinic that patients with intra-abdominal cancer had periumbilical nodules. Therefore, the presence of Sister Mary Joseph's nodes, periumbilical adenopathy, is indicative of peritoneal spread of disease. Similarly, the presence of Virchow's node, supraclavicular adenopathy, is indicative of migration of disease above the diaphragm and Bloomer's shelf nodules suggests peritoneal implants anterior to the rectum which are sometimes palpable on rectal examination.

EGD is the best modality for diagnosing gastric adenocarcinoma. EGD allows one to biopsy the gastric tissue in question, which is critical to providing a diagnosis. Additionally, EGD allows one to assess the location and size of the tumor. Endoscopic ultrasound is evolving as a critical tool in staging gastric cancer,[17] since the depth of invasion and nodal status are key elements in the staging system (Table 9-7). Once a histologic diagnosis of gastric cancer has been made, a staging workup must be initiated. A CT scan of the chest, abdomen, and pelvis will establish patients who are obviously unresectable due to the presence of extragastric disease (i.e., liver, lung, and peritoneal metastasis). Because CT scans are limited in their ability to detect small, less than 5 mm, peritoneal or hepatic metastasis, some surgeons prefer to start with a laparoscopic exploration looking for obvious peritoneal or hepatic disease prior to converting to a formal laparotomy.

In the absence of extragastric disease, aggressive surgical resection of gastric cancers is the objective. Surgical resection involves a wide margin

Table 9-7 **Gastric Cancer Staging**

Evaluation of the primary tumor (T)

TX	Primary tumor cannot be assessed
T0	No evidence of primary tumor
Tis	Intraepithelial tumor without invasion of lamina propria
T1	Tumor invades lamina propria or submucosa
T2	Tumor invades muscularis propria or subserosa
T2a	Tumor invades muscularis propria
T2b	Tumor invades subserosa
T3	Tumor penetrates serosa into visceral peritoneum
T4	Tumor invades adjacent organs

Evaluation of regional lymph nodes (N)

NX	Regional lymph nodes cannot be assessed
N0	No regional lymph node metastasis
N1	Metastasis in 1–6 regional lymph nodes
N2	Metastasis in 7–15 regional lymph nodes
N3	Metastasis in more than 15 regional lymph nodes

Evaluation of distant metastasis (M)

MX	Distant metastasis cannot be assessed
M0	No distant metastasis
M1	Distant metastasis

Stage	T	N	M
0	Tis	0	0
IA	1	0	0
IB	1	N1	0
	2a/b	0	0
II	1	2	0
	2a/b	1	0
	3	0	0
IIIA	2a/b	2	0
	3	1	0
	4	0	0
IIIB	3	2	0
IV	4	1–3	0
	1–3	3	0
	Any T	Any N	M1

encompassing lymph nodes and any adherent organs. A gross margin of 6 cm is usually necessary to ensure an adequate negative margin by final histologic analysis.[18] Tumors located in the proximal to midgastric region are best managed with total gastrectomy. Tumors located in the distal stomach can be managed with a subtotal gastrectomy as long as a 6-cm gross margin can be obtained. The extent of lymph node dissection during resection of gastric tumors is a hotly debated topic. The source of debate stems from the fact that a multitude of Japanese studies have demonstrated a survival advantage to more extensive lymphadenectomies. Early studies in Western countries did not observe the same advantage to aggressive nodal dissections. However, subsequent studies in the United States and Europe have demonstrated an advantage to more extensive nodal dissection when performed at specialized referral centers.[19,20] Following resection, the continuity of the intestinal tract is reestablished in a variety of ways. After a total gastrectomy for a proximal or midgastric tumor, a Roux-en-Y esophagojejunostomy provides good functional outcomes. Alternatively, following a subtotal gastrectomy, the continuity can be reestablished with a Billroth I, Billroth II, or Roux-en-Y gastrojejunostomy.

Since many patients have unresectable disease at the time of diagnosis and since recurrence appears to be the rule rather than the exception, finding an effective systemic or local regional therapy to treat patients with unresectable disease or recurrence is very appealing. Unfortunately, systemic and intraperitoneal therapy has only demonstrated very modest effects and in some cases there are conflicting results. Small series with neoadjuvant therapy has demonstrated some promising results. Although exciting, these small trials will need to undergo the rigors of a large, prospectively randomized trial to demonstrate both safety and efficacy before this strategy can be applied as a standard of care.

GASTRIC LYMPHOMA

Although gastric lymphomas represent less than 5 percent of gastric malignancies, the stomach is the most common site of GI lymphomas. Tumors are considered primary GI lymphoma when lymphoma is confirmed histologically, there is no palpable adenopathy or splenomegaly, there is no evidence of lymphoma by radiographic workup, and when the blood smear and bone marrow assessment are normal. H. pylori infection has also been implicated in the development of gastric lymphoma and mucosa-associated lymphoid tissue (MALT) lymphoma.[21,22] Chronic gastritis secondary to H. pylori infection is considered a major predisposing factor for MALT lymphoma. Common symptoms of gastric lymphoma include abdominal pain and weight loss. Patients can also present with bleeding and perforation as a complication of their gastric lymphoma. Like with gastric adenocarcinoma, the diagnosis of gastric lymphoma is commonly made with EGD and tissues biopsies. A CT scan of the chest, abdomen, and pelvis is also obtained in order to stage the extent of disease.

Controversy remains regarding the best treatment for early stages of this disease. Antibiotic therapy with eradication of *H. pylori* has been associated with remissions of low-grade lymphomas.[23,24] However, some investigators have found that some patients who experienced complete remission still harbor monoclonal B cells questioning the true effectiveness of antibiotic therapy. Chemotherapy, surgery, and combinations have been studied and share comparable results with survival rates of 70–90 percent. Since no clear differences are observed between the most common therapies in patients with early stage disease, and since early stage lymphoma has a high response rate to salvage treatment with surgery and radiotherapy, chemotherapy alone is an effective and safe therapeutic approach. Chemotherapy has an added advantage of preserving gastric anatomy. Advanced stage IIIE and IVE disease is treated primarily with chemotherapy and surgical resection has been reserved for patients with bleeding or perforation.

GASTROINTESTINAL STROMAL TUMORS

Gastrointestinal stromal tumors (GIST) are derived from mesenchymal cells in the stomach. The specific cells of origin are the interstitial *cells of Cajal*. The cells of Cajal are the intestinal pacemaker and responsible for initiating peristalsis in the stomach and small bowel. Approximately 60 percent of GISTs are seen in the stomach with a smaller proportion developing in the small intestine and colon. The gene liable for the development of GISTs is responsible for encoding a tyrosine kinase transmembrane receptor derived from the KIT protein which is expressed on the cells of Cajal. Mutations of KIT are common in malignant GISTs and lead to constitutional activation of tyrosine kinase function, which causes cellular proliferation and resistance to apoptosis.[25] GISTs are most commonly manifested in the sixth decade of life and have a broad spectrum of presentations. Often, GISTs are incidental findings during physical examination or at exploration. GISTs cause symptoms by local compression and can be the cause of vague discomfort and pain. Like other lesions in the stomach, GISTs may also present with bleeding and even perforation.[26]

The diagnosis of a GIST is usually only suspected at the time of laparotomy for an abdominal mass. Patients with vague abdominal complaints will frequently have a CT scan of the abdomen that demonstrates a large mass that is usually associated with the stomach. This suspicion is confirmed by pathology as it is characterized by the expression of the KIT protein product on immunohistochemistry. Patients with no obvious metastatic disease should undergo complete segmental resection of the mass with a 1- to 2-cm margin while exercising great care not to spill tumor fragments. Patients who ultimately receive a pathologic diagnosis of GIST should have regular surveillance as they are at risk for recurrence. Patients whose tumors are larger than 10 cm and/or have more than 5 mitoses per 50 high-power fields are at greatest risk for recurrence. Since GISTs arise from the constitutional activation of tyrosine kinase function, molecular inhibitors of the tyrosine kinase function offers patients with recurrence or unresectable disease measurable hope. Treatment with imatinib mesylate (Gleevec), a recently discovered selective inhibitor of tyrosine kinases is associated with an objective response rate between 60 and 70 percent. This is a tremendous clinical benefit for patients who previously had no better than 30 percent 1-year survival.[27]

REFERENCES

1. Moore KL. *The Digestive System in Before We Are Born*, 9th ed. Philadelphia, PA: W.B. Saunders, 1989.

2. Owen D. In Sternberg SS, ed., *Stomach in Histology for Pathologists*. New York: Raven Press, 1992.

3. Kirkwood KS, Debas HT. In Miller TA, ed., *Physiology of Gastric Secretion and Emptying in Modern Surgical Care*, 2nd ed. St. Louis, MO: Quality Medical Publishing, Inc., 1998.

4. Sirinek KR, Bingener J, Richards ML. In Cameron JL, ed., *Benign Gastric Ulcer and Stress Gastritis in Current Surgical Therapy*, 8th ed. St. Louis, MO: Mosby, 2004.

5. Murayama KM, Miller TA. In Dempsey DT, ed., *Gastric Ulcer in Shackelford's, Surgery of the Alimentary Tract*, 5th ed. Philadelphia, PA: W.B. Saunders, 2002.

6. Megraud F, Burette A, Glupczynski Y, et al. Comparison of tests for assessment of Helicobacter pylori eradication: results of a multi-centre study using centralized facility testing. *Eur J Gastroenterol Hepatol* 12(6):629–633, 2000.

7. de Boer WA, Tytgat GN. Treatment of *Helicobacter pylori* infection. *BMJ* 320:31–34, 2000.

8. Jaffe BM, Florman SS. In Nyhus LM, Baker RJ, eds., *Postgastrectomy and Postvagotomy Syndromes in Mastery of Surgery*, 2nd ed. New York: Little, Brown and Company, 1992.

9. Meilahn JE, Dempsey DT. In Cameron JL, ed., *Postgastrectomy Problems: Remedial Operations and Therapy in Current Surgical Therapy*, 8th ed. St. Louis, MO: Mosby, 2004.

10. Fisher WE, Brunicardi FC. In Cameron JL, ed., *Zollinger-Ellison Syndrome in Current Surgical Therapy*, 8th ed. St. Louis, MO: Mosby, 2004.

11. Alexander HR, Kelsen DG, Tepper JC. In Devita VT, Hellman S, Rosenberg SA, eds., *Cancer of the Stomach in Cancer, Principles and Practice of Oncology*, 5th ed. Philadelphia, PA: Lippincott-Raven, 1997.

12. Crawford JM. In Cotran RS, Kumar V, Collins T, eds., *The Gastrointestinal Tract in Robbins, Pathologic Basis of Disease*, 6th ed. Philadelphia, PA: W.B. Saunders, 1999.

13. Henson DE, Dittus C, Younes M, et al. Differential trends in the intestinal and diffuse types of gastric carcinoma in the United States, 1973-2000: increase in the signet ring cell type. *Arch Pathol Lab Med* 128(7):765–770, 2004.

14. Ericson K, Nilbert M, Bladstrom A, et al. Familial risk of tumors associated with hereditary non-polyposis colorectal cancer: a Swedish population-based study. *Scand J Gastroenterol* 39(12):1259–1265, 2004.

15. Crowe SE. Helicobacter infection, chronic inflammation, and the development of malignancy. *Curr Opin Gastroenterol* 21(1):32–38, 2005.

16. Wong B, Lam S, Wong W, et al. Helicobacter pylori eradication to prevent gastric cancer in a high-risk region of China. *J Am Med Assoc* 291:187–194, 2004.

17. Moreto M. Diagnosis of esophagogastric tumors. *Endoscopy* 37(1): 26–32, 2005.

18. Parikh AA, Mansfield PF. In Cameron JL, ed., *Gastric Adenocarcinoma in Current Surgical Therapy*, 8th ed. St. Louis, MO: Mosby, 2004.

19. Roviello F, Marrelli D, Morgagni P, et al. and Italian Research Group for Gastric Cancer. Survival benefit of extended D2 lymphadenectomy in gastric cancer with involvement of second level lymph nodes: a longitudinal multicenter study. *Ann Surg Oncol* 9(9):894–900, 2002.

20. Volpe CM, Driscoll DL, Douglass HO Jr. Outcome of patients with proximal gastric cancer depends on extent of resection and number of resected lymph nodes. *Ann Surg Oncol* 7(2):139–144, 2000.

21. Kahl BS. Update: gastric MALT lymphoma. *Curr Opin Oncol* 15(5):347–352, 2003.

22. Marshall BJ, Windsor HM. The relation of Helicobacter pylori to gastric adenocarcinoma and lymphoma: pathophysiology, epidemiology, screening, clinical presentation, treatment, and prevention. *Med Clin North Am* 89(2):313–344, viii, 2005.

23. Carlson SJ, Yokoo H, Vanagunas A. Progression of gastritis to monoclonal B-cell lymphoma with resolution and recurrence following eradication of Helicobacter pylori. *JAMA* 275(12):937–939, 1996.

24. Inagaki H, Nakamura T, Li C, et al. Gastric MALT lymphomas are divided into three groups based on responsiveness to Helicobacter Pylori eradication and detection of API2-MALT1 fusion. *Am J Surg Pathol* 28(12):1560–1567, 2004.

25. Connolly EM, Gaffney E, Reynolds JV. Gastrointestinal stromal tumors. *Br J Surg* 90(10):1178–1186, 2003.

26. Kitabayashi K, Seki T, Kishim oto K, et al. A spontaneously ruptured gastric stromal tumor presenting as generalized peritonitis: report of a case. *Surg Today* 31(4):350–354, 2001.

27. de Mestier P, Guetz GD. Treatment of gastrointestinal stromal tumors with imatinib mesylate: a major breakthrough in the understanding of tumor-specific molecular characteristics. World J Surg 2005.

INTESTINE & COLON

Rebekah R. White, MD
Danny O. Jacobs, MD, MPH

SMALL INTESTINE

Introduction

ANATOMY

The small intestine is not just a passive tube but a complex organ that plays several active roles in the process of enteral nutrition. The small intestine measures between 12 and 20 ft from pylorus to the ileocecal valve. As food leaves the pylorus, it enters the duodenum, which is a fixed, retroperitoneal organ approximately 1 ft in length. The second portion of the duodenum is intimately associated with the pancreas and biliary tree where their secretions enter the intestine through the ampulla of Vater. The jejunum begins and the intestine reenters the peritoneum at the ligament of Treitz, which is a commonly referred clinical landmark separating the *upper* from the *lower* gastrointestinal tracts. There is no structure clearly defining the transition from jejunum (proximal 40 percent) to ileum (distal 60 percent), although the ileum is characterized by clusters of lymphoid tissue known as Peyer patches.

FUNCTION

Digestion begins in the stomach, where acid and pepsin begin to break down protein. In the duodenum and proximal jejunum, activated pancreatic enzymes and the brush border enzymes of the intestinal mucosa carry out most of the process of digestion. The majority of absorption of fats, proteins, carbohydrates, and vitamins occurs in the jejunum. In the ileum, the majority of almost 10 L of fluid that is either ingested or secreted into the proximal intestine is reabsorbed. In addition, the distal ileum is the site of absorption of vitamin B_{12} and of reabsorption of bile salts into the enterohepatic circulation. This entire process is dependent on the propulsion of intestinal contents (chyme) by intestinal motility, which is regulated by an intrinsic nervous system as well as by local hormones such as motilin and cholecystokinin.

Meanwhile, the intestinal mucosa provides a selective barrier function and secretes immunoglobulins against gut pathogens.

SHORT GUT SYNDROME

Otherwise healthy adults can generally tolerate resection of up to 50 percent of their small intestine, although specific deficiencies can result from resection of the duodenum (iron) and terminal ileum (B_{12} and bile salts). Massive small bowel resection results in *short gut syndrome*, with malnutrition, dehydration, electrolyte abnormalities, and vitamin deficiencies. The minimum bowel length required for maintenance of enteral nutrition is generally between 40 and 60 cm but depends on factors such as the site of resection, the quality of the remaining bowel, and the age of the patient. The preservation of the ileocecal valve and the colon may help to decrease intestinal transit time and reduce fluid losses. The intestine has a limited potential to adapt and increase absorptive ability, although it is controversial how to best *rehabilitate* the intestine.[1,2] Patients with short gut syndrome are often reliant on lifelong total parenteral nutrition (TPN), with its associated morbidities, as the results of surgical therapies such as small intestine transplantation and intestinal lengthening procedures have so far been disappointing.[3]

Small Bowel Obstruction: Management Greatly Influenced by Surgical History

ETIOLOGY

Mechanical small bowel obstruction (SBO) is one of the most common problems for which the general surgeon is consulted. Although incarcerated groin hernias were the most common cause of SBO in the past, the increase in elective hernia repairs as well as laparotomies over the last several decades have led to adhesions being by far the most common cause of SBO in adults. Hernias are still a common cause of SBO as are Crohn's disease, small bowel neoplasms, radiation enteritis, and miscellaneous other causes such as volvulus, foreign bodies, and gallstone *ileus*[4] (Table 10-1). Ileus, or functional bowel obstruction, is also in the differential diagnosis of many patients. In addition to dehydration and electrolyte abnormalities from fluid losses, the most important complication of SBO is small bowel strangulation due to closed loop obstruction.

DIAGNOSIS

Clinically, patients usually present with crampy abdominal pain, nausea, vomiting, and either decreased or absent stool and flatus. SBO is often characterized as being either complete—when there is no stool or flatus—or partial—when stool may be decreased, normal, or increased (diarrhea). Emesis is often bilious or even feculent, indicating stasis in long-standing SBO. The degree of distention on abdominal examination is greater in patients with distal obstruction. The presence of hyperactive bowel sounds, resulting from

Table 10-1 **Common Causes of SBO**

Mechanical SBO	Ileus
Adhesions	Laparotomy
Hernia	Inflammation
Crohn's disease	Pancreatitis
Neoplasms	Diverticulitis
Radiation enteritis	Appendicitis
Volvulus	Pneumonia
Foreign bodies	Medications
Gallstone *ileus*	Narcotics
	Calcium channel blockers
	Anticholinergic agents
	Electrolytes
	Hypokalemia
	Hyponatremia
	Mesenteric ischemia
	Shock

strong peristaltic contractions, is suggestive of mechanical SBO; however, bowel sounds are often absent in long-standing SBO and in the presence of strangulation. Although mild diffuse tenderness secondary to distention is expected, the presence of severe, focal, or rebound tenderness or of involuntary guarding should raise suspicion for strangulation. Unfortunately, there are no clinical signs that are good enough to reliably rule ischemia in or out.[5] Plain films reveal dilated loops of bowel with air-fluid levels. The absence of distal gas suggests a complete SBO, while the presence of distal gas implies either partial or early complete SBO. The presence of pneumatosis or portal venous gas suggests ischemia, although these are notoriously late and insensitive signs. Computed tomography (CT) is more sensitive for ischemia than plain films and very good at distinguishing SBO from paralytic ileus.[6,7]

TREATMENT

"Never let the sun set or the sun rise on a small bowel obstruction" used to be an often-quoted surgical adage. For patients without a history of abdominal surgery, this statement still holds true, as the obstruction is unlikely to resolve without surgery and is more likely to be associated with strangulation. For patients suspected to have SBO secondary to adhesions and without signs of strangulation, a trial of nonoperative management is appropriate, as many such obstructions will resolve without operation, particularly partial SBO. Nonoperative management includes maintaining the patient nil per os, nasogastric decompression, and intravenous hydration. If signs of ischemia develop or if the patient fails to show signs of improvement after 24–48 h, surgical exploration is warranted. One exception to this is the special case of early postoperative obstruction, which can usually be safely managed non-operatively for at least 10 days to 2 weeks.[8] In addition to the risks associated with operation itself, the benefits of avoiding operation include the fact that the risk of recurrent SBO increases with each operation.[9] When exploration is indicated, the surgeon *runs* the entire length of the intestine, looking for a transition point between dilated proximal and decompressed distal bowel. All sources of obstruction are corrected. After a brief period of observation, all nonviable or marginally viable bowel is resected. In situations where the viability of the bowel is in question or when resection will leave the patient with an inadequate length of small bowel (described earlier), a *second-look* exploration 24 or 48 h later may be indicated.

Ileus: The Response of Normal Intestine to an Abnormal Situation

ETIOLOGY

For many patients presenting with signs and symptoms of SBO, the differential diagnosis includes functional rather than mechanical SBO, also known as paralytic ileus. By far the most common cause of ileus is laparotomy, and some degree of ileus is normal in the first few days following surgery. In patients who are not postoperative, a number of conditions can cause ileus and mimic mechanical SBO (Table 10-1). Inflammation or infection in the peritoneum, retroperitoneum, or thorax, such as pancreatitis, diverticulitis, appendicitis, or pneumonia, can affect adjacent bowel and cause a focal ileus, as can mesenteric ischemia. Sepsis or shock due to any cause can be expected to cause a generalized ileus. Electrolyte abnormalities, particularly hypokalemia, and medications that affect bowel motility, such as narcotics, calcium channel blockers, and anticholinergic agents, are common contributing factors to if not causes of ileus.

DIAGNOSIS

In the early postoperative patient, the distinction between mechanical SBO and ileus may not be critical, as the treatment of both is nonoperative. However, in patients who are not postoperative presenting with SBO, the distinction between the two becomes important, as the treatment of one is generally nonoperative and the other operative. Clinically, ileus can be presented similarly to mechanical SBO, although the history may suggest one of the conditions described earlier, such as focal pain, fever, or medication use. On physical examination, bowel sounds are typically decreased, unlike mechanical SBO. Plain films will reveal dilated loops of bowel and air-fluid levels, but the dilatation is generally less severe and more diffuse than mechanical SBO. If the diagnosis is unclear, CT scan is often very helpful, both in ruling out potential causes of ileus and in the identification of a transition point between dilated proximal and decompressed distal bowel, which is virtually diagnostic of mechanical SBO.[6]

TREATMENT

The treatment of ileus is largely supportive by maintaining the patient nil per os, intravenous hydrations, and parenteral nutrition, if prolonged. Contributing factors should be sought out and corrected. Nasogastric decompression should be used for symptoms of nausea, vomiting, or distention but does not prevent or shorten ileus.[10] The avoidance of systemic narcotics through the use of epidural analgesia and/or nonnarcotic medications does help to reduce ileus. A number of pharmacologic approaches to restoring bowel motility have been investigated but none has been proven effective.

Acute Mesenteric Ischemia: Signs and Symptoms Nonspecific Until Late

ETIOLOGY

A recurring theme in the management of surgical diseases of the intestine is the importance and difficulty of identifying bowel ischemia. The classic presentation of acute mesenteric ischemia is severe abdominal pain *out of proportion* to the physical examination. However, the diagnosis is also frequently entertained when critically ill patients have unexplained ileus, metabolic acidosis and/or sepsis, and the history and physical examination are often limited. Acute mesenteric ischemia occurs when bowel perfusion is compromised by one of four distinct conditions. Emboli originate usually from cardiac thrombi in patients with atrial fibrillation and occlude the mesenteric vasculature anywhere from the superior mesenteric artery to its distal branches, depending on size. Arterial thrombosis typically occurs in the setting of underlying mesenteric atherosclerotic disease, and collateral circulation is often present. Nonocclusive mesenteric ischemia occurs during *low-flow* states, such as shock, and can dramatically exacerbate acidosis. Mesenteric venous thrombosis is generally secondary to a hypercoagulable state and results in decreased perfusion due to venous congestion.

DIAGNOSIS

The cause is often suggested by the history (Table 10-2). A history of *intestinal angina* and weight loss is present in arterial thrombosis, and the onset may be insidious, whereas the lack of collateral circulation in embolic occlusion results in a sudden onset of symptoms. Patients with mesenteric venous thrombosis may also have an insidious onset of symptoms and may or may not have a known hypercoagulable condition. In patients with severe abdominal pain and peritonitis, no further diagnostic workup is necessary; these patients have irreversible bowel ischemia, and surgical exploration is warranted. However, patients with the presentation of severe abdominal

Table 10-2 **Acute Mesenteric Ischemia**

Cause	Past Medical History	Clinical Presentation
Arterial thrombosis	Atherosclerotic disease	Prior intestinal angina, weight loss; insidious onset of severe pain
Arterial embolus	Atrial fibrillation, congestive heart failure	Sudden onset of severe pain
Venous thrombosis	Hypercoagulable conditions	Insidious onset of vague pain
Nonocclusive ischemia	Shock	Metabolic acidosis, sepsis

pain *out of proportion* to their physical examination are often challenging to diagnose. There are no sensitive and specific markers for mesenteric ischemia. The white blood cell count is usually elevated, as it is in many other conditions that cause abdominal pain. Metabolic acidosis, specifically lactic acidosis, is highly suggestive of irreversible ischemia but—like peritoneal signs—is not present until late.[11] Conversely, critically ill patients may have several other potential causes of metabolic acidosis that are unrelated to the bowel. CT scan is more sensitive than plain films for signs of bowel ischemia such as pneumatosis, edema, or free fluid, and CT may also reveal a cause such as arterial or venous thrombosis.[12]

TREATMENT

Regardless of the etiology, surgery is indicated in patients with peritonitis or with other signs of irreversible ischemia. The treatment of suspected embolic occlusion is usually surgical with resection of nonviable bowel and/or embolectomy to restore blood flow to viable bowel followed by systemic anticoagulation to prevent further embolic events. For patients with arterial thrombosis, revascularization can be accomplished surgically by bypass or endarterectomy. For patients without the evidence of irreversible bowel ischemia, percutaneous techniques such as thrombolytic therapy, angioplasty, and vasodilator infusion can be employed. The treatment of mesenteric venous thrombosis is usually nonsurgical with systemic anticoagulation unless there is evidence of nonviable bowel. The treatment of nonocclusive mesenteric ischemia is correction of the low-flow state, if possible, as mucosal ischemia may be reversible.

Intestinal Fistulae: Most Will
Close Spontaneously

ETIOLOGY

A fistula is an abnormal communication between two epithelialized organs. Fistulization of the intestine usually is a result of an iatrogenic injury, although spontaneous fistulae may develop in inflammatory conditions such as Crohn's disease or diverticulitis. Fistulae frequently involve the small bowel and may develop among the bladder, vagina, other segments of bowel, or—most commonly—the skin. Regardless of the cause or location, fistula closure is inhibited by a number of conditions, which are often remembered by students and residents with the mnemonic FRIEND (Table 10-3): Foreign body, Radiation, Inflammatory bowel disease, Epithelialization, Neoplasm, and Distal obstruction.

TREATMENT

The first priority in the management of fistula is to control any undrained abscess associated with the bowel injury. Drainage can usually be accomplished percutaneously, and fistulae rarely require urgent surgical repair. Most fistulae will eventually close spontaneously if adequate nutrition can be provided and inhibiting conditions can be addressed. Even if a fistula is unlikely to close spontaneously, early takedown without nutritional optimization often results in recurrent fistulization. Therefore, other priorities are to correct fluid and electrolyte losses, to provide adequate nutrition, and to avoid skin breakdown in cutaneous fistulae. A basic tenet of surgery is: *if the gut works, use it.* However, whether adequate nutrition can be accomplished via the enteral route depends on the fistula output and the location. Proximal fistulae often are *high output* (more than 500 cc/day) and may require bowel rest and TPN to avoid excessive fluid and electrolyte losses. Treatment with octreotide, a long-acting somatostatin analog, may help to control fistula output while awaiting fistula closure but does not appear to increase the likelihood of spontaneous fistula closure.[13] If the fistula output is manageable or if a feeding tube can be safely positioned distal to the fistula, enteral nutrition is preferable to TPN, as the latter is more expensive

Table 10-3 **Conditions that Inhibit Fistula Closure**

Foreign body
Radiation
Inflammatory bowel disease
Epithelialization
Neoplasm
Distal obstruction

and associated with a higher incidence of complications, including infections, cholestasis, and hyperglycemia.

The likelihood and rate of fistula closure are related more to the presence or absence of inhibiting conditions and to nutrition than to the characteristics of the fistula itself, although a small enteral defect with a long, nonepithelialized fistula tract is more likely to close than is a complete disruption of the bowel that forms an epithelialized end fistula at the skin. Generally, a trial of at least 6 weeks of nonoperative management is recommended prior to considering surgical repair. In patients with Crohn's disease, treatment with infliximab, an antitumor necrosis factor antibody, may help promote and maintain fistula closure.[14] If surgical repair is undertaken, takedown of the fistula with resection of the involved bowel is usually necessary. Care must be taken to correct any sources of distal obstruction and, of course, to avoid injuries that may lead to recurrent fistulization.

LARGE INTESTINE

Introduction

ANATOMY

The large intestine receives much attention as the site of many of the most common problems for which patients are seen by general surgeons. The large intestine is approximately 3–4 ft in length from the ileocecal valve to the anus. The right (ascending) and left (descending) colons are retroperitoneal structures, whereas the transverse and sigmoid colons are located more anteriorly within the peritoneal cavity. The large intestine through the midtransverse colon is of *midgut origin* and receives its blood supply from the superior mesenteric artery. The large intestine from the distal transverse colon through the rectum is of *hindgut origin* and supplied by the inferior mesenteric artery. The *rectum* is a highly specialized organ that is fixed within a cone of muscles comprising the pelvic floor; it is richly supplied by both mesenteric and hypogastric (internal iliac) blood flow and by autonomic innervation that helps to control defecation.

FUNCTION

The major functions of the large intestine are *absorption* of fluid and *storage* of fecal matter. The volume of fluid that passes through the ileocecal valve each day is approximately 1.5 L. Transit through the colon is significantly slower than through the small intestine, and most of this fluid is absorbed in the right colon. The contents of the large intestine therefore become more solid and higher in bacterial count as they move distally. The large intestine can accommodate a large amount of stool, and the anus provides continence. Although this allows us the convenience of being able to control when we have bowel movements, many patients can and do live relatively normal lives without their large intestines. The ileum can adapt to a limited extent (as discussed earlier), and patients with long-term ileostomies may have outputs of less than 1 L/day. With preservation of the anal sphincter, patients who are candidates for ileoanal pouch procedures may be able to retain continence although with more frequent bowel movements.

Large Bowel Obstruction: Very Different Etiology Than Small Bowel Obstruction

ETIOLOGY

While they may present with similar symptoms, SBO and large bowel obstructions (LBO) usually have very different etiologies. Unlike SBO, LBO due to adhesions or incarcerated hernia is uncommon. The most common causes of LBO in adults by far are cancer and inflammatory strictures due to diverticulitis or ischemic colitis. The differential diagnosis also includes volvulus and colonic pseudoobstruction (Ogilvie syndrome).

DIAGNOSIS

With the most common causes being malignant or benign strictures and large bowel contents being more solid than small bowel, LBO tends to present in a less acute fashion than does SBO. Patients with LBO typically describe a gradual onset of abdominal distention and decreased or absent stool. An antecedent history of change in bowel habits can usually be elicited. Nausea and vomiting are less prominent than in SBO, but, due to the large capacity of the colon, abdominal distention is more marked. Plain films will reveal a dilated colon with air-fluid levels, and, if the ileocecal valve is competent, small bowel dilatation may be absent. As in SBO, CT is useful in identifying the level of obstruction and often the etiology of the obstruction. In colonic pseudoobstruction, analogous to paralytic ileus of the small bowel, generalized distention will be observed without a transition point. Contrast enema may be necessary for clearly delineating the extent of distal colonic or rectal obstructions. If a malignant etiology is suspected and a tissue diagnosis will affect the surgical management, lower endoscopy is appropriate for biopsy.

TREATMENT

Unlike SBO, LBO will rarely resolve with nonoperative management, and the treatment of LBO is almost exclusively surgical. The risk of colonic ischemia and perforation increases with diameter greater than 12–14 cm, but gradual, chronic dilatation is tolerated better than acute dilatation. Therefore, with the exception of sigmoid volvulus, the risk of ischemia is less than in SBO, and urgent rather than emergent surgical intervention is usually indicated. The first priority of surgery is decompression, which can be accomplished relatively easily with a diverting ostomy in unstable patients or in patients with unresectable tumors. Otherwise, definitive treatment requires resection of the involved colon. Whether to attempt a primary reanastomosis depends on the location of the obstruction and the condition of the bowel. Reanastomosis is generally safe in right-sided (ileocolic) resections, even in unprepped bowel.[15] In left-sided resections, the traditional approach is a two-stage procedure with unprepped colon due to the high morbidity associated with leak. Reanastomosis can be performed with a protective diverting ileostomy, or the proximal colon can be fashioned as an end colostomy and the distal colon oversewn (Hartmann procedure). Many patients, however, will not complete the second stage (ostomy reversal) due to complications related to the first,[16] and many surgeons advocate a one-stage procedure even for left-sided resections. Otherwise, if a left-sided LBO is not complete, gentle preoperative bowel preparation may help to convert a two-stage to a one-stage procedure.

Lower Gastrointestinal Bleeding: The Importance of Localization

ETIOLOGY

Lower gastrointestinal bleeding can range in presentation from a positive fecal occult blood test to massive bright red blood per rectum, and the differential diagnosis, evaluation, and therapy are appropriately determined by the character and severity of bleeding. In the outpatient setting, hemorrhoids and other benign anorectal diseases are the most common causes of bleeding per rectum, usually bright red blood in small quantities associated with bowel movements. At the other extreme, the differential diagnosis of massive lower gastrointestinal hemorrhage (hemochezia) includes vascular malformations, diverticulosis, and tumors of the small or large intestine. In between the differential diagnosis of bleeding per rectum—ranging from occult blood to frank melena—includes a wide variety of upper gastrointestinal as well as lower gastrointestinal tract sources.

DIAGNOSIS

The evaluation of a patient with lower gastrointestinal bleeding begins with the stabilization of the patient, including obtaining adequate intravenous access, fluid resuscitation, and correction of coagulopathy. Rectal examination and nasogastric lavage can quickly rule out lower rectal and upper gastrointestinal sources, respectively. If bleeding is not massive, rapid bowel prep followed by colonoscopy is the diagnostic procedure of choice. If bleeding is too brisk to visualize by colonoscopy, a technetium-99m-labelled red blood cell scan may detect bleeding as low as 0.1 mL/min and may help guide segmental resection.[17] However, many surgeons believe that this technique is not accurate enough and should be used only as a screening study for selective mesenteric angiography.[18] In addition to more accurately localizing the source of bleeding, angiography may be therapeutic with either embolization or intra-arterial vasopressin infusion.

TREATMENT

Even without percutaneous intervention, most lower gastrointestinal bleeds will stop.[19] Many surgeons establish a *transfusion threshold* above which they will operate, usually of 4–6 units of packed red blood cells but obviously dependent on the patient, whether the bleeding has been localized, and the suspected etiology. If the bleeding stops, elective colonoscopy should be performed to rule out malignancy; if colonoscopy confirms a benign source, such as vascular malformation or diverticulosis, the decision to perform an elective resection depends on the patient's operative risk and risk of recurrent bleeding. If the bleeding does not stop, emergent resection is indicated. If preoperative localization was not successful, intraoperative endoscopy can be attempted. Otherwise, *blind* total abdominal colectomy is usually necessary, as the source of bleeding is rarely obvious at laparotomy.

Colon Versus Rectal Cancer: Location Affects Biology and Treatment

ETIOLOGY

Both environmental and genetic factors have been implicated in the etiology of colorectal cancer. The high incidence in Western populations has been attributed in part to a high-fat low-fiber diet, and there are numerous inherited and acquired genetic alterations that have linked to colorectal cancer. There are two pathways, in particular, that have been well characterized. *Alterations in mismatch repair genes* lead to genetic instability, are associated with spontaneous cancers as well as nonpolyposis cancer syndromes, and are more common in right-sided colon cancers. In contrast, *alterations in the adenomatous polyposis coli (APC) gene* lead to hyperproliferation, are associated with spontaneous cancers as well as familial adenomatous polyposis, and are more common in left-sided colon and rectal cancers.[20] In both pathways, adenomatous polyp formation is usually an intermediate step, and the value of screening for colorectal cancer is largely due to this well-established adenoma-adenocarcinoma sequence.

DIAGNOSIS

The most common presenting sign of colorectal cancer is bleeding, ranging from positive fecal occult blood test to hemochezia. Right-sided colon cancers usually present with bleeding, while left-sided colon cancers also commonly present with changes in bowel habits, due to the stool being more formed than in the right colon. Although many rectal tumors are palpable on physical examination, the diagnosis is usually either made or confirmed endoscopically. The high incidence of concurrent colon polyps or cancers in patients with rectal cancer requires that patients undergo clearance of the entire colon either endoscopically or by contrast enema prior to elective surgery for rectal cancer.

TREATMENT

Stage for stage (Table 10-4), cancers of the colon and rectum have similar survival rates but different patterns of recurrence.[21] In colon cancer, local resectability is not usually an issue. Anatomic resection based on blood supply of the involved segment of colon generally provides ample proximal and distal margins, and resection of the mesentery generally includes the primary lymph nodes that drain the tumor. Involvement of adjacent organs or abdominal wall can usually be treated by en bloc resection. Local recurrence is relatively uncommon, and the most common site of recurrence by far is the liver, due to the hematogenous spread of tumor cells via the portal venous drainage. Adjuvant chemotherapy significantly reduces the risk of recurrence in patients with stage 3 (lymph node positive) disease (Table 10-5).[22] The role of radiation therapy is limited.

The proximity of the anal sphincter and the anatomy of the pelvis make local resectability and local recurrence much bigger issues for rectal cancer. The combined portal and systemic venous drainage of the rectum also make liver and pulmonary metastases common sites of recurrence. The traditional treatment of rectal cancer included resection of the entire rectum and anus (abdominoperineal resection) with permanent end ileostomy. It is now accepted that distal margins of 2 cm (or even less) are sufficient,[23] and low anterior resection of the rectum with sphincter preservation is much more common. Local transanal excision may be suitable for small, mobile tumors within 8 cm of the anal verge. Radiation therapy with or without chemotherapy is widely accepted to reduce local recurrence in patients with stage 2 or 3 disease (Table 10-5). Whether radiation therapy should be delivered preoperatively or postoperatively is controversial, but preoperative radiation therapy has

Table 10-4 **TNM Staging of Colorectal Cancer**

Stage	Tumor Depth	Nodal Status	Distant Metastasis
1	T1 (into submucosa) or T2 (into muscularis propria)	N0	M0
2	T3 (through muscularis propria) or T4 (through serosa)	N0	M0
3	Any T	N > 0	M0
4	Any T	Any N	M > 0

Table 10-5 **Treatment of Colon and Rectal Cancer by Stage**

Stage	Colon Cancer	Rectal Cancer
1	Surgical resection	Surgical resection
2	Surgical resection	Surgical resection plus preoperative or postoperative radiation or chemoradiotherapy
3	Surgical resection plus postoperative chemotherapy	Surgical resection plus preoperative or postoperative radiation or chemoradiotherapy
4	Dependent on extent of metastatic disease	Dependent on extent of metastatic disease

several potential advantages over postoperative radiation therapy, including increased resectability and sphincter preservation.[24] The potential disadvantages of preoperative therapy are that some early stage cancers may be overtreated and that surgical complications may be increased. In most modern practices, tumors are staged by endoscopic ultrasound, and locally advanced tumors—invasion through the muscularis propria (T3 or greater) or evidence of lymph node involvement—are treated preoperatively with radiation or chemoradiation therapy.

Diverticular Disease: Surgery Reserved for Complications

ETIOLOGY

Diverticulosis is endemic in our society, likely as a result of our high-fat low-fiber diet. Pulsion pseudodiverticuli develop secondary to increased intraluminal pressure. The rectum is spared, while the sigmoid colon is almost always involved. Diverticulosis is usually asymptomatic. Symptoms may occur due to bleeding (described earlier), when the diverticulum erodes into the vasa recta, or due to diverticulitis, when the diverticulum becomes obstructed and perforates. The presentation of diverticulitis can range from microscopic perforation with localized inflammation to contained perforation with abscess to free intraperitoneal perforation with peritonitis (Table 10-6). Perforation may result in fistulization to adjacent organs, typically bladder, vagina, or skin, and chronic diverticulitis may lead to stricture and LBO (described earlier).

DIAGNOSIS

The classic symptoms of acute diverticulitis include constant, nonradiating left lower quadrant pain and fever. Nausea and vomiting are common, and

Table 10-6 **Complications of Diverticular Disease**

Bleeding
Free perforation (peritonitis)
Localized perforation (abscess)
Fistula (bladder, vagina, small bowel, skin)
Obstruction

some sort of change in bowel habits is almost always present, usually diarrhea. On physical examination, left lower quadrant tenderness is expected often with associated mass effect or focal peritoneal signs. The presence of diffuse peritoneal signs or free air on plain films indicates free perforation, and no further diagnostic workup is necessary. Otherwise, contrast CT is the study of choice to help triage patients toward medical or surgical management.

TREATMENT

Patients with only inflammation or intramural abscess on CT are considered to have *uncomplicated* diverticulitis and respond well to medical therapy, including bowel rest and antibiotics. Most patients with uncomplicated diverticulitis will never require surgery. Young patients (under age 40), however, are believed to have more aggressive disease, higher rates of recurrence, and higher rates of *complicated* diverticulitis.[25] The morbidity of complicated diverticulitis is high enough that traditional surgical teaching has been that young patients should be offered elective resection after their first episode of even uncomplicated diverticulitis, although this view has more recently been challenged.[26]

Abscesses should be drained percutaneously (or transrectally or transvaginally), if possible, followed by bowel preparation and elective resection as a one-stage procedure. A fistula is essentially an abscess that has spontaneously drained and may similarly be addressed after bowel preparation as a one-stage procedure. Patients with free perforation require urgent exploration and, at least, diversion and drainage but, ideally, resection. Whether elective or urgent, resection should extend distally to the proximal rectum in order to prevent recurrence and proximally to uninflamed, soft bowel.[27] A two-stage procedure is considered necessary in the setting of extensive infection or unprepped bowel due to the risk of anastomotic leak. Reanastomosis can be performed with a protective diverting ileostomy, or the proximal colon can be fashioned as an end colostomy and the distal colon oversewn (a Hartmann procedure).

Ulcerative Colitis and Crohn's Disease: Similar Presentations but Different Prognoses

ETIOLOGY

Inflammatory bowel disease typically manifests as one of two separate disease entities: *Crohn's disease* and *ulcerative colitis* (UC). The etiology of inflammatory bowel disease is unknown, but genetic and autoimmune factors have been implicated. Crohn's disease is a transmural process that can affect the entire gastrointestinal tract and is characterized by *skip lesions*. In contrast, UC is a mucosal process that affects only the colon and rectum and is characterized by continuous involvement. Both are associated with extraintestinal manifestations affecting the skin, eyes, and joints.

DIAGNOSIS

Diarrhea and abdominal pain are common presenting symptoms of colitis due to inflammatory bowel disease. In many cases, the distinction between Crohn's disease and UC is obvious (Table 10-7). Patients with concurrent small intestine, perianal, or fistulizing disease in any location have Crohn's disease. Endoscopically, aphthous ulcerations, fibrotic strictures, and rectal sparing are highly suggestive of Crohn's disease; microscopically, granulomata are diagnostic but are not usually seen on endoscopic biopsy. In contrast, UC is characterized endoscopically by friable mucosa with symmetric, pancolonic involvement. *Indeterminate colitis* is diagnosed in 10–15 percent of cases.

Table 10-7 **Comparison of UC and Crohn Colitis**

	UC	**Crohn Colitis**
Clinical presentation	Bloody diarrhea	Bloody diarrhea, concurrent small bowel, perianal, or fistulizing disease
Endoscopic appearance	Continuous involvement, always including rectum; friable mucosa	Skip lesions, *cobble stoning* due to deep ulcerations
Gross appearance	Relatively normal serosa, shortening of bowel	Thickened bowel wall, *creeping fat* on serosa
Microscopic appearance	Mucosal and submucosal involvement only	Full-thickness involvement, granulomata, lymphoid aggregates

TREATMENT

The initial, acute treatment of the two diseases overlaps significantly and features immunosuppression, although surgery is required for complications such as perforation, hemorrhage, and toxic colitis. The distinction between Crohn's disease and UC is important, as they require very different chronic treatment approaches. Due to the time-dependent risk of carcinoma in UC,[28] resection is strongly recommended for patients with steroid-dependent disease, frequent recurrence, and for almost all young patients. Total proctocolectomy is curative, with reconstruction as an end ileostomy or as an ileal pouch-anal anastomosis, now the standard operation for UC.[29] In urgent situations or in poor surgical candidates, total abdominal colectomy with or without anastomosis is an option, although this requires close surveillance of the rectum left behind. In contrast, surgery is reserved for complications of Crohn's disease, and much greater effort is expended to avoid surgery, as the natural history of Crohn's disease is recurrence. When surgery is necessary, the key surgical principle is the preservation of as much bowel length as possible. Only grossly involved bowel is resected, as microscopic disease at the resection margin does not affect recurrence.[30]

REFERENCES

1. Byrne TA, Morrissey TB, Nattakom TV, et al. Growth hormone, glutamine, and a modified diet enhance nutrient absorption in patients with severe short bowel syndrome. *JPEN J Parenter Enteral Nutr* 19(4):296–302, 1995.

2. Scolapio JS. Effect of growth hormone and glutamine on the short bowel: five years later. [comment]. *Gut* 47(2), 2000.

3. Thompson JS, Langnas AN, Pinch LW, et al. Surgical approach to short-bowel syndrome. Experience in a population of 160 patients. *Ann Surg* 222(4):600–605, 1995.

4. Miller G, Boman J, Shrier I, et al. Etiology of small bowel obstruction. *Am J Surg* 180(1):33–36, 2000.

5. Sarr MG, Bulkley GB, Zuidema GD. Preoperative recognition of intestinal strangulation obstruction. Prospective evaluation of diagnostic capability. *Am J Surg* 145(1):176–182, 1983.

6. Frager D, Medwid SW, Baer JW, et al. CT of small-bowel obstruction: value in establishing the diagnosis and determining the degree and cause. [see comment]. *AJR Am J Roentgenol* 162(1):37–41, 1994.

7. Frager D, Baer JW, Medwid SW, et al. Detection of intestinal ischemia in patients with acute small-bowel obstruction due to adhesions or hernia: efficacy of CT. *AJR Am J Roentgenol* 166(1):67–71, 1996.

8. Sajja SB, Schein M. Early postoperative small bowel obstruction. [see comment]. *Br J Surg* 91(6):683–691, 2004.

9. Fevang BT, Fevang J, Lie SA, et al. Long-term prognosis after operation for adhesive small bowel obstruction. [see comment]. *Ann Surg* 240(2):193–201, 2004.

10. Wolff BG, Pembeton JH, van Heerden JA, et al. Elective colon and rectal surgery without nasogastric decompression. A prospective, randomized trial. *Ann Surg* 209(6):670–673, 1989.

11. Park WM, Gloviczki P, Cherry KJ Jr, et al. Contemporary management of acute mesenteric ischemia: factors associated with survival. *J Vasc Surg* 35(3):445–452, 2002.

12. Kirkpatrick ID, Kroeker MA, Greenberg HM. Biphasic CT with mesenteric CT angiography in the evaluation of acute mesenteric ischemia: initial experience. *Radiology* 229(1):91–98, 2003.

13. Sancho JJ, di Costanzo J, Nubiola P, et al. Randomized double-blind placebo-controlled trial of early octreotide in patients with postoperative enterocutaneous fistula. [see comment]. *Br J Surg* 82(5):638–641, 1995.

14. Sands BE, Anderson FH, Bernstein CN, et al. Infliximab maintenance therapy for fistulizing Crohn's disease. [see comment]. *N Engl J Med* 350(9):876–885, 2004.

15. Miller FB, Nikolov NR, Garrison RN. Emergency right colon resection. *Arch Surg* 122(3):339–343, 1987.

16. Deans GT, Krukowski ZH, Irwin ST. Malignant obstruction of the left colon. *Br J Surg* 81(9):1270–1276, 1994.

17. Suzman MS, Talmor M, Jennis R, et al. Accurate localization and surgical management of active lower gastrointestinal hemorrhage with technetium-labeled erythrocyte scintigraphy. [see comment]. *Ann Surg* 224(1):29–36, 1996.

18. Hunter JM, Pezim ME. Limited value of technetium 99m-labeled red cell scintigraphy in localization of lower gastrointestinal bleeding. *Am J Surg* 159(5):504–506, 1990.

19. McGuire HH Jr. Bleeding colonic diverticula. A reappraisal of natural history and management. *Ann Surg* 220(5):653–656, 1994.

20. Allen JI. Molecular biology of colon polyps and colon cancer. *Semin Surg Oncol* 11(6):399–405, 1995.

21. Obrand DI, Gordon PH. Incidence and patterns of recurrence following curative resection for colorectal carcinoma. *Dis Colon Rectum* 40(1):15–24, 1997.

22. Moertel CG, Fleming TR, Macdonald JS, et al. Fluorouracil plus levamisole as effective adjuvant therapy after resection of stage III colon carcinoma: a final report. *Ann Intern Med* 122(5):321–326, 1995.

23. Pollett WG, Nicholls RJ. The relationship between the extent of distal clearance and survival and local recurrence rates after curative anterior resection for carcinoma of the rectum. *Ann Surg* 198(2):159–163, 1983.

24. Anonymous. Improved survival with preoperative radiotherapy in resectable rectal cancer. Swedish Rectal Cancer Trial. [see comment] [erratum appears in *N Engl J Med* 1997 May 22;336(21):1539]. *N Engl J Med* 336(14):980–987, 1997.

25. Ambrosetti P, Robert JH, Witzig JA, et al. Acute left colonic diverticulitis in young patients. *J Am Coll Surg* 179(2):156–160, 1994.

26. Salem L, Veenstra DL, Sullivan SD, et al. The timing of elective colectomy in diverticulitis: a decision analysis. *J Am Coll Surg* 199(6):904–912, 2004.

27. Benn PL, Wolff BG, Ilstrup DM. Level of anastomosis and recurrent colonic diverticulitis. *Am J Surg* 151(2):269–271, 1986.

28. Ekbom A, Helmick C, Zack M, et al. Ulcerative colitis and colorectal cancer. A population-based study. *N Engl J Med* 323(18):1228–1233, 1990.

29. Parks AG, Nicholls RJ. Proctocolectomy without ileostomy for ulcerative colitis. *Br Med J* 2(6130):85–88, 1978.

30. Fazio VW, Marchetti F, Church M, et al. Effect of resection margins on the recurrence of Crohn's disease in the small bowel. A randomized controlled trial. *Ann Surg* 224(4):563–571, 1996.

HEPATOBILIARY SURGERY

David Sindram, MD, PhD
Janet E. Tuttle-Newhall, MD

INTRODUCTION

Hepatobiliary surgery is a challenging subspecialty in General Surgery. The liver and gallbladder have complex anatomy and associated physiology. The manner in which disease affects this organ system is often complicated. This chapter is not an attempt to be a complete overview of hepatobiliary surgery; however, it should serve as an introduction into this fascinating subspecialty of General Surgery. In the following sections, we will discuss common issues involving anatomy, physiology of the hepatobiliary system, pathologic states, interpretation of common lab tests, and potential interventions.

ANATOMY

An understanding of the hepatic anatomy is mandatory for anyone consider-ing intervention on the hepatobiliary system. Although the importance of the liver and the biliary system has been acknowledged since antiquity, it was not until the second half of the previous century that liver and bile duct surgery became survivable options for patients. Until surgeon scientists correctly translated anatomic research performed on animals to the human situation, surgery on the liver remained a dangerous and often lethal undertaking.[1]

Due to their joined embryologic origin, liver and bile duct anatomy are inseparable. The role of the liver is to interface between the gut and blood stream and its anatomy reflects this priority. As the human body develops, the liver buds from the foregut and incorporates the earliest blood supply, the vitelline and umbilical veins. A portion of the blood supply becomes the portal venous system and establishes blood flow from the gut to the liver. The portal vein is a major link between the gut and liver carrying any-thing that is absorbed or diffused by the bowels into the liver for processing, distribution, or storage. At the same time, the liver receives blood from the corporeal circulation, initially via the umbilical vein, and after birth via the hepatic artery. The blood and its contents are processed by the interfacing hepatocytes and the blood is subsequently pooled and collected by the hepatic veins which drain into the vena cava.

The liver also fulfills a role in detoxification of products absorbed into the gut. Some of the detoxified by-products are returned to the gut via the biliary system. Anatomically, it makes sense that the bile ducts are closely related to the inflow system. Portal venules, small arterial branches, and bile ducts form the portal triad. The combination of these three systems and the smallest microscopic functional units of the liver can be followed macroscopically from the outside of the liver. Although the adult liver is one solid organ, the branching tree-like structure, with the branches consisting of ever smaller bile ducts, portal veins, and hepatic arteries, allows the liver to be divided in functional units and facilitates surgical dissection (Fig. 11-1). Outflow of

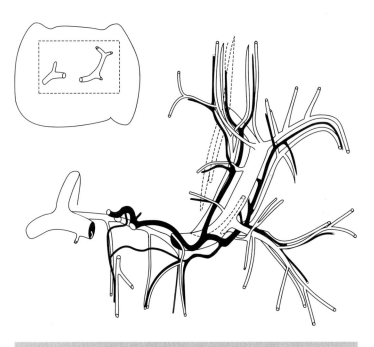

Figure 11-1 **Early detailed anatomic drawings of intrahepatic anatomy (clear portion indicates the portal vein, shaded portion indicates the biliary tree, black portions indicate hepatic artery).** (*Source:* Used with permission from Sutherland F, Claude Couinaud HJ. A passion for the liver. *Arch Surg* 137:1305–1310, 2002.)

blood from the liver into circulation is arranged in a similar fashion, collecting smaller veins into larger hepatic veins, ultimately reaching a left, middle, or right hepatic vein. Applying the known branching structure of the liver, Dr. Couinaud described segmental units and divisional systems that revolutionized hepatobiliary surgery and is used to date to facilitate resection planes in the liver (Fig. 11-2).[2]

Of note, human biliary anatomy, unlike animals, has one additional feature —a gallbladder. Bile is used in the gut to facilitate in the uptake of fat, by breaking fat up like detergent into micelles. Connected to the common bile duct via the cystic duct, bile is collected in the gallbladder to store until it is needed. An intricate hormonal signaling system is in place to signal the gallbladder to contract in order to eject bile into the duodenum as needed at the time of gastric distention with food.

The external anatomy of the liver allows for identification of some landmarks. The umbilical vein becomes obsolete after birth, but remains as the ligamentum Teres, which can be found in the falciform ligament. This ligament,

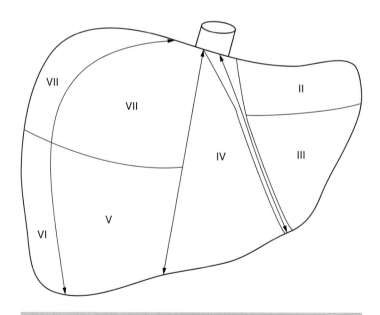

Figure 11-2 **Couinaud's early diagram of the segmental anatomy of the liver. Segments are numbered clockwise with Roman numerals. Segment I is the caudate lobe, not seen underneath.** (*Source:* Used with permission from Sutherland F, Claude Couinaud HJ. A passion for the liver. *Arch Surg 137*:1305–1310, 2002.)

historically has been used to divide the liver into a left and a right lobe; however, using known segmental anatomy, an imaginary line can be drawn from the fossa of the gallbladder to the middle hepatic vein/vena cava, dividing the liver into the anatomic right and left lobe (Fig. 11-3). This imaginary line will often follow the course of the middle hepatic vein.

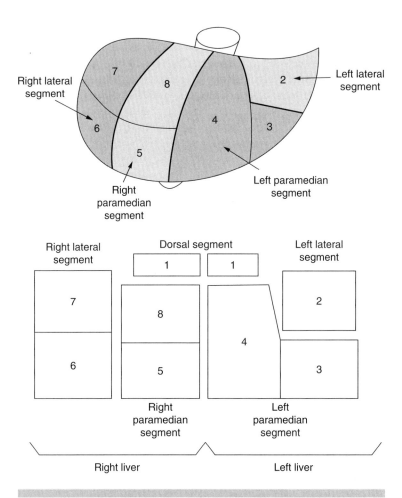

Figure 11-3 ***The three anatomic segmentations with respect to hemiliver (right and left liver), Goldsmith and Woodburne (lateral, paramedian, and dorsal right or left segments), and Couinaud (numbers).*** (*Source*: Used with permission from Soler L, Delingette H, Malandain G, et al. Fully automatic anatomical, pathological, and functional segmentation from CT scans for hepatic surgery. *Comput Aided Surg* 6:131–142, 2001.)

As the middle hepatic vein is within the liver parenchyma, it cannot be visualized without the aid of modern imaging studies such as computed tomography (CT) scans, magnetic resonance imaging (MRI), ultrasound (US), and angiography. The *right* liver is defined as segments 5, 6, 7, and 8 and is made up of the right lateral segment and right paramedian segment. The *left* liver is defined as segments 2, 3, and 4 and consists of the left lateral segment and the left paramedian segment. Segment 1 is the caudate lobe and stands alone anatomically as its venous drainage is not dependent on the right, middle, and left hepatic veins. It drains directly into the vena cava by small venous branches.[3] The unique venous drainage of the caudate lobe becomes very important when discussing disorders of the hepatic venous system such as Budd-Chiari syndrome. Imaging of the liver and bile ducts and the identification of the segments are essential in planning operations on the liver (Fig. 11-4).

One important aspect of liver and bile duct anatomy is its highly variable composition. Both intra- and extrahepatic biliary ducts, as well as the arterial blood supply to liver and gallbladder are highly variant. Even *simple* procedures such as laparoscopic cholecystectomies can become treacherously difficult because of aberrant anatomy.[4] One of the more common anatomic variants is the right hepatic artery either being completely replaced or with an accessory branch, arising from the superior mesenteric artery. Likewise, the left hepatic artery can be replaced completely or with an accessory branch, arising from the left gastric artery. A *replaced* or accessory right hepatic artery will be found in the porta hepatis posterior to the common bile duct and the *replaced* or accessory left hepatic artery will be found coursing through the gastrohepatic ligament. Presence of these arterial variations may affect the surgeon's ability to perform specific procedures (i.e., pancreaticoduodenectomy) or facilitate planned resections (i.e., a right hepatectomy).

PHYSIOLOGY AND FUNCTION

In general, the liver is the biochemical engine of metabolism. The liver receives one-third of the total cardiac output. The hepatic artery carries 25 percent, the portal vein 75 percent, with the liver subsequently receiving 1.5 L of blood per minute.[5] All blood traverses the liver via the portal triads and travels via the hepatic sinusoids to ultimately arrive in the hepatic veins and vena cava. Under normal circumstances, pressure in the portal vein is low, 9–12 mmHg; however, a pressure gradient still exists toward the vena cava, where the central venous pressure generally reaches zero. To allow for the large volume of blood to disperse through the liver, the vascular resistance in the hepatic sinusoids is low. In diseased states, the resistance conversely can increase resulting in high-portal pressure and shunting of blood around the liver via collaterals. Portal hypertension results from any condition that increases prehepatic venous pressures greater than 12 mmHg.

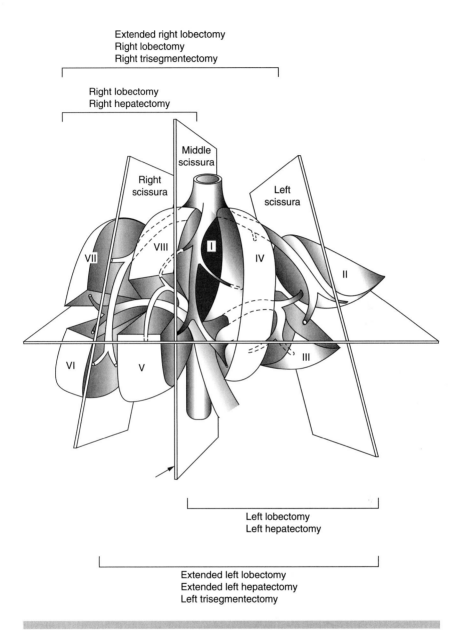

Figure 11-4 **Resection planes for hepatic resections with alternative nomenclatures.** (*Source:* Used with permission from Vauthey JN. Liver imaging: a surgeon's perspective. *Rad Clin North Am* 36:445–457, 1998.)

Portal hypertension can be divided into three main causes: *presinusoidal,* *intrasinusoidal,* or *postsinusoidal.* The most common causes of each respectively are portal vein thrombosis, cirrhosis, and hepatic vein occlusion (Budd-Chiari syndrome). Complications of portal hypertension the include esophageal and gastric varices, encephalopathy, and ascites. Ascites (or accumulation of intra-abdominal fluid) is thought to be secondary to the effects of portal hypertension on increasing splanchnic blood volume as well as the increased secretion of aldosterone.[6]

Nutrients such as proteins, sugars, and fats are metabolized by the liver, but toxins such as various ingested poisons (alcohol, medications, and so on) and gut bacteria translocating through the bowel wall are cleared by the liver as well. Ultimately, the hepatocyte is the core unit of the metabolic machinery. The filtering proportions of sinusoidal endothelial cell, and specialized liver macrophages, Kupffer cells, aid the hepatocyte. The specific role of the hepatocyte is determined by the position of the cell in the hepatic architecture relative to the distance from the portal triad or the hepatic venule. It has become clear that hepatocytes in one area of the liver can be recruited to fulfill tasks in an adjacent area, essentially providing for a continuum, with each hepatocyte capable of providing the full spectrum of necessary functions based on demand.

Detoxification is one of the major functions of the liver, and important enzyme systems exist to break down substances that are toxic to the body. One of the main systems is the cytochrome p450 system, which aides in oxidative break down of toxic metabolites. Certain medications can induce the cytochrome p450 system, as they are toxic, or inhibit the enzyme system and thereby influence the metabolism of other drugs. This can be very important clinically as patients with histories of substance abuse (i.e., alcohol) will have an induced cytochrome p450 system, which increases the metabolism of pain medications, and some anesthetics affecting their clinical management.

Carbohydrate metabolism is one of the core functions of the liver. As energy supply is not constant, the body has to adapt to irregular food intake by devising a system whereby energy can be stored and called upon on demand. The liver provides this function by storing glucose in the form of glycogen in hepatocytes. In situations where the body needs more energy than is currently being ingested or during times of fasting, glycogen is used for neogenesis of glucose. Even in unfavorable situations such as anaerobic metabolism, the liver will continue to provide energy by recycling lactic acid, a product of anaerobic metabolism, into glucose via the Cori cycle.[7] The liver is also a key structure in fat and protein metabolism. Maintaining close communications with adipocytes via cell signaling pathways, the liver regulates fat storage and reabsorption as a more long-term storage of energy. By producing and breaking down amino acids, the liver is primarily responsible for maintaining nitrogen balance in the body. The liver produces more than 5000 proteins, varying from albumin to clotting factors. The importance of the liver as a protein factory becomes relevant in diseased states, when severe hypoalbuminemia and increased clotting times complicate clinical care of the patient with liver disease.

As discussed earlier, the liver produces bile, both as a route to eliminate waste as well as to aid in digestion. One of the main components is bilirubin, derived from the breakdown of hemoglobin. In the systemic circulation bilirubin is bound to albumin, taken up by the liver and conjugated with glucuronic acid in the hepatocyte. Next, the bilirubin is secreted into bile and transported away from the hepatocytes, ultimately to the duodenum. For the most part bilirubin is eventually reabsorbed downstream in the intestinal tract after it has been deconjugated and converted into urobilinogen. Only 5 percent of the bilirubin, converted to urobilinogen by gut bacteria, is excreted with feces, giving it its characteristic brown color. Some of the reabsorbed urobilinogen is excreted with urine, coloring it yellow. Based on where the bilirubin pathway is interrupted, due to liver disease, stones, or reabsorption, either conjugated, or unconjugated bilirubin concentrations will rise in serum and cause jaundice. At concentrations of 2.5 mg/dL initially the sclerae become yellow, but at higher concentrations the skin and entire body will become discolored. An important caveat when examining patients with liver disease is that fluorescent lighting can lead to an erroneous diagnosis of *scleral icterus*; examinations of patients in natural lighting will remove this potential for error.

Normally, there is uninterrupted flow of bile from the liver to the gallbladder and subsequently, the duodenum. There is an intricate interaction between the gallbladder and duodenum, via nervous and hormonal pathways. Based on the amount and consistency of food delivered into the duodenum by the stomach, a certain amount of bile will be excreted from the gallbladder. The *migrating myoelectric complex (MMC)* is a nervous electrical wave essentially propulsing food downstream, mediated by hormonal signals (Motilin). It also induces gallbladder contraction. Another mechanism to release bile into the duodenum is *cholecystokinin (CCK)*, a hormone that directly induces gallbladder contraction and is released by the duodenum. By virtue of the sphincter of Oddi, the sphincter at the end of the common bile duct, as it enters the duodenum, a fairly constant pressure of 15 mmHg is maintained in the bile ducts. Opening and closing of the sphincter of Oddi is also closely regulated by CCK and Motilin.[8]

Bile consists of three major components: *bile salts*, *cholesterol*, and *water*. An equilibrium among these components exists, allowing for the maintenance of flow and the proper digestive properties of bile. Any imbalance in the three components can lead to insolubility resulting in stones and their related disease states.

Of the thousands of proteins the liver produces, the proteins that comprise the coagulation system are of utmost importance. Various proteins are involved in a cascade-like fashion to produce a rapid response to injury. A detailed description of the proteins produced by the liver is beyond the scope of this text; however, a common finding in patients with severe disorders of the liver is an elevated prothrombin time (PT).

PATHOLOGY AND DYSFUNCTION

The previous paragraphs stressed the normal anatomy and function, and touched on the problems one might encounter with hepatobiliary disease. The systematic review of all liver diseases is beyond the scope of this chapter; however, our focus will be on surgical pathologic states and the most commonly encountered problems on clinical rotations. What soon will be apparent is that many diseases converge in common pathways. Infectious diseases such as hepatitis B and C lead to hepatocytes damage and subsequent destruction of the liver architecture. Cholestasis as a result of obstructing stone disease, but also secondary to tumors, autoimmune disease or cystic disease leads to destruction of hepatocytes and liver architecture as well. With the loss of normal hepatic architecture and function, characteristic signs of liver failure surface can easily be understood based on the anatomy and function as discussed previously. For the sake of this chapter, we will divide liver disease in four broad categories: *infections, stones, tumors,* and *chronic liver disease.*

The liver is a major filter of pathogens, mainly originating from the gut but any other connection to the liver may be a portal of entry as well, including the blood supply, biliary tree, and even direct-penetrating trauma. Hepatitis is the common liver disease worldwide. Hepatitis B is indigenous to many parts of the world and is a common risk factor for primary malignancies of the liver. Hepatitis C is the most common infectious hepatitis currently in the United States. It affects 1 percent of the total population in the United States (10 million persons) and is currently the most common cause of end-stage liver disease resulting in liver transplantation.[9] Hepatitis A-, B-, or C-associated liver disease is a medical problem, until complications of the disease result in a complication such as hepatocellular carcinoma (HCC) that can be surgically addressed. Hepatitis B or C is common risk factor for primary hepatic neoplasm, as well as cirrhosis, portal hypertension, and its sequela. Surgical therapies exist for some hepatic neoplasms in the form of resection or transplantation as well as medical refractory complications from portal hypertension.

Another common infectious entity in the liver is hepatic abscess. Once the physiologic clearance of bacteria is outmatched by the influx, localized liver infection can ensue. Commonly, when stasis of fluids occurs, an abscess is formed. Abscesses can result from biliary obstruction, trauma, or secondary to intraperitoneal processes such as diverticulitis or appendicitis. Probably because of the constant assault from the gut with bacteria, the microbial flora found in hepatic abscesses is often mixed with a predominance of gram-negative rods and anaerobic organisms. *Escherichia coli* and *Klebsiella pneumoniae* are common, but *Staphylococcus aureus* and enterococcus species are often found as well. Broad-spectrum antibiotic coverage is required. Prolonged treatment with antibiotics alone does not absolve the problem, and percutaneous drainage is the therapy of choice. Failure of percutaneous drainage is an indication for open surgical drainage and this should be pursued aggressively if percutaneous drainage fails to resolve the processes. Amebic abscesses are the exception to this rule. They usually respond to antibiotic treatment and percutaneous drainage is contraindicated. Amebic abscesses, however, are not very common in the United States and a simple blood test for antiamebic antibodies will be positive in 95 percent of patients with this condition.[10]

One of the more common causes of stasis and thus infection in the United States is gallstone disease. Bile salts, cholesterol, and calcium salts usually are found in perfect solution in bile; however, when an imbalance occurs, the bile salts come out of solution and precipitate into sludge or stones. Hemolytic states, such as due to sickle cell disease, results in the formation of pigmented stones, whereas high cholesterol states result in cholesterol stones, the most common form of gallstones. Mostly, these stones are formed where natural stasis of bile occurs in the gallbladder. Stones are, however, rarely formed in the bile ducts or intrahepatically. Stones are generally asymptomatic until they cause obstruction. Biliary pain can be caused by contraction of the gallbladder, but severe disease typically does not appear until a stone occludes the bladder or a duct. A gallbladder with stones is called *cholelithiasis*. Obstruction of the outflow of the gallbladder by a stone, results in cholecystitis inflammation of the gallbladder. When a stone has passed into the common bile duct, choledocholithiasis, it can result in stasis of bile inside the liver and result in a condition called cholangitis. *Cholangitis* can lead to sepsis and death if left untreated. If the stone obstructs the biliary tree at the site of the ampulla of Vater, this can result in stasis of pancreatic secretions and lead to pancreatitis.

For symptomatic cholecystitis and asymptomatic cholecystolithiasis in high-risk patient populations (i.e., diabetics), surgical removal of the gallbladder is indicated, which is one of the most commonly performed surgical procedures. A rare, but important complication of stone disease in elderly patients is *gallstone ileus*—a bowel obstruction secondary to the passing of a stone into the small bowel through a biliary-enteric fistula. This disease requires open surgical removal of the stone and cholecystectomy with repair of the fistula.

Likewise, neoplasms are commonly found in the liver. It is key to make the distinction between benign and malignant disease as well as true primary hepatic malignancies and metastatic disease from tumors of extrahepatic origin. The three most common benign primary liver tumors are *hepatic adenomas*

(HA), focal nodular hyperplasia (FNH), and *hemangiomas*. These tumors generally are asymptomatic, but diagnostic uncertainty may warrant resection in selected cases.[11] HAs are more common in women and are thought to be associated with hormonal stimulation, most commonly oral contraceptives. These lesions mandate resection due to the risk of spontaneous rupture and hemorrhage as well as the very small risk of malignant transformation. While the size of the lesion may decrease with hormonal withdrawal, the risk of malignant transformation does not and resection is still warranted. Diagnosis of this lesion during pregnancy is problematic as the hormonal stimulation will not cease until delivery and risk of rupture is high. When possible, they should be resected at the safest time for both mother and fetus. FNH on the other hand, if asymptomatic, can be followed with sequential imaging (CT scan, MRI, and US). If the patient becomes symptomatic or the tumor enlarges, local ablation or resection is warranted. The key is the difference between the adenoma and FNH (Table 11-1). Each tumor has distinct characteristics on various forms of imaging that help in the diagnostic dilemma.

HCC or hepatoma is the most common primary hepatic malignancy.[12] HCC is a cancer that is primarily found with chronic liver injury secondary to viral disease (hepatitis B and C), alcohol abuse, or other causes of cirrhosis.

Table 11-1 **FNH Vs. HA**

Imaging Study	FNH	Adenoma
MRI	Low signal central scar on T1-weighted image that enhances with gadolinium	No central scar
Nuclear medicine scan	Increased uptake of sulfur colloid and gallium	Decreased uptake of sulfur colloid and gallium
CT scan	Increased hypervascularity with *spoke wheel* appearance of vasculature	Arterial enhancement with presence of fat and hemorrhage
Clinical parameter		
Malignant degeneration	No	Yes
Hormonally sensitive	⇑	⇑⇑

Source: Adapted from Cho BY, Ngyuen MH. The diagnosis and management of benign liver tumors. *J Clin Gastroenterol* 39(5):401–412, 2005.

Because of this relationship between liver disease and the occurrence of malignancy, the survival of the disease is equally related to the underlying liver disease and degree of hepatic dysfunction as it is to the stage of the tumor. Treatment consists largely of local control by various means (e.g., ablation therapy, embolization, and radiation or chemotherapy), where cure is only offered by resection or transplantation.[13,14] The latter options are limited by location of the tumor and the disease in the remaining liver portion after resection and the lack of sufficient donor organs.

The liver is a common site for metastatic disease. In fact, most hepatic tumors are metastic. Metastatic disease is in general not amendable to surgical treatment. Ablative therapy has been shown to be of some benefit in selected cases. However, one exception has evolved out of extensive research; isolated hepatic metastases in colorectal cancer. Although most metastatic colorectal cancer has spread beyond the liver, solitary lesions in the liver, in absence of extrahepatic spread of the disease can be resected with an important survival benefit in some patients.[15] Currently, several trials are incorporating chemotherapy prior to or after surgery in these lesions, as well as using selective hepatic artery infusion with chemotherapeutic agents in order to make unresectable disease resectable.[16,17]

The biliary system, both intra- and extrahepatic, can also give rise to tumors. Benign lesions are rare. Choledochal cysts and gallbladder polyps are examples of benign tumors. Gallbladder cancer presents similarly to gallstone disease, and a strong association exists with the presence of stones. Cancer is most common in elderly patients, found during workup for right upper quadrant pain, or on cholecystectomy. All gallbladders should be sent to pathology to be examined after cholecystectomy. The classic presentation is that of an elderly patient with painless jaundice. Unfortunately, more than 50 percent of gallbladder malignancies have already metastasized at the time of resection and, consequently, the survival rate is dismal. There may be some survival advantage for a local resection of the gallbladder bed but data are mixed. Malignant tumors arising from the bile ducts are called *cholangiocarcinomas*. These tumors are rare and associated with very poor outcome as well. Despite aggressive surgical treatment, such as hepatic resection with bile duct resection, survival is limited.[18]

Finally, chronic liver disease can be divided into two categories: *synthetic dysfunction* and *complications of portal hypertension*. Both arise from complications of long-term liver damage. Long-term exposure to hepatotoxins can lead to chronic changes in the hepatic architecture. Initially, in response to injury, hepatocytes will form fatty acid vacuoles inside their cytoplasm, eventually leading to a condition known as *steatohepatitis*. Hepatocytes containing large amount of fat is far more susceptible to injury, which can result in dysfunction of the liver as toxic injury continues. Eventually, loss of hepatocytes leads to scar formation, fibrosis and nodular regeneration, or cirrhosis. Cirrhosis can be caused by a myriad of insults: viral disease (e.g., hepatitis

B and C), gene defects (e.g., alpha$_1$-antitrypsin deficiency and Wilson disease), autoimmune diseases (e.g., lupus, primary biliary cirrhosis [PBC], and primary sclerosing cholangitis [PSC]), alcohol, other toxins, or chronic infection. Synthetic dysfunction from cirrhosis requires a large loss of functional hepatocytes. It is the final clinical stage prior to end-stage liver failure and death. More commonly, patients with cirrhosis suffer from the complications of portal hypertension. With the liver receiving 75 percent of its blood supply via the portal vein, one can envision the need for diversion of flow in case the resistance in the liver increases due to cirrhosis secondary to disease. The resulting portal hypertension forces blood to find other ways to escape the portal system. There are five major decompression pathways available to decrease portal pressure by diversion of blood flow: (1) recanalization of blood flow via the umbilical vein, through the ligamentum Teres, resulting in varicosities in the periumbilical veins (clinically, caput medusae); (2) esophageal varices via the left gastric (coronary vein); (3) rectal varices via the hemorrhoidal plexus; (4) retroperitoneal varices; and (5) gastric varices via the splenic vein. The portal vein is composed of the splenic vein and superior mesenteric vein. Increased portal pressure leads to increased pressure in the splenic vein resulting in gastric varices (via the short gastric veins), as well as splenomegaly. It is often the splenomegaly that leads to platelet and leukocyte entrapment giving patients with portal hypertension the characteristic findings on complete blood count (CBC) of low platelet counts and low white blood cells in the presence of an elevated PT.[19]

LABS AND STUDIES

There are many blood tests that one can order to assess the status of the liver. As the liver produces enormous amount of proteins, one may simply follow the production of some key proteins to assess for liver function; however, protein production is multifactorial and may depend on provision of substrate as well as intrinsic hepatic functions. For instance, the production of albumin is largely dependent on intake of nutrients, and albumin levels in turn can be very low with adequate production in severe proteinuria. It becomes increasingly clear that hepatic function is not easily determined by laboratory tests alone.[20]

Liver function tests (LFTs) are a panel of liver enzymes that are released in the blood by hepatocytes. These LFTs, a misnomer, are in fact measurements of enzymes that are released from hepatocytes when they die—they do not reflect liver *function*. We measure these enzymes in hopes that the plasma levels of these enzymes correlate with a certain amount of cell destruction, which in turn is thought to inversely reflect remaining liver function. The two enzymes that are most frequently measured in plasma are aspartate aminotransferase (AST) and alanine aminotransferase (ALT), often in conjunction with bilirubin. AST is not very specific. ALT is more so, but hepatic cell death causes an immediate rise in plasma concentrations of these enzymes. Likewise, one can measure alkaline phosphatase (AP), gamma-glutamyltranspeptidase (GGT), or lactate dehydrogenase (LDH) with similar limitations. The latter markers are more sensitive rather than organ specific for cell death; none of the previous markers, including AST and ALT, will help to predict outcome. To be more accurate one could measure several factors that signify hepatic cell injury as well as some liver functions to assess a patient's clinical status. For example, a prolonged bleeding time as a result of lack of production of clotting factors, together with a rise in AST and ALT, and an increase in conjugated bilirubin may for instance suggest, and certainly not diagnose, liver disease secondary to cholestasis.

The liver is the manufacturer of most of the proteins involved in the clotting cascade. Abnormal bleeding time and other abnormalities of parameter of coagulation are often reflective of liver dysfunction. One of the most important ways to determine the degree of liver function in the body is by measuring the PT or international normalized ratio (INR). A prolonged INR is an important marker of liver disease.

Several other tests are available to assess for specific enzyme deficits (e.g., alpha$_1$-antitrypsin), the presence of tumor cells (e.g., carcinoembryonic antigen [CEA] and alpha-fetoprotein [AFP]), or the presence of specific antibodies to components of liver cells (e.g., antineutrophil antibodies in primary sclerosing cholangitis and antimitochondrial antibodies in primary biliary cirrhosis). Although some methods to test the function of hepatic enzyme systems such as the p450 enzyme system (MEGX test) and (indocyanine green metabolic excretion test) exist, these tests do not provide additional diagnostic assistance to standard blood work or imaging.

In order to overcome a dependable method to assess true liver function in an individual patient, scoring systems have been devised that try to *weigh* various measurements as well as clinical symptoms to better classify liver injury. A scoring system that has found widespread clinical use is the *Child-Pugh* scoring (Table 11-2). It gives points for bilirubin level, albumin, PT, and the severity of the presence of ascites or encephalopathy. Although this scoring system was not developed for any particular liver disease, it does allow for grading of the severity of the disease. Other scoring systems are being used such as model end-stage liver disease (MELD) score in the allocation of livers for transplantation.[21] New systems are being evaluated on a regular basis, signifying the lack of satisfying LFTs to aid in adjusting for severity and prognosis.

In daily practice, we can often arrive at the proper diagnosis and stage of disease by assessing the various laboratory values as well as the results of radiologic studies. A wide array of possible radiologic studies such as US imaging, plain films, MRI, CT scan, angiography, and positron emission tomography (PET) scans are available to aid in the diagnostic process. Often

Table 11-2 **Child-Pugh Turcotte Scoring**

Clinical Parameter	Rank	Score
Bilirubin (mg/dL)	<2	1
	2–3	2
	>3	3
Albumin (g/dL)	>3.5	1
	2.8–3.5	2
	<3.5	3
Prothrombin ratio (%)	>50	1
	30–50	2
	<30	3
Encephalopathy	Absent	1
	I°–II°	2
	III°	3
Ascites	Absent	1
	Mild	2
	Tense	3
Child A: 5–6 points	Child B: 7–9 points	Child C: >10 points

Source: Adapted from Pugh RNH, Murray-Lyon IM, Dawson JL, et al. Transection of the oesophageal varices. *Br J Surg* 60:646–664, 1973.

the combination of imaging studies is superior to any one test alone in discerning liver pathology and the associated involved anatomy. For example, US is very good at detecting gallstones, but lacks the anatomic detail of a CT scan, as stones are often missed on CT scan. MRI identifies certain intrahepatic tumors better than CT scan, but does not outline anatomic borders as well as CT; however, due to unique aspects of MRI, it may give histologic differentiation of benign tumors, such as hemangiomas, FNH, and HA. PET scans are sensitive in picking up metastatic disease, but lack the resolution to define specific anatomy. Similarly, angiography is the gold standard to evaluate the intrahepatic vasculature, but does not show the tissues through which the blood vessels flow. One will often see combinations of these studies, especially when planning surgical resolution of hepatic problems, to provide diagnostic and anatomic insight.[22]

INTERVENTIONS AND OPERATIONS

Once a diagnosis has been made of liver or biliary tree pathology via clinical examination, laboratory data in combination with radiologic imaging, a care strategy to relieve symptoms and address the pathology is made. Often, this strategy involves radiologic interventions, surgery, or a combination of these two modalities. Careful planning and a clear understanding of the underlying disease must guide the choice of intervention. A thorough discussion of all potential invention strategies is beyond this text but we will discuss the more common procedures seen on the clinical wards.

Gallstones and their related complications are one of the most common hepatobiliary abnormalities seen in the clinical wards. As previously discussed, all symptomatic cholelithiasis and asymptomatic cholelithiasis in high-risk groups such as the elderly and diabetics, should be surgically addressed. However, in case of a common duct stone, choledocholithiasis, endoscopic retrograde pancreatography (ERCP), or interventional radiology techniques (percutaneous transhepatic cholangiogram [PTC] with percutaneous biliary drainage [PBD] catheter placement) are favored as first-line therapy for duct drainage and stone retrieval over surgical bile duct exploration. Open common duct exploration has been associated with much higher morbidity and mortality than ERCP for common duct stones. Surgery is strongly indicated for removal of the gallbladder once the common duct stone has been addressed. In the case of cholangitis in the presence of choledocholithiasis, immediate bile duct drainage is required either endoscopically, via PBD or surgically as well as broad-spectrum antibiotic coverage.

For uncomplicated gallstone disease, the laparoscopic approach for removal has become standard in most patient populations. While previous surgery is not always a contraindication for laparoscopy, inability to adequately visualize the arterial and biliary anatomy during the procedure is an absolute indication to convert to an open procedure. Cirrhosis, ascites, chronic obstructive pulmonary disease (COPD), previous biliary surgery, and portal hypertension are a few absolute contraindications for laparoscopic cholecystectomy. If a bile duct injury occurs during a cholecystectomy, and is recognized at the time of the procedure, repair by a trained colleague familiar with techniques of biliary reconstruction is recommended. Frequently, the biliary injury occurs as a result of thermal conduction from the electrocautery. Biliary reconstruction via a Roux-en-Y hepaticojejunostomy is usually indicated and preferred. A hepaticojejunostomy is an anastomosis between the side of bowel (usually jejunum) and the common bile duct. Enteral continuity is restored with a side-to-side enteroenterostomy. This technique of biliary reconstruction is commonly used in large liver resections that involve the bile duct as well as in transplantation for specific patient populations such as pediatric patients, procedures such as living donor transplants, and disease states that involve the biliary tree, such as primary sclerosing cholangitis.

For neoplasms of the liver, surgical resection is often warranted. The principles of resection are the same for both benign and malignant disease; resect the lesion with an adequate margin leaving enough functional liver behind to avoid hepatic failure. Although, the liver has regenerative capacity, one should not remove more than 75 percent of the liver parenchyma at the time of resection. This resection threshold may be lower (i.e., even less may be removed) in patients with abnormal liver parenchyma, such as cirrhosis or fatty liver. A clear understanding of liver anatomy is paramount. The hepatectomy can be performed in multiple ways and depends on the anatomy involved with the disease process. Resections can include nonanatomic resections, anatomic segmental resections, anatomic *lobe* or sectoral resections (left lobe segments = II, III, and IV; right lobe = V, VI, VII, and VIII; segment I, the caudate, can be taken with either the left or the right), and complete hepatectomy at the time of transplantation. In order to facilitate the choice of resection, preoperative imaging is mandatory. Once the decision has been made to proceed with resection, some additional staging technique is used in the operating room to assist in the decisions regarding extent of resection and often, to assess resectability in cases of malignancy. These techniques include staging laparoscopy and intraoperative ultrasound (IOUS). While staging laparoscopy can predict resectability in the majority of cases of primary malignant liver tumors, IOUS is more sensitive for detecting occult liver metastasis not found on traditional imaging. Appropriate staging is important if you are resecting patients with colorectal metastases. Surgical principles are constant.

To minimize blood loss during the resection and demarcate the area to be resected, isolation of the inflow vasculature that is relevant to the area to be resected is performed prior to transecting the liver parenchyma. There are multiple methods of liver parenchymal transection. The classic method is the *finger fracture* technique where a clamp, or the surgeon's fingers, is used to bluntly transect the liver tissue with the identified vascular and biliary structures ligated, clipped, or cauterized. There are many other methods of parenchymal transection including using devices such as the ultrasonic cavitron device or a saline enhanced radiofrequency ablation (RFA) device. The choice of transection technique is left to the surgeon. To further minimize blood loss in larger resections, a Pringle maneuver is often performed. The Pringle involves temporary clamping of the porta hepatic. A noncirrhotic liver can tolerate this warm ischemia for up to 30 min. Occasionally, in larger resections, ligation of the hepatic vein responsible for that portion of liver is also ligated prior to parenchymal dissection to further minimize blood loss. At the completion of the parenchymal transaction, hemostasis is obtained and any small biliary leak or bleeding on the parenchymal surface is controlled with suture ligation. Drains are often placed to drain any potential bile leak or to detect bleeding. Complications after liver resection include hemorrhage, abscess, pleural effusions, bile leak, and hepatic failure.

In those patients with colorectal metastasis who are not candidates for traditional resections but have only liver disease, local control techniques offer an alternative to cure. RFA uses high frequency alternating current that destroys tissue via thermal mechanisms. It is delivered to the tumor area either percutaneously under CT guidance, laparoscopically with laparoscopic US, or via the open technique in the operating room assisted by IOUS. Local reoccurrence or persistence of the tumors occurs in 7 percent of patients, usually at the periphery of the ablation field. RFA is often a palliative procedure.[23] Other local techniques of tumor control include microwave coagulation and local alcohol injection. Alcohol injection is reserved for patients where cure is not possible and is a palliative therapy.

Finally, there is the surgical therapy of portal hypertension and end-stage liver disease (Table 11-3). Within the past decade, the available treatment options for patients with bleeding varices and portal hypertension from cirrhosis has changed. Surgical shunts, once the therapy of choice in both the emergency and elective setting, have largely been replaced by endoscopic and interventional radiology techniques. In the emergency setting, endoscopic sclerotherapy or banding have become the interventions of choice to control variceal bleeding.[24] The placement of a transjugular intrahepatic portosystemic shunt (TIPS) is now being performed more commonly than surgical shunts, mainly as a bridge to liver transplantation. The TIPS involves placement of a stent into the suprahepatic cava, through the liver parenchyma, and into the portal vein via interventional radiologic techniques. It is highly effective in decompressing varices in the emergency setting but carries the risk of worsening encephalopathy. Other indications for TIPS in patients with symptoms of portal hypertension resulting from cirrhosis may include refractory ascites, portal gastropathy, and the hepatorenal syndrome.[25] Surgical shunts are warranted only in those patients with refractory bleeding varices who have failed medical therapy and are not candidates for TIPS who have appropriate anatomy. While there are numerous surgical shunts described, the most commonly performed surgical shunt currently is the distal splenorenal shunt or Warren shunt. The Warren shunt entails anastomosing the distal end of the splenic vein with the left renal vein and disconnecting the significant venous collaterals such as the left gastric and gastroepiploic veins. Preoperative angiogram is mandatory to confirm portal vein patency and assess the size of the splenic vein, which should be greater than 1 cm.[26]

Table 11-3 **Model/Mayo End-stage Liver Disease Score: Log-based Score Using PT INR, Bilirubin (mg/dL), and Creatinine (mg/dL)**

Score	3-Month Mortality (%)
<10	2–8
10–19	6–29
20–29	50–76
30–39	62–80
>40	100

Source: Adapted from Malinchoc M, Kamath PS, Gordon FD, et al. A model to predict poor survival in patients undergoing transjugular intrahepatic portosystemic shunts. *Hepatology* 31:864–871, 2000.

Neither TIPS nor shunting procedures have changed survival for patients with end-stage liver disease. Only liver transplantation has improved survival and quality of life of those patients that warrant transplantation. Liver transplantation is currently indicated for patients with complications of end-stage liver disease, a MELD greater than 15, who have no medical contraindications for surgery after an exhaustive workup. Liver transplants require lifelong immunosuppression, requiring the patient to have no contraindications for immunotherapy and socioeconomic support to pay for those medications. In the United States currently, end-stage liver disease resulting from hepatitis C is the most common indication for liver transplantation. Long waiting lists and lack of organ availability has translated into deaths on the waiting list such that being listed for an organ transplant is no guarantee of receiving one in time.

CONCLUSION

Hepatobiliary surgery is a fascinating and complex subspecialty of General Surgery. Appropriate therapies for specific hepatic or biliary pathologies is dependent on the practitioner having a reasonable knowledge of anatomy and physiology, as well as imaging modalities and other intervention strategies in addition to surgical management.

REFERENCES

1. Fortner JG, Blumgart LH. A historic perspective of liver surgery at the end of the millennium. *J Am Coll Surg* 193:210–220, 2001.

2. Sutherland F, Harris J. Claude Couinaud: A passion for the liver. *Arch Surg* 137:1305–1310, 2002.

3. Soler L, Delingette H, Malandain G, et al. Fully automatic anatomical, pathological, and functional segmentation from CT scans for hepatic surgery. *Comput Aided Surg* 6:131–142, 2001.

4. Healey JE, Schroy PC. Anatomy of the biliary ducts within the human liver: analysis of the prevailing pattern of branchings and the major variations of the biliary ducts. *Arch Surg* 66:599–616, 1953.

5. Bradley EL III. Measurement of hepatic bloodflow in man. *Surgery* 75:783, 1974.

6. Benoit JN, Granger DN. Splanchnic hemodynamics in chronic portal hypertension. *Semin Liver Dis* 6:287–298, 1986.

7. Zakim D. Metabolism of glucose and fatty acids by the liver. In Zakim D, Boyer TD, eds., *Hepatology: A Textbook of Liver Disease*. Philadelphia, PA: W.B. Saunders, 2003: 49–80.

8. Muller M, Jansen PLM. Mechanisms of bile secretion. In Zakim D, Boyer TD, eds., *Hepatology: A Textbook of Liver Disease*. Philadelphia, PA: W.B. Saunders, 2003: 271–290.

9. Seeff LB, Hoofnagle JH. The National Institutes of Health Consensus Development Conference Management of Hepatitis C 2002. *Clin Liver Dis* 7:261–287, 2003.

10. Barnes PF, De Cock KM, Reynolds TN, et al. A comparison of amebic and pyogenic abscess of the liver. *Medicine* 66:472–483, 1987.

11. Edmondson HA, Henderson B, Benton B. Liver-cell adenomas associated with the use of oral contraceptives. *N Engl J Med* 294:470–472, 1976.

12. Lau WY. Primary hepatocellular carcinoma. In Blumgart LH, Fong Y, eds., *Surgery of the Liver and Biliary Tract*, 3rd ed., Vol. II. London, UK: W.B. Saunders, 2000:1423–1450.

13. Mazzaferro V, Regalia E, Doci R, et al. Liver transplantation for the treatment of small hepatocellular carcinomas in patients with cirrhosis. *N Engl J Med* 334:693–699, 1996.

14. Poon RT, Fan ST, Tsang FH, et al. Locoregional therapies for hepatocellular carcinoma: a critical review from the surgeon's perspective. *Ann Surg* 235:466–486, 2002.

15. Wagner JS, Adson MA, van Heerden JA, et al. The natural history of hepatic metastases from colorectal cancer: a comparison with resective treatment. *Ann Surg* 199:502–508, 1984.

16. Kadry Z, Clavien PA. New treatments with curative intent for metastatic colorectal liver cancer. *Expert Opin Pharmacother* 3:1191–1197, 2002.

17. Kemeny N, Huang Y, Cohen AM, et al. Hepatic arterial infusion of chemotherapy after resection of hepatic metastases from colorectal cancer. *N Engl J Med* 341:2039–2048, 1999.

18. Carriaga MT, Henson DE. Liver, gallbladder, extrahepatic bile ducts, and pancreas. *Cancer* 75:171–190, 1995.

19. Henderson JM, Barnes DS, Geisinger MA. Portal hypertension. *Curr Probl Surg* 35:379–452,1998.

20. Zimmerman H, Reichen J. Assessment of liver function in the surgical patient. In Blumgart LH, Fong Y, eds., *Surgery of the Liver and Biliary Tract*. Philadelphia, PA: W.B. Saunders, 2000:35–64.

21. Wiesner R, Edwards E, Freeman R, et al., and United Network for Organ Sharing Liver Disease Severity Score Committee. Model for end-stage liver disease (MELD) and allocation of donor livers. *Gastroenterology* 124:91–96, 2003.

22. Vauthey JN, Rousseau DL Jr. Liver imaging. A surgeon's perspective. *Clin Liver Dis* 6:271–295, 2002.

23. Bleicher RJ, Allegra DP, Nora DT, et al. Radiofrequency ablation in 447 complex unresectable liver tumors: lessons learned. *Ann Surg Oncol* 10:52–60, 2003.

24. Grace ND. Portal hypertension and variceal bleeding. *Cur Opin Gastro* 9:441–449, 1993.

25. Coldwell D, Ring EJM, Rees CR, et al. Multicenter investigation of the role of transjugular intrahepatic portosystemic shunt in the management of portal hypertension. *Radiology* 196:335–340, 1995.

26. Henderson JM Gilmore GT, Hooks MA, et al. Selective shunt in the management of variceal bleeding in the era of liver transplantation. *Ann Surg* 216(3):248–255, 1992.

PANCREAS

Bradley H. Collins, MD, FACS

INTRODUCTION

The pancreas is a functionally diverse, retroperitoneal organ that is located behind the posterior wall of the upper abdomen. It is situated in close proximity to a number of vital structures including the duodenum, spleen, common bile duct, inferior vena cava, and superior mesenteric vessels. The pancreas functions as both an exocrine and endocrine gland; therefore, disease processes that affect it can have life-altering and even life-threatening effects. Medical conditions such as intestinal malabsorption and impaired glucose homeostasis are representative of pancreatic pathophysiology and require daily medications for the management of symptoms. In addition, because of its location and complex lymphatic drainage, malignant neoplasms of this organ represent some of the most lethal cancers encountered.

One must keep in mind that a detailed discussion of the development and function of the pancreas as well as diseases that affect the gland is beyond the scope of this text. The purpose of this chapter is to briefly outline the anatomy, physiology, pathophysiology, and major neoplasms of the pancreas. It is meant to serve as an introduction to the organ and prompt readers to pursue more detailed accounts. An emphasis will be placed on those disease processes that require surgical management.

EMBRYOLOGY

The pancreas is endodermal in origin and develops from two buds. The *ventral bud* derives from the hepatic diverticulum and *dorsal bud* arises from the nascent duodenum. Clockwise rotation of the ventral bud then occurs around the duodenum, and the buds fuse during the sixth week of gestation to form the gland (Fig. 12-1). The ventral bud becomes the inferior head and the uncinate process, and the dorsal bud develops into the remainder of the gland (superior head, neck, body, and tail), as described in the Anatomy section. Failure in the rotation and/or fusion processes results in specific congenital

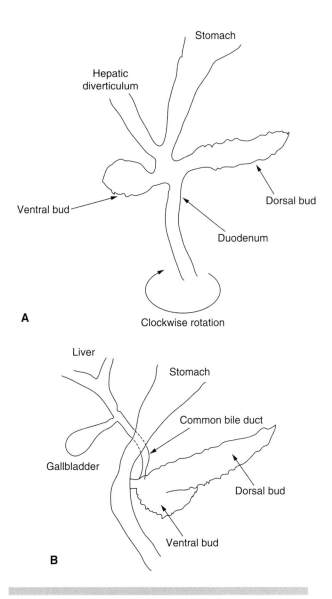

Figure 12-1 **(A) The pancreas develops from two distinct buds of endodermal origin. The ventral bud originates from the hepatic diverticulum and the dorsal bud from the nascent duodenum. The foregut undergoes clockwise rotation resulting in fusion of the pancreatic buds during the sixth week of gestation. (B) The ventral bud develops into the inferior pancreatic head and the uncinate process. The dorsal bud becomes the superior pancreatic head as well as the neck, body, and tail.**

abnormalities that may have clinical consequences (e.g., pancreas divisum, annular pancreas, and pancreatic heterotopia).

One of the most fascinating aspects of pancreatic embryology is the development of the ductal system via which the gland's exocrine secretions enter the gastrointestinal tract. Each of the pancreatic buds (ventral and dorsal) contains a main duct that spans the length of the bud. The duct of the ventral bud, commonly referred to as the *duct of Wirsung*, drains into the second portion of the duodenum through the major papilla (ampulla of Vater). It should be noted that the common bile duct also empties into the duodenum through the ampulla of Vater. Autopsy studies have revealed that the distal pancreatic and common bile ducts share a short, common channel as they exit the ampulla in 85 percent of individuals.[1] The pancreatic and common bile ducts exit the ampulla via separate orifices in 5 percent of cases. The duct of the dorsal bud, also known as the *duct of Santorini*, drains separately into the duodenum via the minor papilla.

As the ventral bud rotates and then combines with its dorsal counterpart, the proximal aspect ventral duct fuses with the distal third of the dorsal duct to form the major pancreatic duct of Wirsung that runs the length of the gland (Fig. 12-2). In most instances, the distal third of the dorsal duct (Santorini) remains in continuity with the major duct and drains the superior head of the

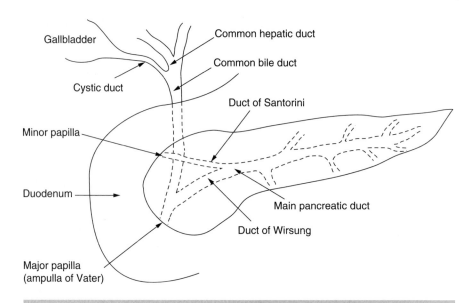

Figure 12-2 **The main duct of the ventral bud fuses with the main duct of the dorsal bud to form the main pancreatic duct (duct of Wirsung) that runs into the duodenum via the ampulla of Vater. The proximal segment of the dorsal bud becomes the duct of Santorini which drains through the minor papilla.**

pancreas into the duodenum via the minor papilla (Fig. 12-2). In a smaller percentage of individuals, the minor duct of Santorini is obliterated; therefore, the entire pancreas drains via the major duct. Five percent of individuals exhibit nonfusion of the pancreatic ducts, a condition known as *pancreas divisum*. In these patients, the majority of the pancreas drains via the minor duct, a structure that is not often suited to accommodate this volume of secretions. Chronic abdominal pain due to recurrent bouts of acute pancreatitis often ensues (see section Acute Pancreatitis).

ANATOMY

Gross

GLAND

The pancreas is an encapsulated, retroperitoneal structure of the posterior, upper abdomen that is situated behind the peritoneal layer lining the base of the lesser sac. Intra-abdominal organs overlying the pancreas include the stomach and transverse colon. The gland weighs approximately 100 g and ranges from 20 to 25 cm in length and tapers in diameter from 5 to 3 cm as one progresses distally. It is divided anatomically into four sections that correspond with the gross appearance of the gland as opposed to functional components: the (1) head and uncinate process, (2) neck, (3) body, and (4) tail (Fig. 12-3). The uncinate process is the inferior portion of the pancreatic head and corresponds to the ventral bud following rotation and fusion with the dorsal bud.

The head of the pancreas is located within the C-loop of the duodenum and is adherent to it through the first, second, and third portions (D1–D3). The pancreatic head and duodenum share a common blood supply; therefore, surgeons contemplating operations involving either structure must account for the adjacent organ. Approximately 50 percent of the pancreatic mass is located in the head and its uncinate process. The neck of the pancreas lies anterior to the origin of the portal vein as it derives from the junction of the superior mesenteric and splenic veins. The body of the pancreas extends from the left of the portal vein and is the portion of the gland that is exposed if the floor of the lesser sac is divided. Anterior to the left kidney is the tail of the pancreas. The pancreatic tail is actually positioned in close proximity to the splenic hilum; therefore, great care must be exercised to avoid the complications of pancreatic injury when splenectomy is performed. On the other hand, the spleen is usually included with the specimen during distal pancreatic resections due to a common blood supply.

DUCTAL SYSTEM

In most individuals, the exocrine pancreas is drained by the main duct of Wirsung that lies in the center of the gland and spans the length of the organ. It is 1 mm in diameter in the tail and gradually increases to approximately

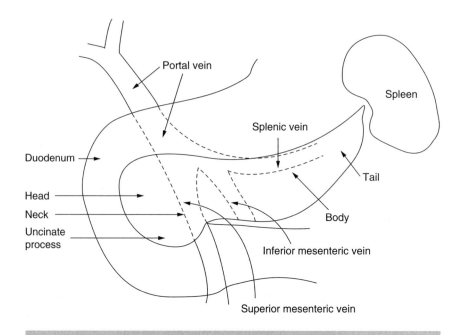

Figure 12-3 **The figure depicts the anatomic sections of the pancreas. The head is located within the C-loop of the duodenum. The uncinate process represents the embryologic ventral bud. The neck lies anterior to the origin of the portal vein. The body extends lateral to the portal vein. The tail is in close proximity to the splenic hilum.**

3.5 mm in the head. Numerous secondary ducts join the major duct along its length, thereby draining the tail, body, neck, and uncinate process. The majority of pancreatic exocrine products exit via the main duct and enter the duodenum through the ampulla of Vater, located 10–12 cm distal to the pylorus. The superior head of the pancreas is drained by the minor duct of Santorini that, in most, is in continuity proximally with the main pancreatic duct and empties distally into the duodenum via the minor papilla, which is situated a couple of centimeters proximal to the ampulla of Vater (Fig. 12-2).

The release of pancreatic exocrine secretions into the gastrointestinal tract is controlled by a series of sphincters. The distal main pancreatic duct has an individual sphincter, as does the distal common bile duct prior to merging to form the aforementioned common channel. The *sphincter of Oddi* surrounds the common channel at the ampulla of Vater and prevents the reflux of duodenal contents into the pancreaticobiliary tree. Complex neural and hormonal signals control each of the sphincters.

ARTERIAL SUPPLY

The pancreas has a rich blood supply that is derived from major branches of the aorta, specifically the celiac and superior mesenteric arteries.[2] The head of the gland is supplied by a series of arcades that often collateralize with other vessels. The anterior and posterior pancreaticoduodenal arcades are supplied directly by the gastroduodenal artery from above and the inferior pancreaticoduodenal artery from below. Arterial blood flow to the body and tail of the pancreas originates from the splenic artery which courses along the superior aspect of the gland en route to the spleen. Numerous branches of the splenic artery enter the gland along the body and tail including the dorsal, great, and caudal pancreatic arteries that exit along the inferior surface of the gland and collateralize with the inferior pancreaticoduodenal artery.

VENOUS DRAINAGE

As with most organ systems, venous drainage of the pancreas generally mirrors the arterial supply. The head is drained by the anterior and posterior venous arcades, which empty into the suprapancreatic portal vein. Drainage of the body and tail occurs via venous tributaries that enter the splenic vein. It is of note that all venous blood exiting the pancreas eventually enters the portal vein; therefore, endocrine products of the gland are subject to first pass effect by the liver.

INNERVATION

Both sympathetic and parasympathetic components of the autonomic nervous system innervate the pancreas. The former originates from the thoracic sympathetic chain, and the latter from the vagus nerves. Both the exocrine and endocrine functions of the pancreas are under sympathetic and parasympathetic control. Although a detailed account of the interactions between the nervous system and pancreas is beyond the scope of this text, in general, parasympathetic nerves *stimulate* pancreatic secretion (exocrine and endocrine), whereas the sympathetic system *inhibits* these functions.[3]

The pancreas also has a complicated intrinsic nervous system that influences control over exocrine and endocrine functions by means of a group of peptide neurotransmitters.[3] In addition, afferent sensory fibers are present and are thought to mediate abdominal pain associated with chronic pancreatitis and pancreatic cancer.

LYMPHATIC DRAINAGE

The lymph nodes and channels that drain the pancreas comprise an intricate network that empties into several regional lymphatic groups. Drainage of the pancreatic head occurs through the celiac and superior mesenteric nodes. The body and tail are drained by nodes that lie adjacent to the splenic blood vessels as they course along the superior border of the gland. These lymphatics then empty into larger, named nodal groups. The complex nature of the pancreatic lymphatic system renders curative resection of pancreatic malignancies an uncommon occurrence because of lymphatic metastases noted at laparotomy as well as undetected, residual lymphatic disease left in situ during pancreatectomy.

Microscopic

EXOCRINE PANCREAS

The pancreas has separate systems for its exocrine and endocrine functions. At least 80 percent of the pancreatic mass is devoted to synthesizing, secreting, and delivering exocrine products to the gastrointestinal tract. The significant components include acinar and centroacinar cells as well as the ductal apparatus. An acinus is a terminal ductule and is lined by centroacinar cells and surrounded by acinar cells. The centroacinar cells regulate fluid and electrolyte secretion, whereas the acinar cells secrete digestive enzymes (see Physiology). The terminal ductules combine to form first the *intralobular* ducts and then the *interlobular* ducts, the latter draining into the main pancreatic duct.

ENDOCRINE PANCREAS

Although the endocrine component of pancreatic function is considered the most vital aspect of the gland, merely 2 percent of the pancreatic mass is devoted to this function. Named after the German pathologist who discovered them in 1869, the *islets of Langerhans* contain the cells that are responsible for the production and release of pancreatic hormones. The 10^6 islets found in the average human pancreas are dispersed throughout the gland, although most are located in the body and tail.

Islets of Langerhans contain five major cell types, each of which produces at least one significant hormone: α (alpha), β (beta), δ (delta), $\delta1$ (delta 1), and pancreatic-polypeptide-producing (PP) cells. The most abundant cells are the insulin-producing β cells which comprise 75 percent of an islet's mass and are located in the core of the islet. The glucagon-producing α cells occupy a peripheral position and represent approximately 20 percent of an islet's mass. Glucose homeostasis is controlled by both α and β cells which generate glucagon and insulin, respectively (see Physiology). Hormonal products of the other cell types include somatostatin from δ cells, vasoactive intestinal peptide (VIP) from the $\delta1$ population and pancreatic polypeptide from PP cells. Interestingly, the concentration of β and δ cells in islets throughout the pancreas is consistent, whereas the concentration of the α and PP populations varies as a function of location.[4]

PHYSIOLOGY

The disparate functions of the pancreas can be divided into two distinct categories: *exocrine* and *endocrine*. Despite the seemingly unrelated nature of these functions, there is considerable interplay between the exocrine and endocrine processes.

Exocrine Pancreas

BICARBONATE

The centroacinar and ductular epithelial cells collectively secrete between 500 and 2000 mL of a clear, alkaline fluid into the duodenum per day. The pH ranges from 7.5 to 9.0 and is determined by the concentration of bicarbonate which is generated from carbonic acid by the enzyme carbonic anhydrase, a process controlled by centroacinar cells. Interestingly, the concentration of bicarbonate correlates directly with the rate of pancreatic secretion (Fig. 12-4). Secretin, a product of duodenal mucosal cells, is the primary stimulant of bicarbonate release; however, hormones such as cholecystokinin and gastrin also play a role. The appearance of acidic contents from the stomach in the duodenum is the prime stimulus for secretin release. The ensuing flux of bicarbonate serves the important role of neutralizing the stomach acid, thus protecting the mucosa of the duodenum and proximal jejunum. Although the explanation above is straightforward, the control of bicarbonate release

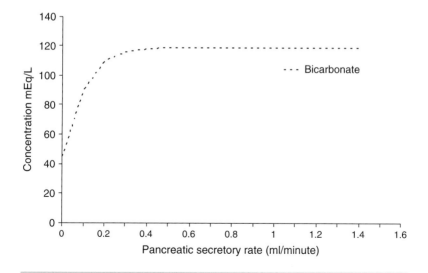

Figure 12-4 **As the pancreatic flow rate increases, the concentration of bicarbonate in the pancreatic effluent increases dramatically.**

by the pancreas is tightly governed by a series of neural and hormonal regulatory and counterregulatory pathways.

ENZYMES

The acinar cells' contribution to the pancreatic effluent is a set of enzymes responsible for the digestion of ingested materials (i.e., carbohydrates, fats, and proteins). Like the bicarbonate component of pancreatic juice, enzyme secretion is regulated by a number of neural and hormonal factors, with cholecystokinin serving as the primary stimulant. The enzyme products are amylase, multiple lipases, and several proteases. Amylase hydrolyzes glycogen and starch to simpler sugars such as glucose, whereas the lipases hydrolyze fat. Protein products are hydrolyzed by the proteases including trypsin, chymotrypsin, and the carboxypeptidases to name a few.

Because of its potent products, the pancreas would be at considerable risk for autodigestion were it not for protective mechanisms. Interestingly, with the exception of amylase, pancreatic enzymes are released into the duodenum as zymogens (inactive configurations). One of these enzymes, trypsinogen, is converted to its active form trypsin on entry in the duodenum by enterokinase, an enzyme synthesized by the duodenum. Trypsin then cleaves the other pancreatic enzymes to their active forms in the duodenum. Other pancreatic protective mechanisms include the presence of protease inhibitors within the gland that can inactivate trypsin as well as the other proteases.

Pancreatic exocrine insufficiency is a clinical syndrome occasionally encountered by general surgeons and is manifested by intestinal malabsorption. It is certainly present in patients who undergo total pancreatectomy; however, individuals with chronic pancreatitis or those who have undergone major pancreatic resection are at considerable risk.[5] In addition, several disorders are associated with pancreatic exocrine insufficiency including cystic fibrosis, Crohn's disease, and other autoimmune diseases.[6,7] Symptoms of malabsorption include diarrhea (abnormally foul smelling and fatty stools) and weight loss. Physical findings are consistent with malnutrition. Pancreatic enzyme replacements are available in tablet formulations that contain amylase, lipase, and protease components.

Endocrine Pancreas

INSULIN

As previously mentioned, the pancreas secretes a number of hormones that play an integral role in physiologic equilibrium. The most well known of these is insulin, a product of the β cell that is critical for the maintenance of glucose homeostasis. Insulin was discovered by the Canadian surgeon Frederick Banting for which he was awarded the 1923 Nobel Prize in Physiology/ Medicine.[8,9] Beta cells are stimulated to secrete insulin by glucose as well as hormonal and neural activity. The initial protein synthesized by β cells is proinsulin which is converted into its active form on the proteolytic cleavage of C-peptide. Insulin is released into the portal circulation where at least 50 percent is cleared during this first pass through the liver. The remaining insulin binds to insulin receptors which promote the *active* transport of glucose across the membranes of most cells, especially of the muscle and adipose tissue compartments. In addition, insulin stimulates the storage of glucose in the form of glycogen within the liver, as well as promotes fatty acid and protein synthesis.

GLUCAGON

Glucagon is a product of the α cells whose primary function is, in a general sense, to counter the effects of insulin by increasing glucose levels. Like insulin, it is synthesized in an inactive form, proglucagon, that requires cleavage to glucagon prior to release. The principal stimulator of glucagon secretion is hypoglycemia, whereas the prime inhibitor is insulin.

OTHERS

The physiologic role of somatostatin (δ cells) is generally inhibitory. Within the pancreas, it serves to inhibit the secretion of insulin and glucagon. It also functions as an inhibitor of biliary, gastric, and exocrine pancreatic secretion. VIP ($\delta 1$ cells) enhances the secretion of water into pancreatic juice and bile as well as promotes smooth muscle relaxation. PP cells plays a role in the inhibition of pancreatic exocrine secretions as well as other functions yet to be fully elucidated.

CONGENITAL ABNORMALITIES

Pancreas Divisum

Failure of the pancreatic ducts to fuse during rotation of the embryonic ventral and dorsal buds results in *pancreas divisum*, a condition found in approximately 5 percent of individualps.[1] In these instances, the majority of the gland's exocrine output drains via the duct of Santorini and into duodenum through the minor papilla. Although the condition is an incidental finding in the vast majority of affected persons, some individuals are plagued by chronic abdominal pain and others have recurrent episodes of acute pancreatitis that may progress to chronic pancreatitis.

It is thought that the symptoms and disease processes associated with pancreas divisum correlate with a relatively stenotic minor papilla. Endoscopic techniques involving minor papillotomy in combination with stenting of the duct of Santorini have produced mixed results.[10] Operative intervention (i.e., sphincteroplasty) may be necessary and involves transduodenal incision of the minor papilla, then tacking the ductal mucosa to the duodenal mucosa, thus *propping* the papilla open.

Annular Pancreas

Annular pancreas is an uncommon congenital anomaly that is usually diagnosed in neonates. It is the consequence of an abnormal connection between the ventral pancreas and the duodenum that on embryologic rotation results in a band of normal pancreatic tissue surrounding the second portion of the duodenum. This can produce duodenal obstruction and intractable, bilious vomiting in the neonatal period. Surgical bypass by side-to-side anastomosis of either the proximal to distal duodenum (duodenoduodenostomy) or proximal duodenum to proximal jejunum (duodenojejunostomy) is indicated for the relief of symptoms. Division of the constricting band of pancreatic tissue is not recommended as the risk of postoperative duodenal and pancreatic fistula formation is prohibitively high. Although primarily a pediatric syndrome, symptomatic annular pancreas has been reported in adults and also requires operative bypass.[11]

Pancreatic Heterotopia

Pancreatic heterotopia is a congenital abnormality that is manifested by ectopic rest of pancreatic tissue in the wall of the stomach, duodenum, jejunum, or ileum, usually in the submucosal layer. Most affected individuals are asymptomatic; however, obstruction, ulceration, bleeding, and malignant degeneration have been reported. In addition, foci of pancreas have been found as the lead points for intussusception within Meckel diverticulum. Surgical intervention is required for each of the aforementioned complications. In most instances, the diagnosis of pancreatic heterotopia is made after histologic evaluation of the resected specimen.

TRAUMA

Because of its retroperitoneal position, the pancreas is somewhat protected from injury; however, this anatomic location can complicate the diagnosis of trauma to the gland. Up to 12 percent of victims of severe abdominal trauma have an associated pancreatic injury.[12] Missed pancreatic injuries due to blunt or penetrating trauma can result in significant morbidity and mortality. Due to its close proximity to vital structures, 90 percent of the victims of pancreatic trauma have at least one associated injury.[12] An isolated injury to the pancreas is unusual. Because the pancreatic injury is often discovered at the time of surgical exploration for another injury, the trauma surgeon must be adept at their management. Early deaths of trauma victims with an identified pancreatic injury are usually due to hemorrhage from large blood vessels (e.g., aorta, inferior vena cava, portal vein, and superior mesenteric artery/vein). Late deaths are the result of a combination of sepsis and multisystem organ failure.

Mechanisms

Pancreatic injuries can range from contusions to complete transection of the gland. Because of its fixed position over the first lumbar vertebral body, the pancreas is susceptible to fracture and even disruption during blunt abdominal trauma. Deceleration injuries that occur during motor vehicle collisions due to contact with either the steering wheel or a functioning seat belt can yield this type of injury. Penetrating trauma of the pancreas is the result of projectiles or stab wounds and can occur anywhere in the gland.

Diagnosis

Hemodynamically unstable victims of blunt abdominal trauma usually require expeditious laparotomy for stabilization. During that time, evaluation of the pancreas should occur to rule out occult injury. Of course, obvious intraoperative signs of potential pancreatic injury (e.g., central retroperitoneal hematoma, edema in the lesser sac, and peripancreatic edema) mandate formal evaluation and definitive management. Hemodynamically stable, blunt abdominal trauma patients are routinely evaluated by abdominal computerized axial tomography (CAT) scanning which can identify signs associated with a pancreatic injury including fluid in the lesser sac, hematoma of the gland, central retroperitoneal hematoma, and fracture of the pancreas. Depending on their severity, these findings should prompt further evaluation of the pancreas, which may range from serial CAT scanning to endoscopic retrograde cholangiopancreatography (ERCP) to determine the integrity of the pancreatic duct.

Gunshot wounds to the abdomen are routinely explored; therefore, assessment of the pancreas should occur at that time. The surgeon's index of suspicion should be heightened if structures in the vicinity of the pancreas are injured or if the trajectory of the projectile is in the vicinity of the gland.

Management

The management of pancreatic injuries depends on the extent of the injury. Contusions and minor lacerations of the gland without ductal injury can usually be managed by closed suction drains placed during laparotomy. More significant trauma involving parenchymal injury with ductal disruption, including distal transaction of the gland, should be managed with distal pancreatectomy with attempts made to preserve the spleen in hemodynamically stable patients without associated splenic injury.[12,13] In patients with no prior pancreatic disease, 80 percent of the gland can be resected without affecting glucose homeostasis.

Proximal pancreatic injuries involving the duct are more difficult to manage and usually require subtotal pancreatectomy with wide drainage of the pancreatic stump.[12] Likewise, combined injuries of the pancreas and duodenum are challenging due to the proximity of vital structures. Occasionally, removal of both the pancreatic head and duodenum is required (see Whipple procedure); however, overall mortality rates approach 50 percent in some series.[12] Another option involves diverting stomach contents from the duodenum by pyloric exclusion and wide, external drainage of the pancreas.

PATHOPHYSIOLOGY

Diabetes Mellitus

Diabetes mellitus (DM) is the disease state marked by the inability to metabolize insulin properly due to the absence of insulin or a decreased sensitivity to insulin. *Type 1 DM*, formerly know as juvenile onset or insulin-dependent DM, is due to the development of antibodies against islets cells and insulin. This autoimmune response is thought to be initiated by some combination of viral infection and genetic factors. Patients with type 1 DM lack insulin production, so their survival is dependent on insulin replacement therapy. Insulin is administered by either intermittent subcutaneous injection or continuously via a pump. Conversely, *type 2 DM*, formerly know as non-insulin- dependent DM, develops when patients exhibit a significant decrease in insulin sensitivity. In fact, these patients are initially hyperinsulinemic and respond to such measures as diet control and weigh loss. In a significant number of type 2 diabetics, the insulin requirements eventually exceed the ability to increase insulin synthesis and the patient requires exogenous insulin therapy.

Diabetes is routinely managed by internists; however, general surgeons are frequently requested to participate in the management of complications of the disease. Late complications include vasculopathy (both micro- and macroangiopathy), nephropathy, retinopathy, peripheral neuropathy, and a host of autonomic, neuropathic abnormalities including gastroparesis, chronic diarrhea, and orthostatic hypotension. Diabetes quadruples one's risk for myocardial infarction or stroke. Although the incidence of some diabetic complications is virtually universal in long-term diabetics (retinopathy, neuropathy), others occur less frequently. For example, less than 40 percent of diabetics ever develop clinically significant nephropathy. The etiology of these complications is likely multifactorial, although high tissue levels of sorbitol, a glucose breakdown product and known tissue toxin, has been implicated. Glucose is degraded to sorbitol by aldose reductase, and it has been demonstrated that increased aldose reductase activity can lead to oxidative stress in the tissues at risk.[14]

Peripheral Vascular Disease

Diabetics have a 10 percent lifetime risk of major extremity amputation. In fact, 80 percent of major amputations are performed in diabetics. Peripheral vascular disease in this population is due to large or small vessel lesions or a combination of both. The lower extremities are most commonly affected. Large vessel, atherosclerotic lesions associated with rest pain, tissue loss, or life-altering claudication that are not amenable to percutaneous management require operative bypass with either saphenous vein or prosthetic grafts. In the absence of proximal lesions, small vessel disease cannot be treated with bypass techniques. In these cases, amputation (toe, transmetatarsal, below knee, or above knee) may be necessary for the management of diabetic foot infections and/or tissue loss. The efficacy of antibiotics is decreased in these regions due to diminished blood flow.

Nephropathy

The most common indication for kidney transplantation in the United States is renal failure secondary to diabetic nephropathy (types 1 and 2). Kidneys for transplant recipients were generally obtained from deceased donors; however, the advent of the *laparoscopic* donor nephrectomy technique has resulted in living donors supplying greater than 50 percent of kidneys at many transplant centers. Following successful kidney transplantation, diabetics remain at risk for allograft loss due to recurrent diabetic nephropathy.

PANCREAS TRANSPLANTATION

For those type 1 diabetics with minimal medical comorbidities, pancreas transplantation has been performed successfully with excellent long-term results. Type 2 diabetic patients are not candidates for transplantation as their metabolic defect is due to insulin insensitivity as opposed to a complete absence of the hormone. The differentiation between types 1 and 2 is imperative prior to consideration for pancreas transplantation and may be accomplished by serum C-peptide sampling (type 1 diabetic patients lack the endogenous insulin breakdown product C-peptide due to a complete absence of insulin). Currently, whole organ pancreas transplantation represents the only *cure* for type 1 diabetes as recipients have normal glucose tolerance. The Diabetes Control and Complications Trial Research Group demonstrated that intensive blood glucose control resulted in a delay in the onset and progression of the secondary complications of diabetes, specifically nephropathy, retinopathy, and neuropathy when compared to the standard therapy of twice daily insulin injections.[15] Armed with these data, transplant surgeons sought to use pancreas transplantation as means of preventing and/or treating the secondary effects of the disease.

Because the incidence of secondary complications in diabetics is unpredictable, pancreas transplantation is usually reserved for those patients who have developed renal failure secondary to diabetic nephropathy. In most instances, patients receive simultaneous pancreas and kidney transplants from the same deceased donor. A less common scenario involves deceased donor pancreas transplantation into the recipient of a long-term kidney transplant from either a living or deceased donor. The least used approach is solitary pancreas transplantation in those brittle, type 1 diabetics who have failed insulin pump therapy and experience life-threatening episodes of hypoglycemia.

The long-term results of simultaneous pancreas/kidney transplantation are excellent with greater than 60 percent of recipients demonstrating excellent pancreatic function at 10 years.[16] The role of successful pancreas transplantation in the treatment of the secondary complications of diabetes cannot be overstated. Numerous studies have demonstrated that pancreas transplantation improves native nephropathy (in solitary pancreas recipients), microangiopathy, and neuropathy, both peripheral and autonomic.[17-20] Although retinopathy does not improve, it has been shown to stabilize in most recipients of successful pancreas transplants.[21]

ISLET CELL TRANSPLANTATION

One of the most exciting areas of clinical and research innovation in the field of transplantation has been the recent evolution of pancreatic islet cell transplantation. Prior to the application of modern techniques and medications, 1-year survival for clinical islet cell transplants was less than 10 percent. Some of the most commonly used immunosuppressants, such as steroids and tacrolimus, have adverse effects on the pancreatic β cell function. Shapiro and colleagues of the University of Alberta developed a protocol of islet cell isolation, purification, and implantation that incorporated an immunosuppression regimen that was not toxic to β cells.[22] Current protocols entail the infusion into the portal venous circulation either percutaneously or by minilaparotomy via a mesenteric vein. Ultimately, the islets reside intrahepatically where they release insulin in response to blood glucose levels.

The major advantage of islet cell transplantation is that it is relatively noninvasive and can be performed as an outpatient procedure. Whole organ pancreas transplantation requires a generous laparotomy and carries the attendant risks of major surgery (hemorrhage, abscess, graft pancreatitis, and so on). In addition, several weeks of recuperation are required for a patient to return to their normal level of function. The disadvantages of islet cell transplantation have limited its widespread application. Facilities to process pancreases into transplantation-grade islets are expensive. Most recipients require the islets of more than one donor pancreas to achieve and maintain insulin independence, a problem that only exacerbates an already critical organ shortage. In addition, the recipients of *successful* islet cell transplants have been shown to have impaired glucose tolerance. Theoretically, this has the potential to reduce the impact of transplantation on the secondary complications of diabetes that is observed in whole organ pancreas recipients.

Acute Pancreatitis

Inflammation of the exocrine pancreas can produce the clinical syndrome known as acute pancreatitis, a common cause of abdominal pain. Most patients have reversible glandular injury that follows a self-limited course and responds to supportive measures; however, 15 percent of victims develop a severe form of the disease that affects multiple organ systems and tests the limits of critical-care medicine. Because patients with acute pancreatitis usually present with abdominal pain, surgeons are usually involved in their evaluation. In addition, surgeons are intimately involved in the management of patients with routine cases as well as those who develop complications of disease.

Etiology

Estimates indicate that 0.5 percent of the population in the United States will experience an episode of acute pancreatitis during their lifetimes.[23] A number of etiologic factors have been associated with the development of acute pancreatitis. The final common pathway is inflammation secondary to autodigestion of the gland by the activated pancreatic enzymes described earlier in this chapter. Regardless of the cause, all patients are at risk for progressing to the life-threatening form of the disease.

ETHANOL

In the United States, ethanol use is the leading cause of acute pancreatitis, accounting for at least 50 percent of cases. Elucidation of the mechanism by which ethanol leads to acute pancreatitis is the subject of a number of hypotheses. Some investigators believe that ethanol induces spasm of the sphincter of Oddi which, in the presence of a common pancreaticobiliary channel, can lead to bile reflux into the pancreatic duct.[24] In addition, spasm of the sphincter can lead to hypertension of the pancreatic duct which may promote the leakage of pancreatic enzymes and activating proteases into the gland. The role of ethanol as a direct pancreatic toxin has also been investigated.[25] Although the association between ethanol use and the incidence of pancreatitis is linear, only 5 percent of alcoholics will ever develop the disease.[26]

GALLSTONES

Biliary tract stone disease accounts for approximately 30 percent of cases of acute pancreatitis in the United States. Pancreatic ductal hypertension secondary to transient obstruction of the ampulla by a migrating gallstone or impaction of a stone in the ampulla have been implicated as etiologies, the former occurring much more frequently. Only 5 percent of patients with cholelithiasis will ever develop acute pancreatitis.[27]

POSTPROCEDURAL

Hyperamylasemia occurs commonly following imaging of the pancreaticobiliary tree via ERCP; however, approximately 1 percent of patients undergoing the procedure develop acute pancreatitis. Measures such as limiting the pressure of contrast injection into the pancreatic duct likely contribute to the minimal incidence.

Although uncommon, acute pancreatitis can complicate operative procedures. Patients undergoing upper abdominal operations develop pancreatitis secondary to manipulation or injury of the gland or the usage of contrast injection in the biliary system. Operations in regions remote to the pancreas, such as cardiac procedures, may induce pancreatitis through perturbations in blood flow to the gland. Abdominal trauma victims can develop pancreatitis by direct injury of the gland or duct or from extrinsic compression by edema, collection of fluid, or hematoma.

PHARMACOLOGIC AGENTS

A number of medications have been implicated in the development of acute pancreatitis: thiazide diuretics, tetracyclines, corticosteroids, estrogen preparations, azathioprine, pentamidine, procainamide, methyldopa, and valproic acid. The pathogenesis of drug-induced pancreatitis is unknown.

INFECTION

A variety of infectious agents have been linked to the development of acute pancreatitis. Assorted bacteria, fungi, viruses, and parasites have been implicated.

CLINICAL SYNDROMES

Clinical syndromes known to be associated with acute pancreatitis include hyperparathyroidism, hypertriglyceridemia, autoimmune disease, and pancreas divisum. Of course, there are those patients in whom a cause is never identified, that is, idiopathic.

Presentation

Ninety percent of patients with acute pancreatitis complain of abdominal pain.[28] It is usually a continuous, midepigastric sensation that ranges from mild to excruciating. In 50 percent of cases, the pain radiates to the back.[28] Inflammation of the pancreas can induce ileus, so it is not surprising that approximately 70 percent of patients have nausea and vomiting.[28] There is often a delay in the diagnosis of acute pancreatitis in the postoperative setting as abdominal pain, nausea, and vomiting frequently complicate abdominal procedures.

Surgeons are routinely involved in the evaluation of patients with abdominal pain and become involved in the care of patients ultimately diagnosed with acute pancreatitis during the evaluation stage in the emergency department or in consultation. Typical vital signs included low-grade fever and tachycardia, the latter due to pain or dehydration secondary to third-space fluid losses into the retroperitoneum. Patients with severe cases can present in shock (hypotension, oliguria, and mental status changes). The abdomen is often distended with diminished bowel sounds secondary to ileus. Abdominal examination is variable and can range from mild epigastric tenderness to frank peritonitis. Approximately 3 percent of patients will have one or both of the classic signs associated with severe, hemorrhagic pancreatitis: Cullen sign (periumbilical bruising) and Grey Turner sign (bilateral flank bruising).[29–31]

Diagnosis

The diagnosis of acute pancreatitis is based on the patient's history and physical findings in the setting of hyperamylasemia. One must be cognizant that no symptom, physical sign, biochemical marker, or radiographic finding is universal to acute pancreatitis.

LABORATORY

Increased serum amylase levels were first associated with acute pancreatitis in 1929 by surgeons Robert Elman and Evarts Graham.[32] During an attack of acute pancreatitis, amylase is released from the pancreatic acinar cells. In fact, hyperamylasemia usually develops within a few hours of the onset of symptoms and peaks within 24–48 h of the attack. The amylase level normalizes over the next 5–7 days unless the course is complicated by abscess, pseudocyst, or ongoing pancreatic injury (see section Complications). Greater than 80 percent of patients with acute pancreatitis develop hyperamylasemia; however, there is *no* correlation between the serum amylase level and severity of the episode.[33]

Since less than half of the absolute serum amylase level is of pancreatic origin, the presence of hyperamylasemia is not always attributable to acute pancreatitis. A number of other disease processes are associated with this finding including salivary gland disease (mumps, parotitis), perforated peptic ulcer, diabetic ketoacidosis, acute appendicitis, mesenteric vascular occlusion, ruptured aortic aneurysm, renal dysfunction (diminished amylase clearance), and a host of others. Serum amylase is actually composed of a number of isoamylases that can be fractionated. These determinations are especially useful in differentiating salivary gland amylase from other sources. Although pancreatic isoamylase is a product of the pancreas, it has been shown to be elevated in some of the aforementioned disease processes in the absence of pancreatic inflammation. In summary, hyperamylasemia is a fairly sensitive marker of acute pancreatitis in the setting of the appropriate symptoms and physical signs; however, it is not specific for the disease.

Lipase is another acinar cell enzyme that is used in the diagnosis of acute pancreatitis. Since its primary source is the pancreas, it was once thought to be more specific for acute pancreatitis than amylase; however, a number of other disease processes can produce hyperlipasemia. Lipase does have a unique role in the diagnosis of acute pancreatitis. Like amylase, its level rises and peaks soon after an attack; however, normalization of serum lipase levels occurs over at least 2 weeks. Patients who present to medical attention late in the course of the disease may still have hyperlipasemia, thus lending credence to the suspected diagnosis.

In general, care must be exercised when interpreting serum pancreatic enzyme levels in the absence of a patient's medical history and physical findings. Investigators continue to search for the ideal serum marker for acute pancreatitis.[34]

RADIOLOGIC

Radiographic studies have been shown to be quite valuable in confirming the diagnosis of acute pancreatitis. Although plain film findings are not specific for the disease, they certainly support the diagnosis in most of the severe cases. The evaluation of any patient with abdominal pain should include a chest x-ray as well as an abdominal series. Although patients with acute pancreatitis may exhibit a left pleural effusion, left basilar atelectasis, or elevation of the left hemidiaphragm, the most vital role of the chest film in this population is to rule out other pathology, especially surgical emergencies as evidenced by pneumoperitoneum. Abdominal films may demonstrate the sentinel loop sign in the upper abdomen, a focally dilated segment of proximal jejunum secondary to ileus.

Ultrasonography represents a noninvasive method of evaluating the pancreas that is usually readily available and can be performed rapidly. In a significant number of the patients with acute pancreatitis, the pancreas cannot be visualized due to overlying bowel gas. Findings consistent with acute pancreatitis include pancreatic enlargement and edema in the lesser sac, whereas glandular necrosis or pancreatic hemorrhage is indicative of more severe cases. The most significant role for ultrasonography in the evaluation of patients with acute pancreatitis is determining whether the biliary tree played a role in the development of the disease as indicated by the presence of stones.

The gold standard for diagnosing and grading acute pancreatitis is CT scan. Findings confirming mild cases of the diagnosis include glandular enlargement, parenchymal edema, and inflammation of the peripancreatic fat. Hemorrhage and glandular necrosis are manifestations of more severe forms of the disease. Using various grading systems, CT radiologists can serve a role in predicting prognosis.[35]

ERCP is generally avoided due to the risk of exacerbating the disease process with contrast injection into the pancreatic duct.

Prognostication

On presentation, it is difficult to predict which patients with acute pancreatitis will progress to the life-threatening form of the disease unless they have evidence of multisystem involvement (shock) or necrosis of the gland documented on CT scan. A number of methods have been developed to assist clinicians in determining which patients are at increase risk for disease progression that are based on clinical criteria readily available on presentation or soon thereafter.

The classic system, developed by surgeon John Ranson and reported in 1974, is still used today.[36] It is composed of 11 factors that are determined during the initial 48 h of medical care (Table 12-1). Note that serum amylase level is not a criterion since it does not correlate with severity illness. There is a linear relationship between the number of criteria present and the mortality rate. For instance, those patients with two or fewer signs have a mortality rate of approximately 1 percent, whereas those with seven or more signs have a mortality rate that approaches 100 percent. Other severity of illness stratification methods have been applied to acute pancreatitis, such as the acute physiology and chronic health evaluation (APACHE) and the Glasgow system.[37]

Treatment

The diagnosis of acute pancreatitis warrants admission to a hospital as the clinical picture on presentation may deteriorate dramatically over a period of hours to a couple of days. Patients with severe attacks should be managed in an intensive care unit.

GENERAL

Most cases of acute pancreatitis are self-limited and respond to supportive measures. These include intravenous resuscitation to counteract fluid losses due to third spacing into intestines affected by ileus and the inflamed retroperitoneum and as well as other factors such as emesis. Initially, crystalloid solutions are generally used; however, colloids may be necessary to maintain the oncotic pressure. Adequacy of hydration should be confirmed

Table 12-1 **Ranson's Criteria**

At admission
1. Age >55 years
2. White blood cell count >16,000 cells/mm3
3. Blood glucose >200 mg/dL
4. Aspartate aminotransferase (AST) >250 IU/dL
5. Serum lactate dehydrogenase (LDH) >350 IU/L

During initial 48 h
6. Decrease in hematocrit of >10%
7. Serum calcium <8 mg/dL
8. Arterial PaO2 <60 mmHg
9. Increase in blood urea nitrogen (BUN) >5 mg/dL
10. Base deficit >4 meq/L
11. Estimated fluid sequestration >6 L

by hourly urine output assessments via a Foley catheter (greater than 0.5 mL/kg/h for adults and greater than 1.0 mL/kg/h for children). Central venous monitoring may be necessary for those patients in whom resuscitative measures are unsuccessful. Patients with prolonged shock may develop renal failure secondary to acute tubular necrosis and require dialysis.

Electrolyte abnormalities should be identified and corrected. Hypocalcemia frequently accompanies severe, acute pancreatitis and is likely due to deposition into areas of fat necrosis. Intravenous replacement therapy is the treatment of choice. Hyperkalemia secondary to tissue necrosis or renal insufficiency should be treated acutely with intravenous insulin/glucose, inhaled bronchodilators, exchange resin enemas, or dialysis. Hyperglycemia can exacerbate hypovolemia due to osmotic diuresis; therefore, insulin therapy should be initiated early, and an insulin drip should be used to control labile blood glucose levels.

Nasogastric suctioning benefits those patients with acute pancreatitis who have vomiting due to ileus. In the early stages of acute pancreatitis, clinicians usually recommend the avoidance of oral intake so as not to stimulate the exocrine pancreas in an attempt to achieve a state of pancreatic rest. In fact, it was once thought that total parenteral nutrition (TPN) was *necessary* to offset the effects of catabolism associated with acute pancreatitis. The results of recent studies have contradicted this adage as patients have been shown to benefit from the early addition of enteral nutrition administered via the jejunum or even by nasogastric tube.[38,39]

Severe cases of acute pancreatitis necessitating management in an intensive care unit may require support of individual organ systems: ventilator, hemodialysis, pressors, blood products, and so on.

GALLSTONE PANCREATITIS

The management of gallstone pancreatitis deserves special mention. Because of the significant risk of recurrent pancreatitis due to additional gallstones, patients should undergo cholecystectomy, preferably via the laparoscopic approach, during the index admission. Surgeons will usually defer cholecystectomy until the amylase normalizes or there is a consistent downward trend in the serum level. Intraoperative imaging of the common bile duct is usually performed by cholangiography. The identification of ductal stones mandates common bile duct exploration at the time of cholecystectomy or subsequent stone retrieval by ERCP with or without concomitant sphincterotomy.

Complications

Although the majority of cases of acute pancreatitis resolve spontaneously without sequelae, disease-specific complications are associated with significant morbidity and mortality. Frequently, these complications require surgical intervention. Early deaths are usually due to hemodynamic issues, whereas late deaths are the result of infection leading to sepsis and multisystem organ failure.

INFECTED PANCREATIC NECROSIS

Patients with pancreatic necrosis demonstrated on CT scan are at highest risk for the development of complications of the disease. For those patients who continue exhibiting clinical deterioration despite maximal supportive care, early operative debridement of the necrotic tissue is indicated. During these operations, formal pancreatic resection is avoided in favor of debriding nonviable tissues.

The use of antibiotics in the early stages of acute pancreatitis has been debated in the past. These agents are usually avoided in the absence of documented infection (pancreatic or otherwise); however, patients with glandular necrosis are at risk for the development of pancreatic infection and would likely benefit from systemic antibiotics, although the debate continues.[40] Microbiologic sampling of the pancreas and associated collections by CT-guidance may differentiate sterile from infected necrosis so that antibiotic therapy may be initiated and tailored appropriately. The conversion of pancreatic necrosis from sterile to infected is often heralded by clinical deterioration and is associated with increased mortality. This subset of patients benefits from early operative debridement with wide drainage.[41] Some patients require multiple trips to the operating room for staged debridement, whereas others benefit from leaving the initial abdominal wound open and performing dressing changes at the bedside to permit healing by secondary intent. Pancreatic fistulae occasionally complicate operative debridement and usually close without specific intervention, although octreotide administration may accelerate the process by inhibiting exocrine secretion. There are reports in the literature of successful, nonoperative management of infected pancreatic necrosis.[42]

Briefly, *pancreatic abscess* may be managed by percutaneous drainage techniques or operative debridement with wide drainage as described earlier. Antibiotic coverage is determined by the results of microbiologic assays.

PANCREATIC PSEUDOCYSTS

Pancreatic pseudocysts are fluid-filled collections of pancreatic secretions that complicate episodes of acute pancreatitis most commonly secondary to ethanol use. As the name implies, a pancreatic pseudocyst does not have a true epithelial lining. It is the result of disruption of some portion of the pancreatic duct or radical, and its wall is formed by the adjacent viscera (stomach, colon, small intestinal loops). Symptoms and signs of pancreatic pseudocysts are caused by the displacement of affected organs as the collections enlarge (pain, dysphagia, nausea, vomiting, ileus, jaundice, abdominal mass, and persistent hyperamylasemia).

The management of pancreatic pseudocysts is dependent on a number of factors.[43] Acute pseudocysts can be observed, provided the symptoms are not debilitating, and followed radiologically until they resolve. Symptomatic cysts may be treated with indwelling drains placed by CT-guidance since simple aspiration is associated with a high rate of recurrence. Over period of weeks, cysts that do not resolve usually develop thickening of the wall. A variety of methods have been used to treat symptomatic pseudocysts once they have *matured*. Those that abut the stomach may be chronically drained into the stomach by endoscopic or open, transgastric techniques. The duodenum and jejunum are also potential targets for operative drainage, provided that anatomic considerations are conducive. Laparoscopic approaches have also been used. An antecedent episode of acute pancreatitis usually implies the benign nature of pseudocysts; however, during operative intervention, a biopsy of the pseudocyst wall should be obtained to rule out cystadenocarcinoma.

HEMORRHAGE

Hemorrhage is an uncommon complication of acute pancreatitis. The most common source is the gastrointestinal tract, and etiologies include peptic ulcer disease, gastritis, and stress ulceration. Prophylaxis with proton pump inhibitors should be employed for all patients. The pancreatic enzymes liberated during an attack of acute pancreatitis can also erode arteries resulting in free hemorrhage or pseudoaneurysmal formation. The most commonly affected vessels in descending order are the splenic, gastroduodenal, inferior pancreaticoduodenal, and the superior pancreaticoduodenal arteries. Pseudoaneurysms can also develop when a pseudocyst erodes into an artery and blood fills the cavity. Patients with hemodynamic instability unresponsive to blood replacement warrant emergent laparotomy. Those exhibiting hemodynamic stability may undergo angiography and embolization.[44]

Erosion of visceral veins by pancreatic enzymes can result in thrombosis. The splenic vein is most commonly involved. A long-term sequela of this complication is the development of gastric varices which may be a source of massive upper gastrointestinal bleeding. Splenectomy is the treatment of choice and is curative.

Chronic Pancreatitis

Progressive and irreversible destruction of the exocrine pancreas produces the clinical syndrome of chronic pancreatitis. Ongoing injury of the gland secondary to chronic ethanol excess or obstruction of the pancreatic duct leads to fibrosis of the parenchyma. Other etiologies include autoimmune disease and chronic malnutrition as well as hereditary and idiopathic causes.

Presentation

In the United States, the typical clinical scenario is a patient with a long history of alcohol abuse associated with previous attacks of acute pancreatitis.

Initially, patients have intermittent abdominal pain that coincides with the acute attacks; however, the pain becomes constant as the gland fibroses. For most patients with chronic pancreatitis, pain is the foremost symptom. It is a visceral sensation that is located in the epigastric area and radiates to the upper back between the shoulder blades. Because the pain is exacerbated by eating, patients with advanced disease are often malnourished. Fatty stools are indicative of exocrine insufficiency. It is of note that clinically significant pancreatic endocrine insufficiency, as defined by insulin dependence, occurs in less than half of the patients suffering from chronic pancreatitis.

Diagnosis

Serum biochemical measures do not contribute to the diagnosis of chronic pancreatitis. Amylase levels are usually normal due to the contribution from the salivary glands. They are elevated if the patient develops concomitant acute pancreatitis or has a pseudocyst.

Imaging studies play a major role in the evaluation of chronic pancreatitis. Approximately 50 percent of patients have calcification of the gland that can be seen on abdominal plain films or CT scans. Other CT findings consistent with the diagnosis include glandular atrophy and dilatation of the pancreatic duct. The tests of greatest utility in the evaluation of chronic pancreatitis and the status of the duct are ERCP and, more recently, the less invasive magnetic resonance cholangiopancreatography (MRCP).[45] Findings can range from irregularity of the secondary and tertiary ducts in the earliest stages of the disease to marked dilatation of the duct (in excess of 10 mm) in the latter stages. Patients frequently have pseudocysts, either intra- or extrapancreatic, that are visible on ERCP or MRCP.

Treatment

Because there is no *cure* for chronic pancreatitis, therapeutic options are based on controlling the symptoms. These should include abstinence from alcohol, which has been shown to decrease the degree of pain. Patients require narcotics for relief of abdominal pain, and drug dependence is common in this population. Pancreatic enzyme replacements and dietary fat restriction are used to treat steatorrhea, and diabetes is managed with standard, intermittent insulin injections.

The management of pain tends to dictate the course of treatment options for patients with chronic pancreatitis. Percutaneous celiac plexus blocks have been used with assorted agents; however, the effect is short lived in that subset of patients in whom it works. A number of operative techniques have been developed to manage the intractable abdominal pain associated with chronic pancreatitis. A CT scan should be part of the preoperative workup to rule out a concomitant pancreatic malignancy, as the operative plan would be significantly altered. In general, the operative management of chronic pancreatitis involves either ductal drainage procedures or resectional procedures.

Patients with long-segment pancreatic ductal dilatation of at least 8 mm are candidates for the Puestow procedure, a long, side-to-side anastomosis of the pancreatic duct to a Roux-en-Y limb of jejunum. The anterior surface of the pancreas is exposed through the lesser sac and the duct is identified by aspiration with a small gauge needle. The pancreas is then divided longitudinally including the duct. After the Roux limb is fashioned, the side-to-side anastomosis is performed. Approximately 70 percent of patients have complete or significant pain relief 5 years after the Puestow procedure.[46]

Chronic pancreatitis sufferers with diminutive ductal systems may be candidates for pancreatic resection. The type of resection is dependent on the location of abnormalities as defined by CT scan and ERCP. Disease of the body and tail may be managed by distal pancreatectomy with or without splenectomy.[47] If the spleen is removed, the patient should receive the appropriate immunizations preoperatively. The procedure may be complicated by diabetes if too much pancreas is removed (greater than 60 percent). Disease localized to the pancreatic head may require pancreaticoduodenectomy or some variation thereof (see Whipple procedure).[48,49]

Total pancreatectomy is performed in one of two settings: as the initial operation or as a salvage procedure for those patients who have had prior resection. The resultant diabetes is often difficult to control. Patients have received islet cell autotransplants from their own total pancreatectomy specimens; however, the results have been generally poor due to the difficulties associated with procuring viable islets from a fibrosed gland.

NEOPLASIA

Pancreatic neoplasms can involve the exocrine or endocrine components of the gland. Most of these tumors derive from the exocrine pancreatic ductal system and are quite lethal. The endocrine tumors have less malignant potential, however their physiologic effects can be devastating.

Exocrine Neoplasms

Greater than 90 percent of pancreatic malignancies are adenocarcinomas of ductal origin. This form of cancer is the fifth leading cause of cancer death in the United States. The most significant risk factors appear to be cigarette smoking and high dietary fat consumption. Most victims are in their seventh decade of life, men are affected twice as often as women, and Blacks carry double the risk of Whites. Despite advances in surgical techniques and chemotherapy, it continues to have one of the lowest survival rates of any form of cancer.

Presentation

The symptoms and signs of pancreatic cancer are variable and, in part, are dependent on the location of the tumor. Approximately 70 percent of adenocarcinomas arise in the head of the gland, 15 percent in the body, 10 percent in the tail, and the remainder spread throughout the gland. Unfortunately, due to the location of the pancreas and complex lymphatic drainage, the majority of patients have metastatic disease on presentation; therefore, some of the symptoms and signs are actually indicative of advanced disease.

Patients with tumors of the pancreatic head complain most often of weight loss, jaundice, pain, anorexia, dark urine, acholic stools, nausea, and vomiting, in descending order. Weight loss is likely secondary to a combination of anorexia, vomiting, and metastatic disease. Jaundice, dark urine, and acholic stools are due to obstruction of the bile duct by the tumor. Gastric outlet obstruction by the tumor leads to vomiting. The symptom profile for lesions of the body and tail in descending order include weight loss, pain, weakness, and nausea.

Diagnosis

Serum biochemistry abnormalities in patients with pancreatic cancer are due to extrahepatic obstruction of the bile duct. These include elevations in conjugated bilirubin and alkaline phosphatase. The tumor markers CA 19-9 and carcinoembryonic antigen (CEA) may also be elevated in some patients; however, they have insufficient specificity to serve as screening tests.

Radiographic techniques have proven quite useful in the diagnosis and staging of pancreatic cancer. The CT scan plays a major role in identifying the lesion as well as determining the involvement of major blood vessels that would indicate unresectability, such as the portal vein and superior mesenteric or hepatic arteries. Angiography can also demonstrate vascular involvement, but is usually unnecessary. Endoscopic ultrasound has shown to be of benefit in locating small tumors, determining vascular involvement, identifying regional lymph node involvement, and enabling fine-needle aspiration of lesions to confirm the diagnosis.[50]

The tumor/node/metastasis (TMN) staging system has been applied to adenocarcinoma of the pancreas and is useful in determining prognosis. Intraoperatively, the stage frequently worsens due to findings not noted on preoperative imaging studies.

Treatment

Complete surgical resection represents the only chance for cure in patients with pancreatic adenocarcinoma. Unfortunately, approximately 90 percent of patients are determined to have unresectable disease during the evaluation phase. A thorough preoperative evaluation that includes radiographic findings such as vascular invasion or metastatic disease (liver, lymph nodes) rules out most of these individuals. At some centers, patients who are deemed resectable undergo laparoscopy just prior to attempted open resection to rule out metastatic disease such as peritoneal or serosal implants or liver lesions not noted on CT scans.

Patients with tumors of the pancreatic head who are ultimately determined to be resection candidates undergo pancreaticoduodenectomy, a complex and time-consuming operation also known as the Whipple procedure.[51] Although Dr. Whipple's original report in 1935 described resection of tumors of the ampulla of Vater, the technique was applied to pancreatic head masses. The procedure is performed through either a generous midline incision or a subcostal incision extended bilaterally (Chevron incision). A thorough inspection of the peritoneal, serosal, and liver surfaces is performed to rule out metastatic implants which would likely result in conversion of the operation to a less demanding palliation procedure. The duodenum and pancreatic head are mobilized so that the extent of the tumor may be ascertained. Many surgeons will perform a needle biopsy at this point to confirm the diagnosis. Others will proceed with the operation given the magnitude of preoperative data supporting the diagnosis. During this time, an assessment is made for enlarged lymph nodes around the pancreas and along the celiac axis. Enlarged nodes should be biopsied and sent for frozen section. In most settings, the presence of lymph node metastases is a contraindication to definitive resection. The plane between the anterior surface of the portal vein and posterior surface of the pancreas is then developed. Most surgeons would consider the tumor unresectable if there is evidence of portal vein invasion. Surgeons at referral centers for pancreas cancer who practice advanced techniques will consider including the involved portal vein and/or superior mesenteric artery with the specimen and then reconstruct the resected vessel with femoral, saphenous, or internal jugular vein.

If the decision is made to proceed with the Whipple procedure, the antrum of the stomach is divided, cholecystectomy is performed, the common bile duct is divided, and the jejunum is divided several centimeters distal to the ligament of Treitz. Some surgeons perform a pylorus-preserving variation of the Whipple procedure as postoperative gastric emptying is improved. The resection is completed on transection of the gland through the neck as it lies over the portal vein. Reconstruction of the gastrointestinal tract requires three anastomoses using the free end of jejunum. The pancreatic stump is anastomosed to the end of the jejunum (pancreaticojejunostomy), the bile duct to the side of the jejunum (hepaticojejunostomy), and the antrum to the side of the jejunum (gastrojejunostomy), several centimeters distal to the aforementioned anastomoses.

Tumors of the pancreatic body and tail are rarely discovered prior to metastasis due to the paucity of symptoms. Resection usually includes the distal pancreas and spleen.

Adjuvant protocols involving chemotherapy and/or intra- or postoperative radiation have been used in the management of pancreatic cancer; however, the results have been relatively inconclusive.

Outcome

Despite medical and surgical advances, the overall mortality rate of pancreatic adenocarcinoma has remained fairly unchanged for decades. Five-year survival following resection remains less than 10 percent, although some high-volume centers report slightly better results which some would attribute to referral patterns and patient selection.[52] Patients whose tumors are resected when they are small (less than 2 cm) have better outcome; however, discovery and resection of a tumor this small is rare.

Palliative Therapy

Patients with unresectable tumors of the pancreatic head are at risk for the development of biliary and/or gastric outlet obstruction. Symptoms of these complications include jaundice/debilitating pruritus and chronic vomiting, respectively. These patients are candidates for palliative double bypass procedures involving formation of Roux limb of jejunum followed by formation of hepatico- and gastrojejunostomies. In those patients who undergo biliary bypass procedures, the risk of developing subsequent gastric outlet obstruction is approximately 20 percent.[53] Some surgeons recommend performing prophylactic gastrojejunostomy in those patients explored for biliary obstruction. Endoscopic technology has improved to such a degree that the endoscopic placement of biliary and duodenal stents has spared patients the morbidity associated with an extensive laparotomy.[54]

Cystic tumors

A number of cystic neoplasms of the pancreas have been described. The lesions are rare, and associated symptoms and operative management depend on the location.[55]

SEROUS CYSTADENOMA

Serous cystadenoma is a benign neoplasm that occurs most often in the pancreatic body and tail, but is occasionally found in the head of the gland. Patients usually present with an abdominal pain or an abdominal mass. Patients undergo resection as a means of differentiating the mass from malignant lesions as well as to control symptoms. Cystadenomas are composed of multiple, small cysts that contain serous fluid. Complete excision is usually curative.

MUCINOUS CYSTADENOMA/CYSTADENOCARCINOMA

Like serous cystadenomas, mucinous cystic neoplasms of the pancreas are usually located in the body and tail of the gland and present with an abdominal mass and abdominal pain. The tumors contain one or a few large cysts that are filled with thick mucous. All of these lesions should be considered malignant as even the mucinous cystadenomas have foci of atypia or carcinoma. An aggressive surgical approach is indicated, even a Whipple procedure for lesions located in the pancreatic head. Five-year survival rate exceeds 50 percent for those lesions found to be malignant on final pathology. The CT scan appearance of mucinous tumors is similar to pseudocysts. An antecedent bout of acute pancreatitis favors the latter diagnosis. Nevertheless, it is imperative to biopsy the wall of any lesion thought to be pseudocyst prior to surgical drainage into the gastrointestinal tract as the surgical management of cystic neoplasms is drastically different.

Periampullary Tumors

There is a subset of malignancies that arise from ampulla of Vater that is distinct from pancreatic adenocarcinoma. It is an uncommon malignancy that, like colon cancer, probably arises in preexisting ampullary adenomas. Ampullary tumors can invade the pancreatic head as well as the duodenum. The treatment of choice is the Whipple procedure which is associated with a 5-year survival rate that approaches 50 percent. Some would argue that a suspicious- appearing polyp of the ampulla should be treated by pancreaticoduodenectomy.

Endocrine Neoplasms

Endocrine tumors of the pancreas are either benign or malignant lesions that are of neuroendocrine origin. They have been subclassified as functional and nonfunctional as defined by the production and release of a hormone product with physiologic effects. *Functioning* endocrine tumors will be briefly discussed below. *Nonfunctioning* tumors are detected incidentally or because of the symptoms of mass effect such as bile duct or duodenal obstruction. CT scan is the imaging method of choice, and care should be exhibited during resection due to their hypervascular nature.

Insulinoma

Insulinomas originate from the β cells of the pancreatic islet and have a malignancy rate of approximately 10 percent.[56] These tumors are generally small (less than 5 mm) and solitary. The identification of multiple insulinomas is consistent with multiple endocrine neoplasia syndrome type 1 (MEN 1). Patients with MEN 1 have associated pituitary and parathyroid tumors. Patients with insulinoma have episodes of hypoglycemia that are induced by exercise or fasting. Nonspecific symptoms include dizziness and confusion. Some patients have exaggerated symptoms that include temporary paralysis, decreased mentation, and unusual, psychiatric disorders. The diagnosis is made by the demonstration of hyperinsulinemia in the presence of hypoglycemia induced by fasting.

Preoperative localization of insulinomas is generally made by pancreatic angiography or endoscopic ultrasonography. The precise location of the tumor is confirmed by palpation during laparotomy. Surgical management involves enucleation if technically possible or pancreatic resection. Symptom control can be achieved in patients with liver metastases by resection of the primary tumor and administration of adjuvant agents.

Gastrinoma

Gastrin is a product of antral G cells of the stomach that promotes the secretion of acid. Gastrinomas are gastrin-secreting tumors and are associated with recurrent ulcer disease. Most gastrinomas are located in the pancreas and are malignant. Gastrinomas have also been identified in the stomach, duodenum, jejunum, and liver. Approximately 90 percent of gastrinomas are located in the gastrinoma *triangle* as defined by the junction of the cystic and common bile ducts, the second and third portions of the duodenum, and the junction of the neck and body of the pancreas.[57] The clinical syndrome associated with gastrin hypersecretion was first described by Zollinger and Ellison for whom the syndrome was named.[58]

Patients with Zollinger-Ellison syndrome present with recalcitrant peptic ulcer disease, unusual ulcer sites along the gastrointestinal tract, and diarrhea. Symptom temporization has been achieved with proton pump inhibitors and histamine$_2$-receptor antagonists. Even in the setting of controlled symptoms, the significant potential for malignancy warrants operative management. Tumors may be identified by a combination of endoscopic ultrasound, CT scanning, and visceral angiography. Enucleation, excision, and pancreatic resection are surgical options. Tumors in the head of the pancreas may require the Whipple procedure. Five-year survival rate exceeds 80 percent for resectable lesions and decrease to 20 percent for patients with metastatic disease.

Others

Other pancreatic endocrine tumors have been identified including glucagonoma, VIPoma, and somatostatinoma. Most of these lesions are malignant; therefore, formal resection is indicated.

REFERENCES

1. Sigfússon BF, Wehlin L, Lindström CG. Variants of pancreatic duct system of importance in endoscopic retrograde cholangiopancreatography. *Acta Radiol Diagn (Stockh)* 24:113–128, 1983.

2. Abdomen. In: Agur AMR, Dalley AF, eds. *Grant's Atlas of Anatomy*. Philadelphia, PA: Lippincott Williams & Wilkins, 2005:91–181.

3. Ahrén B, Taborksy GJ Jr, Porte D Jr. Neuropeptidergic versus cholinergic and adrenergic regulation of islet hormone secretion. *Diabetologia* 29:827–836, 1986.

4. Stefan Y, Orci L, Malaisse-Lagae F, et al. Quantitation of endocrine cell content in the pancreas of nondiabetic and diabetic humans. *Diabetes* 31:694–700, 1982.

5. Forsmark CE. Chronic pancreatitis and malabsorption. *Am J Gastroenterol* 99:1355–1357, 2004.

6. Pencharz PB, Durie PR. Pathogenesis of malnutrition in cystic fibrosis, and its treatment. *Clin Nutr* 19:387–394, 2000.

7. Hegnhoj J, Hansen CP, Rannem T, et al. Pancreatic function in Crohn's disease. *Gut* 31:1076–1079, 1990.

8. Banting FG, Best CH. The internal secretion of the pancreas. *J Lab Clin Med* 7:251–266, 1922.

9. Banting FG, Best CH. Pancreatic extracts. *J Lab Clin Med* 7:464–472, 1922.

10. Gerke H, Byrne MF, Stiffler HL, et al. Outcome of endoscopic minor papillotomy in patients with symptomatic pancreas divisum. *JOP* 5:122–131, 2004.

11. Chen Y-C, Yeh C-N, Tseng J-H. Symptomatic adult annular pancreas. *J Clin Gastroenterol* 36:446–450, 2003.

12. Jurkovich GJ, Carrico CJ. Pancreatic trauma. *Surg Clin North Am* 70:575–593, 1990.

13. Wisner DH, Wold RL, Frey CF. Diagnosis and treatment of pancreatic injuries: an analysis of management principles. *Arch Surg* 125:1109–1113, 1990.

14. Obrosova IG, Pacher P, Szabó C, et al. Aldose reductase inhibition counteracts oxidative-nitrosative stress and poly (ADP-ribose) polymerase activation in tissue sites for diabetes complications. *Diabetes* 54:234–242, 2005.

15. The Diabetes Control and Complications Trial Research Group. The effect of intensive treatment of diabetes on the development and progression of long-term complications in insulin-dependent diabetes mellitus. *N Engl J Med* 329:977–986, 1993.

16. Di Carlo A, Odorico JS, Leverson GE, et al. Long-term outcomes in simultaneous pancreas-kidney transplantation: lessons relearned. *Clin Transpl* 215–220, 2003.

17. Fioretto P, Steffes MW, Sutherland DER, et al. Reversal of lesions of diabetic nephropathy after pancreas transplantation. *N Engl J Med* 339:69–75, 1998.

18. Solders G, Tyden G, Tibell A, et al. Improvement in nerve conduction 8 years after combined pancreatic and renal transplantation. *Transplant Proc* 27:3091, 1995.

19. Hathaway DK, Abell T, Cardoso S, et al. Improvement in autonomic and gastric function following pancreas-kidney versus kidney-alone transplantation and the correlation with quality of life. *Transplantation* 57:816–822, 1994.

20. Abendroth D, Schmand J, Landgraf R, et al. Diabetic microangiopathy in type 1 (insulin-dependent) diabetic patients after successful pancreatic and kidney or solitary kidney transplantation. *Diabetologia* 34:S131–S134, 1991.

21. Scheider A, Meyer-Schwickerath V, Nusser J, et al. Diabetic retinopathy and pancreas transplantation: a 3-year follow-up. *Diabetologia* 34:S95–S99, 1991.

22. Shapiro AM, Lakey JR, Ryan EA, et al. Islet transplantation in seven patients with type 1 diabetes mellitus using a glucocorticoid-free immunosuppressive regimen. *N Engl J Med* 343:230–238, 2000.

23. Greenberger NJ, Toskes PP, Isselbacher KJ. Acute and chronic pancreatitis. In: Wilson JD, Braunwald E, Isselbacher KJ, et al., eds., *Harrison's Principles of Internal Medicine*, 12th ed. New York: McGraw-Hill, 1991: 1373.

24. Singh M, Simsek H. Ethanol and the pancreas: current status. *Gastroenterology* 98:1051–1062, 1990.

25. Noronha M, Salgadinho A, Ferreira De Almeida MJ, et al. Alcohol and the pancreas. I. Clinical associations and histopathology of minimal pancreatic inflammation. *Am J Gastroenterol* 76:114–119, 1981.

26. Dreiling DA, Koller M. The natural history of alcoholic pancreatitis: update 1985. *Mt Sinai J Med* 52:340–342, 1985.

27. Frakes JT. Gallstone pancreatitis: mechanism and management. *Hosp Pract* 25:56–60, 63–64, 1990.

28. Malfertheiner P, Kemmer TP. Clinical picture and diagnosis of acute pancreatitis. *Hepatogastroenterology* 38:97–100, 1991.

29. Cullen TS. A new sign in ruptured extrauterine pregnancy. *Am J Obstet Dis Women Child* 78:457, 1918.

30. Grey Turner G. Local discoloration of the abdominal wall as a sign of acute pancreatitis. *Br J Surg* 7:394–395, 1919.

31. Dickinson AP, Imrie CW. The incidence and prognosis of body wall ecchymosis in acute pancreatitis. *Surg Gynecol Obstet* 159:343–347, 1984.

32. Elman R, Arneson N, Graham EA. Value of blood amylase estimations in the diagnosis of pancreatic disease: a clinical study. *Arch Surg* 19:943–967, 1929.

33. Clavien P-A, Robert J, Meyer P, et al. Acute pancreatitis and normoamylasemia: not an uncommon combination. *Ann Surg* 210:614–620, 1989.

34. Yadav D, Agarwal N, Pitchumoni CS. A critical evaluation of laboratory tests in acute pancreatitis. *Am J Gastroenterol* 97:1309–1318, 2002.

35. Mortele KJ, Wiesner W, Intriere L, et al. A modified CT severity index for evaluating acute pancreatitis: improved correlation with patient outcome. *AJR Am J Roentgenol* 183:1261–1265, 2004.

36. Ranson JH, Rifkind KM, Roses DF, et al. Prognostic signs and the role of operative management in acute pancreatitis. *Surg Gynecol Obstet* 139:69–81, 1974.

37. Eachempati SR, Hydo LJ, Barie PS. Severity scoring for prognostication in patients with severe acute pancreatitis: comparative analysis of the Ranson score and the APACHE III score. *Arch Surg* 137:730–736, 2002.

38. Radenkovic D, Johnson CD. Nutritional support in acute pancreatitis. *Nutr Clin Care* 7:98–103, 2004.

39. Eatock FC, Chong P, Menezes N, et al. A randomized study of early nasogastric versus nasojejunal feeding in severe acute pancreatitis. *Am J Gastroenterol* 100:432–439, 2005.

40. Isenmann R, Henne-Bruns D. Prevention of infectious complications in severe acute pancreatitis with systemic antibiotics: where are we now? *Expert Rev Anti Infect Ther* 3:393–401, 2005.

41. Malangoni MA, Martin AS. Outcome of severe acute pancreatitis. *Am J Surg* 189:273–277, 2005.

42. Runzi M, Niebel W, Goebell H, et al. Severe acute pancreatitis: nonsurgical treatment of infected necroses. *Pancreas* 30:195–199, 2005.

43. Soliani P, Franzini C, Ziegler S, et al. Pancreatic pseudocysts following acute pancreatitis: risk factors influencing therapeutic outcomes. *JOP* 5:338–347, 2004.

44. Bergert H, Hinterseher I, Kersting S, et al. Management and outcome of hemorrhage due to arterial pseudoaneurysms in pancreatitis. *Surgery* 137:323–328, 2005.

45. Czako L, Takacs T, Morvay Z, et al. Diagnostic role of secretin-enhanced MRCP in patients with unsuccessful ERCP. *World J Gastroenterol* 10:3034–3038, 2004.

46. Ihse I, Borch K, Larsson J. Chronic pancreatitis: results of operations for relief of pain. *World J Surg* 14:53–58, 1990.

47. Aldridge MC, Williamson RCN. Distal pancreatectomy with and without splenectomy. *Br J Surg* 78:976–979, 1991.

48. Stapleton GN, Williamson RCN. Proximal pancreatoduodenectomy for chronic pancreatitis. *Br J Surg* 83:1433–1440, 1996.

49. Beger HG, Buchler M, Bittner R, et al. Duodenum-preserving resection of the head of the pancreas—an alternative to Whipple's procedure in chronic pancreatitis. *Hepatogastroenterology* 37:283–289, 1990.

50. Maguchi H. The roles of endoscopic ultrasonography in the diagnosis of pancreatic tumors. *J Hepatobiliary Pancreat Surg* 11:1–3, 2004.

51. Whipple AO, Parsons WB, Mullins CR. Treatment of carcinoma of the ampulla of Vater. *Ann Surg* 102:763–779, 1935.

52. Sohn TA, Yeo CJ, Cameron JL, et al. Resected adenocarcinoma of the pancreas—616 patients: results, outcomes, and prognostic indicators. *J Gastrointest Surg* 4:567–579, 2000.

53. Watanapa P, Williamson RC. Surgical palliation for pancreatic cancer: developments during the past two decades. *Br J Surg* 79:8–20, 1992.

54. Vanbiervliet G, Demarquay JF, Dumas R, et al. Endoscopic insertion of biliary stents in 18 patients with metallic duodenal stents who developed secondary malignant obstructive jaundice. *Gastroenterol Clin Biol* 28:1209–1213, 2004.

55. Moesinger RC, Talamini MA, Hruban RH, et al. Large cystic pancreatic neoplasms: pathology, respectability, and outcome. *Ann Surg Oncol* 6:682–691, 1999.

56. Rothmund M, Angelini L, Brunt LM, et al. Surgery for benign insulinoma: an international review. *World J Surg* 14:393–398, 1990.

57. Stabile BE, Morrow DJ, Passaro E Jr. The gastrinoma triangle: operative implications. *Am J Surg* 147:25–31, 1984.

58. Zollinger R, Ellison E. Primary peptic ulcerations of the jejunum associated with islet cell tumors of the pancreas. *Ann Surg* 142:709–723, 1955.

SPLEEN

Dev M. Desai, MD, PhD

IMPORTANT PRINCIPLES

The spleen is the largest lymphoid organ and occupies the left upper quadrant of the abdomen. The spleen functions as a site of antibody production and initiation of the cellular immune response, as well as a site of removal of red blood cells (RBCs) and platelet storage. The vast majority of conditions that necessitate removal of the spleen are extrinsic in nature. Blunt abdominal trauma is the leading cause of splenectomy, while hematologic and immunologic disorders including hereditary spherocytosis, sickle cell anemia, and idiopathic thrombocytopenic purpura (ITP) are the primary etiologies for elective splenectomy.

The importance of the spleen has been demonstrated in patients with clinical and surgical hyposplenism, as they are at significantly increased risk for bacterial sepsis and death. The infectious morbidity associated with splenectomy has resulted in a major shift toward methods of splenic salvage in case of splenic trauma and increased scrutiny at the indications for elective splenectomy. All patients with functional or anatomic asplenia should be vaccinated against the major encapsulated bacteria—*Streptococcus pneumoniae, Haemophilus influenzae,* and *Neisseria meningitides* either prior to or as early as possible after splenectomy. There is no evidence for any benefit of long-term prophylactic antibiotics in asplenic patients.

ANATOMY

The spleen develops as an outgrowth of numerous anlage of the dorsal mesogastrium resulting in an organ with multiple clefts. The splenic primordium migrates into the left upper quadrant of the abdomen and is present by the fifth to sixth week of gestation. The normal spleen, with its reddish-purple parenchyma and surrounding thin mesothelial cell capsule, weighs 75–150 g. The spleen is not normally palpable as it is located beneath the eight to eleven ribs and surrounded superiorly by the left hemidiaphragm. Inferiorly the spleen is associated with the left kidney and splenic flexure of the colon, while medially the stomach and pancreas are intimately associated with spleen. The spleen is stabilized in its left upper quadrant locations by five peritoneal attachments termed *ligaments*. Medially the splenogastric ligament contains the short gastric vessels, while the splenophrenic ligament runs from the left hemidiaphragm to the superior pole of the spleen. The splenocolic and splenoomental ligaments fix the lower splenic pole with the splenic flexure of the colon and the left lateral aspect of the omentum, respectively. The splenorenal ligament, an anterior traversing segment of the posterior peritoneum, envelops the splenic vessels and tail of the pancreas (Fig. 13-1).

The spleen receives its arterial supply from the splenic artery, a branch of the celiac axis. The splenic artery generally branches into two to four vessels that then enter the spleen at the hilum. These main splenic artery tributaries branch into the trabecular arteries which then branch into the central arteries,

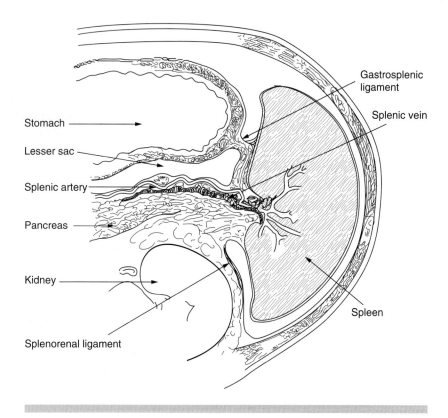

Figure 13-1 **Anatomy of the spleen and surrounding organs.** (*Source*: Adapted from Zollinger RM, Zollinger RM Jr. *Atlas of Surgical Operations*, 7th ed. New York: McGraw-Hill, 1993.)

surrounded by white pulp, that send radial branches into the red pulp consisting of macrophage-lined sinusoids. The sinusoids coalesce into venules that merge to form the splenic vein. The splenic vein courses on the caudal aspect of the pancreas to join the superior mesenteric vein at the level of the head of the pancreas to form the portal vein. Because of the portal venous drainage of the spleen, portal hypertension is one of the most common causes of splenomegaly. The short gastric vessels also provide arterial supply and venous drainage, which provides a conduit between the portal and systemic circulation.

Microscopically and functionally, the spleen is divided into two zones, the *white pulp*, surrounding the central arteries which is composed of T and B lymphocytes and the *red pulp* which is predominantly composed of cells of the reticuloendothelial system. The white pulp is comprised of the periarterial lymphatic sheaths containing T lymphocytes and the more peripheral germinal centers composed of B lymphocytes and antibody-producing plasma cells. The red pulp is composed of vascular sinusoids separated by splenic cords (cords of Billroth). The splenic cords contain macrophages with long dendritic processes that create a labyrinth-like network, through which blood cells slowly percolate (Fig. 13-2).

PHYSIOLOGY

The spleen has two major distinct functions: *immune modulation* and *blood filtration*. The spleen also participates in hematopoiesis and hematologic storage functions, although in the case of hematopoiesis, this function under normal physiologic conditions is lost shortly after birth. However, production of blood elements can be seen in certain pathologic conditions such as myeloid metaplasia. The spleen also functions as a storage compartment for blood components, namely platelets and lymphoid cells. The spleen stores approximately one-third of the body's total platelet mass; however, in the setting of splenomegaly this can increase to over 75 percent.

The spleen is an important immunologic organ and represents the largest collection of lymphoid tissue. The microcirculation of the spleen is central to its immunologic functions. The central arteries are surrounded by the periarterial lymphatic sheaths of the white pulp, which contains T lymphocytes and macrophages that sample the blood for soluble antigens. Presentation of soluble antigen by macrophages to T cells can result in the initiation of a primary or amnestic immune response. After passing the periarterial lymphatic sheath, blood reaches the surrounding lymphoid follicles, containing B cells, which if stimulated by cognate antigen can proliferate forming germinal centers. Plasma cells, mature antibody-producing cells, are formed by terminal differentiation of activated B cells. This is why many disease states mediated by autoantibodies are successfully managed with splenectomy.

The filtration function of the spleen occurs in red pulp, which is a region of open circulation (no endothelial cells) composed of reticuloendothelial cells

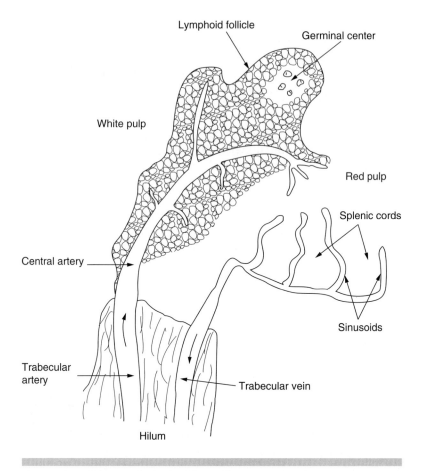

Figure 13-2 **Schematic illustration of the splenic microvascular and lymphoid architecture.**

and specialized macrophages that phagocytose antibody-coated particles. This process called *opsonization* is an effective method to tag harmful objects (e.g., bacteria- and viral-infected cells) for efficient removal. Additionally, injured or old cellular components of the hematopoietic system are also removed from the circulation by the reticuloendothelial cells of the red pulp.

EVALUATION OF THE SPLEEN

Physical Examination

In the normal physiologic state, the spleen is generally not palpable because of its location behind the left costal margin. In the adult, the spleen is approximately 8–12 cm in length and 4–7 cm in width. In the case of an enlarged spleen, it may be palpable below the left costal margin and can extend into the left iliac fossa in cases of severe hypersplenism. The normal spleen can sometimes be palpated under the left costal margin at the end of a deep inspiratory effort as flattening of the diaphragm displaces the spleen inferiorly. Even in situations of extreme splenic enlargement, the spleen is generally not tender with palpation (Fig. 13-3). Splenic pain or tenderness is indicative of splenic infarction, trauma/rupture, or an inflammatory/infective process. Additionally, other sources of left upper quadrant pain can include pathologic processes involving the stomach, distal pancreas, colonic splenic flexure, or left kidney.

Imaging

A number of imaging modalities are available to evaluate and aid in the diagnosis of splenic disorders. Plain abdominal x-rays can be used in the diagnosis of splenomegaly, with depiction of a large splenic shadow, and/or displacement of the stomach, colon, or left hemidiaphragm. Plain radiographs demonstrating fractures involving the lower half of the left rib cage (ribs 6–12) may be the first indication of splenic trauma.

Ultrasound is a very useful rapid, portable, and noninvasive diagnostic modality to evaluate splenic size, traumatic injury, cysts, abscesses, infarcts, masses, and accessory splenules. The use of ultrasound in the emergency

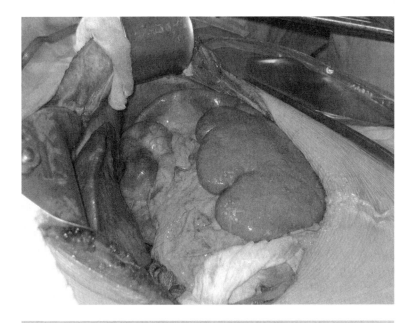

Figure 13-3 **Massive splenomegaly in a patient with hepatic cirrhosis.**

room to evaluate trauma victims for hemoperitoneum has become standard of care. The efficacy of ultrasound may be limited by patient body habitus, overlying bowel gas, and operator proficiency.

Cross-sectional imaging via computed tomography (CT) or magnetic resonance imaging (MRI) scans provide the most detailed information of splenic anatomy and pathologic processes, as well as information about potential disease processes in surrounding organs. Serial cross-sectional imaging studies can be used to monitor therapeutic response and to guide percutaneous catheter-based treatment. The main limitations on the use of cross-sectional imaging are the lack of portability, cost, and exposure to ionizing radiation and intravenous contrast agents in the case of CT scans.

Angiography, another imaging modality using ionizing radiation and catheter-guided contrast injection, has become an important therapeutic modality in addition to its diagnostic utility in evaluating splenic artery aneurysms and splenic vein thrombosis. Splenic artery embolization can be used as an adjunctive or primary treatment modality for the management of splenic trauma and splenomegaly.

Lastly, nuclear medicine scans using colloidal technetium or radiolabeled white blood cells (WBCs) or RBCs have been used to elicit information on splenic function and the presence of accessory spleens.

DISEASE STATES OF THE SPLEEN

The majority of the pathologic states of the spleen are related to its immunologic and filtration functions. Disorders of the spleen can be classified as— too little function (hyposplenism) or too much function (hypersplenism). Hyposplenism is uncommon, with congenital asplenia being extremely rare. The most common cause of hyposplenism is surgical absence of the spleen. Functional hyposplenism can also occur in instances where the spleen involutes from chronic infarcts, most commonly seen with sickle cell anemia.

Splenomegaly

Splenomegaly or clinical hypersplenism is the most common pathologic diagnosis and indication for elective splenectomy. Hypersplenism is characterized predominantly by thrombocytopenia and leukopenia, although anemia may also been seen. Conditions associated with hypersplenism can be categorized into two groups: primary disorders of hematopoietic cells and second, intrinsic disorders of the spleen (Table 13-1).

Benign Lesions
Cysts

Cystic lesions of the spleen are either congenital or acquired due to parasitic infection. *Congenital cysts*, the result of an error during organogenesis, are

Table 13-1 **Disorders Associated with Hypersplenism**

Congestive splenomegaly: cirrhosis, splenic vein thrombosis, cardiac failure (right-sided)
Inflammatory diseases: sarcoid, Felty syndrome, systemic lupus erythematosus
Acute infections: Epstein-Barr virus, cytomegalovirus
Chronic infections: tuberculosis, malaria
Storage diseases: Gaucher disease, glycogen storage disease, Niemann-Pick disease
Hematologic disorders (chronic hemolysis): spherocytosis, thalassemia, elliptocytosis, autoimmune hemolytic anemia, ITP
Myeloproliferative disorders
Other disorders: splenic cysts, amyloidosis, hamartomas

round well-circumscribed lesions on imaging studies. These lesions are usually asymptomatic, however, occasionally in the setting of splenomegaly, they may be associated with left upper quadrant pain.

Infectious cystic lesions of the spleen are usually associated with echinococcal infections. This condition is endemic in the Western United States, Australia, and New Zealand.[1] The treatment for splenic echinococcal disease is similar to that for hepatic echinococcal cysts—albendazole therapy combined with cysts removal through splenectomy. Care must be taken not to allow the cyst contents to spill into the abdominal cavity as it can induce an immediate anaphylactic reaction.

SOLID LESIONS

Hemangioma and hamartomas are the most common benign solid lesions of the spleen and are usually incidental findings after splenectomy or on imaging studies. *Hemangiomas* are well-circumscribed lesions which display delayed filling on intravenous contrast-enhanced CT scans. *Hamartomas* are focal lesions composed of normal cellular components in a dense unorganized cluster. Hemangiomas and hamartomas have no malignant potential and generally do not require any type of intervention.[2]

Malignant Lesions

LYMPHOMA

A number of lymphoproliferative disorders can involve the spleen. Hodgkin lymphoma, with the classic multinucleated Reed-Sternberg cells, is a malignant neoplasm originating in a localized nodal group with subsequent progression to other lymph node basins. Treatment of Hodgkin lymphoma is based on accurate staging.[3] The disease originates and remains localized to lymph nodes above the diaphragm (stages I and II) in 80 percent of patients; however, in those patients with stage III (abdominal nodal involvement) or stage IV (supra- and infradiaphragmatic nodal involvement) disease, the spleen may be a site of tumor involvement. Staging laparotomy was commonly performed in patients with stage III and stage IV disease, but now has significantly decreased because of improvements in coaxial imaging technology and the frequent use of systemic chemotherapeutic agents (regardless of disease stage), thus precluding the need to determine infradiaphragmatic nodal involvement.

Non-Hodgkin lymphoma and leukemia are systemic diseases that may or may not involve the spleen. No survival benefit has been demonstrated for splenectomy in the treatment of these diseases; however, splenectomy is occasionally applicable for management of symptomatic splenomegaly and for management of leukopenia or thrombocytopenia that limits medical therapy.

MYELOPROLIFERATIVE DISORDERS

These disorders are constituted by the deregulated proliferation of hematopoietic lineage cells within the bone marrow, but also may result in proliferation of blood components in former extramedullary sites of hematopoiesis, namely the liver and spleen. Myeloproliferative disorders can result in splenomegaly due to increased splenic blood flow, but can also be secondary to portal hypertension from obstructive hepatic fibrosis due to proliferation of myeloid hematopoietic components in the liver. The treatment of myeloproliferative disorders involves the use of alkylating chemotherapeutic agents and periodic blood product transfusions. Splenectomy is indicated for symptomatic splenomegaly, chronic pain from splenic infarcts, or for the management of severe anemia or thrombocytopenia necessitating frequent transfusions or precluding chemotherapy.

Hematologic Disorders Affecting the Spleen

HEREDITARY SPHEROCYTOSIS

Hereditary spherocytosis is an autosomal dominant genetic defect resulting in the absence of spectrin, an RBC membrane protein, which results in the loss of RBC membrane plasticity. The rigid RBCs are unable to pass through the splenic vasculature, resulting in RBC trapping and increased rate of RBC destruction within the spleen. The RBC trapping in the spleen results in massive splenomegaly, as well as anemia and jaundice from increased bilirubin production from hemoglobin breakdown. The diagnosis of hereditary spherocytosis is readily made by peripheral blood smear.

Splenectomy is the treatment of choice for hereditary spherocytosis.[4] While splenectomy does not alter the underlying genetic defect, it is 100 percent effective in resolution of the symptoms secondary to anemia, reticulocytosis, and jaundice.

THALASSEMIA

Thalassemia is a group of genetic disorders that result in a defect in the synthesis of hemoglobin subunits. Structurally abnormal hemoglobin subunits result in its intracellular precipitation. There is an increased uptake of these abnormal RBCs as well as a higher rate of RBC destruction in the spleen. The increased uptake of RBCs results in splenomegaly as well as splenic infarcts. Thalassemia major (homozygous) is the more severe form of the disease in which patients require frequent blood transfusions and have a decreased life expectancy. Thalassemia minor (heterozygous) on the other hand may be completely asymptomatic and only detectable on peripheral blood smear.

Splenectomy is only indicated in patients with symptomatic splenomegaly or splenic infarcts. Splenectomy results in a decreased transfusion requirement; however, the complication rate from infections is extremely high, thus appropriate patient selection is critical.

SICKLE CELL ANEMIA

Sickle cell anemia is another genetic hemoglobinopathy that results in RBC deformity, especially in the setting of low oxygen tension. These crescent-shaped RBCs become lodged in distal capillary beds leading to tissue ischemia. The episodes of *sickle crisis* related to vascular occlusion can result in severe abdominal and bone pain, hematuria, priapism, skin ulceration, and splenic infarcts. Patients with sickle cell anemia are particularly prone to the development of splenic abscesses in the area of infarction. Splenectomy is beneficial in patients with splenic infarcts or abscesses and helps with splenic sequestration.

IDIOPATHIC AUTOIMMUNE HEMOLYTIC ANEMIA

The spleen is the largest lymphoid organ and serves as a major site of antibody production. Idiopathic autoimmune hemolytic anemia results from the production of antibodies that bind RBC membrane proteins, resulting in the sequestration and destruction of these RBCs in the red pulp of the spleen. Characteristically, the symptoms are anemia and jaundice and in rare severe cases, can result in hematuria and renal failure secondary to acute tubular necrosis. The disease occurs in patients of all ages, but predominantly affects women over the age of 50. Diagnosis is made by blood smear and laboratory evidence of anemia, reticulocytosis, and a positive direct Coombs' test. The main line of therapy is administration of corticosteroids, with splenectomy reserved for patients that have failed steroid therapy or where steroids are contraindicated. Splenectomy is curative in approximately 80 percent of the cases; however, relapses can occur.

IDIOPATHIC THROMBOCYTOPENIC PURPURA

Idiopathic thrombocytopenic purpura results in the sequestration and destruction of platelets in the spleen due to production of antiplatelet antibodies.

Platelet counts generally tend to be less than $50,000/mm^3$ and can even be undetectable. The hallmark of ITP is ecchymosis and purpura with bleeding. Bleeding can present as benign spontaneous epistaxis or gingival bleeding as well as significant potentially life-threatening gastrointestinal hemorrhage or hematuria.

Therapy for ITP consists of corticosteroids for a period of 4–8 weeks. In those with refractory disease, immune globulin infusions and plasmapheresis may also be warranted. Splenectomy is reserved for patients that do not respond with an elevation of their platelet count to more than $75,000/mm^3$ following medical therapy. Additionally, splenectomy may also be performed in patients that develop recurrent disease with reduction of corticosteroids. Medical therapy has approximately a 20 percent permanent cure rate, while surgery approaches approximately 85 percent. Patients who develop recurrent disease after splenectomy require evaluation for accessory spleens by technetium colloid scan or CT scan. In patients with recurrent ITP following splenectomy, identification and removal of an accessory spleen almost universally results in permanent cure.[5]

THROMBOTIC THROMBOCYTOPENIC PURPURA

Thrombotic thrombocytopenic purpura (TTP) is manifested by widespread occlusion of arterioles and capillaries by fibrin strands and hyaline membranes resulting in microangiopathic anemia and thrombocytopenia. The hallmark of TTP is the pentad of clinical features: (1) fever, (2) neurologic changes, (3) renal failure, (4) hemolytic anemia, and (5) thrombocytopenic purpura. Unlike ITP, TTP is a rapidly progressive disease with a significant risk of morbidity and mortality secondary to renal failure and intracerebral hemorrhage. Plasmapheresis and high-dose corticosteroids comprise the first line of therapy, with splenectomy reserved for treatment failure.

Other Disorders

FELTY SYNDROME

Felty syndrome is an autoimmune process consisting of severe neutropenia, rheumatoid arthritis, splenomegaly, as well as possible anemia or thrombocytopenia. Clinically, these patients develop frequent and resistant bacterial infections as a result of the profound neutropenia; however, there also appears to be a poorly characterized neutrophil dysfunction because following splenectomy, there is an improved response to infection even though neutropenia persists. Again as with most autoimmune disorders, corticosteroids are the treatment of choice, with splenectomy reserved for patients with serious recurrent infections or anemia and thrombocytopenia necessitating frequent transfusions. Splenectomy results in improvement in blood counts and response to infections but does not impact the rheumatoid arthritis.

GAUCHER DISEASE

Gaucher disease is a part of the family of lysosomal storage diseases resulting in the accumulation of glucocerebroside in reticuloendothelial cells. It is an autosomal recessive disease caused by an enzymatic deficiency in beta-glucosidase. Glycolipid-laden macrophages accumulate throughout the body, resulting in hepatosplenomegaly, and bone marrow replacement as well as lung infiltration. Enzyme replacement therapy is now available with recombinant acid beta-glucosidase (Cerezyme, Genzyme Corp., Cambridge, MA) with a 25 percent reduction in hepatosplenomegaly after 6 months of therapy. Splenectomy is performed for symptomatic splenomegaly or hypersplenism that does not respond to enzyme replacement therapy.

SARCOIDOSIS

Sarcoidosis is a chronic systemic disorder of unknown etiology characterized by accumulation of T lymphocytes and mononuclear phagocytes as well as noncaseating granulomas in the affected organs. The spleen is affected in a quarter of patients with sarcoidosis, resulting in splenomegaly and hypersplenism. Splenectomy is indicated for symptomatic disease.

Trauma

The leading indicator for splenectomy is splenic trauma, either iatrogenic or accidental. Because of the location, absence of a smooth muscle cell containing capsule and multiple ligamentous attachments, the spleen is the most commonly injured organ following blunt abdominal trauma. The mechanisms of blunt splenic injury include compressive, deceleration, and penetrating injury (rib fracture). Splenic injury is classified into various grades depending on the degree of splenic surface area involved, depth of injury, and location, namely the hilum where the splenic vein and artery reside (Table 13-2).

Evaluation of splenic injury should be performed according to the advanced trauma life support (ATLS) guidelines, as isolated splenic injury occurs in less than 25 percent of trauma patients. In hemodynamically unstable patients or patients with penetrating or other signs of abdominal hemorrhage, prompt celiotomy is required. Hemodynamically stable patients should undergo complete head to toe evaluation according to ATLS guidelines. Signs and symptoms of splenic injury include left upper quadrant tenderness, localized fullness, left shoulder pain, and left-sided rib fractures. Patients should undergo focused assessment with sonography for trauma (FAST) ultrasound to evaluate for intra-abdominal hemorrhage. Stable patients with evidence of splenic injury that do not require celiotomy for other indications should then undergo abdominal CT scan with intravenous contrast enhancement.

Management of splenic injury has greatly evolved over the last 15 years. Traditionally, most splenic injuries were treated with prompt splenectomy;

Table 13-2 **AAST—Spleen Injury Scale**

Grade	Injury Description
I. Hematoma	Subcapsular, <10% surface area
Laceration	<1 cm parenchymal depth
II. Hematoma	Subcapsular, 10–50% surface area; intraparenchymal, <5 cm depth
Laceration	1–3 cm depth, not involving trabecular vessel
III. Hematoma	Subcapsular, >50% surface area or expanding; ruptured subcapsular or parenchymal hematoma
Laceration	>3 cm depth or involving trabecular vessels
IV. Laceration	Involving segmental or hilar vessels producing >25% splenic devascularization
V. Laceration	Completely shattered spleen or hilar injury that completely devascularizes spleen

however, with greater understanding of the immunologic functions of the spleen and demonstration of increased infectious complications not only in the perioperative period, but also long term, has resulted in the primacy of splenic preservation. Splenic preservation can be achieved through both operative and nonoperative methods. Early in the experience of splenic preservation, all techniques involved surgical intervention—splenorrhaphy, partial splenectomy, and the adjunctive use of topical hemostatic agents.[6] More recently, nonoperative methods of splenic preservation, including radiologically guided splenic artery embolization as well as simple close observation with serial laboratory, radiologic, and physical examination have replaced surgical techniques as the treatment of choice. There are well-established criteria for nonoperative management of splenic injury which must all be met: (1) hemodynamic stability, (2) CT scan documentation of the degree of injury, (3) no evidence of active splenic bleeding on CT scan, (4) absence of other intra-abdominal injury requiring celiotomy on CT scan, and (5) limitation of blood transfusion to less than 2 units due to splenic injury. In general, grade I–III splenic lesions can be managed nonoperatively, while most grade IV and V lesions require operative intervention.

SPLENECTOMY

Preoperative Preparation

Preoperative preparation of patients for splenectomy is similar to that of patients undergoing other major abdominal surgical procedures; however, there are some items of importance specifically relevant to patients undergoing elective splenectomy. In general, preoperative bowel preparation is not necessary, but in patients with large splenic tumors or abscesses, consideration should be given to prophylactic bowl preparation due to the proximity of the splenic flexure of the colon. In patients with hypersplenism and thrombocytopenia, platelet infusions should be withheld until ligation of the splenic artery to prevent platelet sequestration.

One of the major functions of the spleen is to help clear infections caused by encapsulated bacteria through the production of antibodies recognizing capsular expressed antigens and subsequent clearance of these antibody-coated organisms. Thus, all patient scheduled to undergo splenectomy should be administered polyvalent pneumococcal, meningococcal, and *H. influenza* vaccines 2 weeks prior to splenectomy.

Surgical Procedure

There are two major techniques for splenectomy: laparoscopic and open. *Laparoscopic splenectomy* is reserved for patient undergoing an elective procedure and one in which the spleen is not massive in size.[7] One means of facilitating successful laparoscopic splenectomy is to preoperatively embolize the splenic artery to decrease the size of the spleen, thus increasing the surgeon's ability to visualize important structures and manipulate the spleen without causing iatrogenic injury and bleeding. Additionally, laparoscopic splenectomy necessitates that the spleen fit into a laparoscopically inserted bag so the spleen can be morcellated to facilitate its extraction from the peritoneal cavity without the creation of a large incision or spillage of splenic tissue into the peritoneal cavity. Intraperitoneal spillage of splenic tissue can result in splenic autotransplantation and a state referred to as *splenosis*, that could result in a recurrent disease state for which splenectomy was initially undertaken. Relative contraindications to laparoscopic splenectomy are trauma or when the histologic architecture of spleen is critical to the pathologic diagnosis or postsurgical management of the underlying disease.

The *open surgical technique* of splenectomy can be approached via a left subcostal or upper midline incision. If the spleen is small, such as in trauma patients or if partial splenectomy is planned then the retroperitoneal attachments to the spleen should be mobilized so it can be brought up into wound. Once that is accomplished, the gastric, colonic, and diaphragmatic attachments can be readily divided. The short gastric vessels are also more accessible at this point and can be safely divided. If there is massive splenomegaly or there are dense attachments to the retroperitoneum due to tumor or infection, then it is safer to ligate the splenic artery and vein prior to mobilization of the spleen. The splenic vessels can be readily identified along the superior border of the pancreas after dividing the gastrocolic ligament to gain access to the lesser sac.

In both the open and laparoscopic technique, it is important to perform a thorough exploration of the left upper quadrant and lesser sac for accessory splenules, especially in the case of splenectomy for hematologic disorders as there is a risk of recurrent disease if an accessory spleen is left behind. Also it is critical to be cognizant of the pancreatic tail during splenectomy, as the tail of the pancreas is intimately associated with the splenic hilum. If a pancreatic injury does occur or is suspected, then it is important to leave a closed system drain in the splenic bed.

Postoperative Care and Complications

Postoperative care is similar to that following other major abdominal operations. Evaluation and prevention of pulmonary complications, deep venous thrombosis, hemorrhage, and wound infections should be undertaken. Persistent left pleural effusion or intractable hiccups should prompt evaluation for a left subphrenic fluid collection or abscess. Inadvertent pancreatic injury, though rare, can result in significant postoperative morbidity including pancreatic fistula, pseudocyst formation, and necrotizing pancreatitis, thus prolonged recovery should prompt thorough evaluation that includes CT imaging of the abdomen.

Postsplenectomy syndrome causing neutrophil-based leukocytosis and thrombocytosis is not uncommon. Generally no specific therapy is required; however, if the platelet count exceeds one million/mm^3, then antiplatelet therapy should be initiated. The leukocytosis and thrombocytosis are usually self-limited and do not pose a long-term problem.[8]

The most serious complication following splenectomy is overwhelming postsplenectomy infection (OPSI). Following splenectomy, there is reduced bacterial clearance from the blood, decreased levels of IgM, and decreased opsonic activity, resulting in a 40-fold greater risk of sepsis than the general population. The potential risk for OPSI is 2–4 percent in the pediatric population and half of that in the adult population. Patients undergoing splenectomy for hematologic disorders seem to be at the greatest risk, while trauma patients are at the least risk, possibly secondary to traumatic splenosis. Additionally, children under 6 years of age also appear to be at greater risk for the development of OPSI, especially within the first 2 years following splenectomy.[9]

Encapsulated bacteria are the typical mediators of OPSIs with S. pneumoniae being the most common, followed by H. influenzae and N. meningitides. Vaccines against all these organisms are widely available and patients undergoing elective splenectomy should be vaccinated 2 weeks prior to surgery. In the case of unplanned splenectomy, patients should receive the vaccinations once they are clinically stable and at the latest immediately prior to hospital discharge.

The use of prophylactic antibiotics to prevent OPSI in adult patients had not been shown to be efficacious due to issues of compliance and development of resistant organisms. Some physicians have advocated that patients in rural or geographically isolated areas keep a supply of penicillin to be taken at the first sign of overwhelming infection while they seek medical attention. Many pediatricians initiate prophylactic penicillin in children until they reach 6 years of age, although there is limited data supporting such therapy. The most effective measure to prevent severe morbidity and mortality from OPSI is patient education and encouragement to seek early medical attention so that prompt evaluation and treatment can be initiated, if necessary.

REFERENCES

1. Dawes LG, Malangoni MA. Cystic masses of the spleen. *Am Surg* 52:333–336, 1986.

2. Morgenstern L, Rosenberg J, Geller SA. Tumors of the spleen. *World J Surg* 9:468–476, 1985.

3. Urba WJ, Longo DL. Hodgkin's disease. *N Engl J Med* 326:678–687, 1992.

4. Swartz SI. Role of splenectomy in hematologic disorders. *World J Surg* 20:1156–1159, 1996.

5. Walters DN, Roberts JL, Votaw M. Accessory splenectomy in the management of recurrent immune thrombocytopenic purpura. *Am Surg* 64:1077–1078, 1998.

6. Cogbill TH, Moore EE, Jurkovich GF, et al. Nonoperative management of blunt splenic trauma: a multicenter experience. *J Trauma* 29:1312–1315, 1989.

7. Phillips EH, Carroll BJ, Fallas MJ. Laparoscopic splenectomy. *Surg Endosc* 8:931–933, 1994.

8. Horowitz J, Smith JL, Weber TK, et al. Postoperative complications after splenectomy for hematologic malignancies. *Ann Surg* 223:290–296, 1996.

9. Davidson RN, Wall RA. Prevention and management of infections in patients without a spleen. *Clin Microbiol Infect* 7:657–660, 2001.

BREAST

RECONSTRUCTION

Michael R. Zenn, MD, FACS

BODY

The purpose of breast reconstruction is to restore body image and to enable patients to wear all types of clothes without restriction. Most women can wear the most revealing styles with complete confidence after breast reconstruction. It is usually impossible to tell which side is the reconstructed side while dressed. The need for an awkward and sometimes embarrassing external prosthesis is eliminated by permanent reconstruction of the breast.[1,2]

No method of breast reconstruction will precisely duplicate a normal breast. It is not possible, for example, to restore normal feeling. Some techniques have limitations in terms of creating a soft breast as well as imitating the natural sag of a mature breast. It is impossible to eliminate the scar that results from mastectomy although it can frequently be integrated into the reconstruction so that it is less obvious. Despite these shortcomings, the vast majority of women are pleased with the results achieved by breast reconstruction.

Reconstruction with Breast Implants

The most common form of breast reconstruction uses a saline-filled or silicone gel implant to rebuild the breast mound. This technique does not add new scars to the body, as the other techniques require. *Implant reconstruction* also requires less extensive surgery than other techniques, but more procedures are required to complete the reconstructive process.[1,2]

Not all women are candidates for implant reconstruction. Those with small-to moderate-sized breasts that do not sag are the best candidates. Extremely small breasts (A cup) or breasts that are excessively large (DD cup or larger) or have a lot of sag are difficult to simulate with an implant. Implants are made in limited sizes and extremely small and excessively large implants do not exist. Women with larger breasts may be candidates for implant reconstruction if a breast reduction is performed on the contralateral side, allowing a match with an implant. Similarly, if a woman with extremely small breasts is willing to undergo contralateral breast augmentation, she may then be a candidate for an implant reconstruction.

Those who have received chest wall radiation prior to reconstruction generally are not candidates for standard implant techniques, with rare exception. The chance of complications requiring removal of the implant is very high in this setting. The effects of radiation on tissues is long lasting and severe, complicating all types of reconstruction. Other alternatives for reconstruction should be sought.

The Role of Tissue Expanders in Implant Reconstruction

A mastectomy normally removes a variable amount of breast skin with the nipple. The amount removed depends on tumor size and also on the location of the biopsy scar. The skin circulation and its healing ability are also compromised by mastectomy. Both of these factors prevent the immediate placement of a permanent implant at the time of mastectomy in virtually all patients. Tissue expansion is a process that replaces the missing skin in preparation for placement of a permanent implant later.

A tissue expander is an inflatable plastic bag that is inserted into a pocket under the skin and muscle of the chest (Fig. 14-1). It is similar in construction to a saline implant but the shape is different, it has an adjustable capacity, and it contains a metal port for fluid injection. The expander is usually placed in its collapsed form at the time of mastectomy (*immediate reconstruction*) or any time after mastectomy (*delayed reconstruction*). Beginning about 2 weeks after placement, fluid is introduced by needle into the tissue expander to partially inflate it. This is repeated during weekly office visits to gradually expand the skin of the chest. Expansion is completed in approximately 8 weeks. Four weeks are then allowed for the skin to stabilize and loosen. After this time the tissue expander is replaced with an implant as a separate surgical procedure. If needed, an augmentation, a reduction, or a lift of the opposite side is usually performed at the same time.

Breast Implant Controversies

Breast implants are thin-walled containers made of hard silicone plastic that are filled with saline (salt water) or silicone gel. They have been in use for 30 years and have an excellent safety record. The Institute of Medicine's recent review of breast implants and their safety found saline and silicone gel implants to be similar. Both types of implants were associated with local complications (rupture, scar formation called *capsular contracture*, and infection) but not with systemic complications as once feared. The decision to use saline implants versus silicone implants is often patient driven or determined by surgeon's preference.

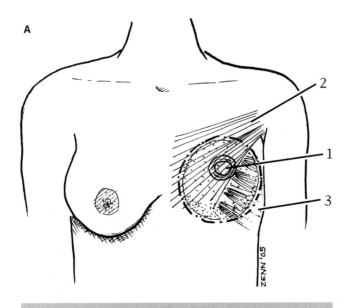

Figure 14-1 **(A) Anteroposterior (AP) view of submuscular tissue expander placed during or after mastectomy. (1) Tissue expander with integrated port, (2) pectoralis muscle, and (3) serratus muscle. (B) Lateral view of submuscular tissue expander. (1) Pectoralis muscle, (2) integrated fill port, (3) tissue expander, and (4) subcutaneous tissue.**

Complications of Implant Reconstruction

The complications associated with breast implant reconstruction are listed in Table 14-1. Of these, scar tissue is perhaps the most problematic for the reconstruction patient as time goes on. The body normally forms a layer of scar tissue around any artificial material implanted beneath the skin. With breast implants, that scar tissue is called a *capsule* and the process of scarring and subsequent deformation of the breast shape is called *capsular contracture*. If the capsule which forms remains thin and pliable, it will be nonvisible and nonpalpable and of little concern to a patient. In some patients the capsule can become quite thick, resulting in a firm breast which can be distorted in shape. The variability in capsule formation is a reflection of each individual's biologic response to an implant as well as responses to infection around the implant and surgical bleeding around the time of surgery. Capsular contracture requires surgery to relieve symptoms. That surgery consists of the removal of the scar tissue and replacement of the breast implant.

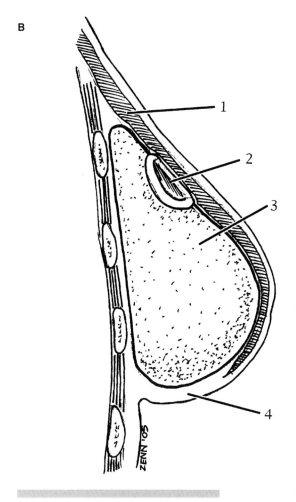

Figure 14-1 (**Continued**)

Despite the less extensive nature of breast reconstruction with implants, complications are common (Table 14-1) and tend to increase over time. It is for this reason that some patients choose to avoid implants and use other methods of reconstruction.

Reconstruction with Body Tissue

A breast mound can also be created with tissue borrowed from another part of the body. Breasts reconstructed in this fashion are soft and have a natural shape. It is therefore much easier to match the remaining breast with this technique. (Fig. 14-2) Fewer procedures are required to complete the reconstruction

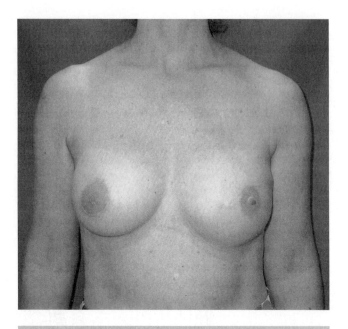

Figure 14-2 **Left breast reconstruction with implant and final nipple reconstruction to match an augmented right breast for best symmetry.**

compared to implant techniques. The reconstruction is permanent, ages naturally, and rarely requires *touch up* procedures later in life. The main disadvantages are that there will be a scar left at the site where the tissue is taken from and that the operative procedure can be lengthy. The most common area used to donate tissue for breast reconstruction is the lower abdomen. This is called a TRAM flap. The term relates to the muscle supplying vascularity to the lower abdominal block of tissue that is transferred (*T*ransverse *R*ectus *A*bdominis *M*yocutaneous flap).[3–6] The back tissues (latissimus myocutaneous flap) can be used in some situations, but often an implant is needed in addition for adequate breast projection. The buttock, hips, and other areas of the body can also be used in special situations.

TRAM Flap Reconstruction

A patient must have sufficient tissue in the lower abdomen to be a candidate for this procedure. The volume of tissue must also match the volume of tissue in the contralateral breast one is trying to match. Surprisingly, little tissue is needed to match an A-cup breast, and a large amount of tissue may be transferred to match a very large breast. The resultant shape in these two

Table 14-1 **Complications of Breast Implant Reconstruction**

Reoperation
Breast pain
Wrinkling
Asymmetry
Replacement/removal
Capsular contracture
Implant malposition
Implant deflation
Bleeding/hematoma
Infection

cases is much more natural than any implant reconstruction. The lower abdomen can also be divided for bilateral simultaneous reconstruction.

Different methods exist to transfer the lower abdominal tissues to the chest for breast reconstruction (Fig. 14-3). The simplest and most common way to do this is to move the tissue to the chest area by sliding it through a tunnel underneath the upper abdominal skin to reach the mastectomy site. This is the *pedicled TRAM flap* where the tissue remains attached to one of the abdominal muscles which is loosened enough to allow the tissue to move upward. The muscle provides blood supply to the skin and fat tissue that will form the breast. The blood supply for the flap ultimately is derived from the superior epigastric vessels. These vessels are a secondary blood supply to the lower abdomen, as they are quite at a distance from the lower abdomen and must exit the chest and travel the length of the rectus muscle before supplying the overlying skin and fat tissue. Some who perform this procedure try to improve the blood supply to the lower abdominal flap by *delaying* the TRAM flap.[7] This maneuver divides the primary blood supply of the lower abdomen, the inferior epigastric vessels, surgically 2 weeks before the TRAM surgery. This maneuver is felt to increase the lower abdominal tissues reliance on the superior epigastric system.

Use of the muscle can result in abdominal weakness because one of the two main abdominal muscles is no longer functional. Bilateral TRAM cases may sacrifice both rectus abdominis muscles. Dissections of and use of the entire muscle is also responsible for much of the abdominal discomfort experienced right after surgery. In this type of reconstruction, muscle function is sacrificed and the transferred muscles are used to carry the blood supply to the transferred tissues.

There is another method of TRAM reconstruction that limits muscle harvest and bases the blood supply to the transferred tissue on primary (inferior

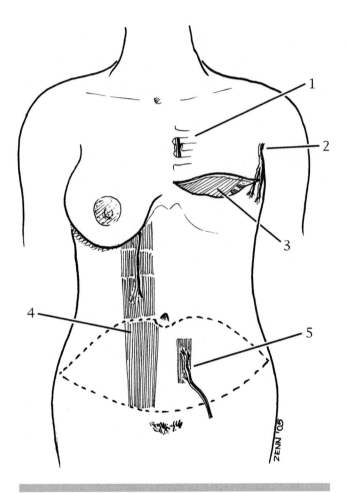

Figure 14-3 **TRAM flap breast reconstruction. The dotted line is the tissue carried with the flap which can be used to replace missing breast skin and fat tissues. (1) Internal mammary vessels exposed after rib removal for recipient site for free flap reconstruction. (2) Thoracodorsal vessels also used for recipient vessels. (3) Mastectomy defect awaiting reconstruction. (4) Muscle pedicle used for pedicled TRAM flaps based on the superior epigastric system. (5) Deep inferior epigastric vessels used to supply TRAM during free and perforator flaps.**

epigastric) blood supply. This technique takes the same skin and fat tissue harvested with a pedicle TRAM but instead of taking a rectus muscle with it, it keeps the inferior epigastric vessels attached. Only a small piece of muscle is needed around the inferior epigastric vessels as they pass through the muscle into the tissues. With this technique, muscle weakness is minimized and recovery is quicker. Instead of sliding the fat and skin tissue still attached by muscle, the entire block of tissue is completely detached from the body, moved to the chest, and then its blood vessels are reattached to vessels in the chest area using an operating microscope. Abdominal muscle function is largely preserved and the circulation to the transposed tissue is actually enhanced with this technique. A large block of tissue that is completely detached from the body in this way is referred to as a *free flap* and in this case, a free TRAM flap. Further refinement of the free TRAM can be done by harvesting no muscle at all with the flap. In this case, the perforating vessels of the deep inferior epigastric system are dissected through the rectus abdominis muscles, leaving the entire rectus muscle intact. These *perforator flaps* are named by their source blood vessels. In this case the deep inferior epigastric perforating vessels supply the flap and hence it is called a *DIEP* flap.[8] The pedicle TRAM, the free TRAM, and the DIEP flap will all have the same donor and reconstructive scars, just differ in the way blood is supplied to the tissues (Fig. 14-4).

Microsurgical free flaps are best performed only at specialized centers with experienced personnel. Even in the best of hands, 1–3 percent of patients will have a complication with the microsurgery limiting blood supply to the flap. If this happens the entire piece of transferred tissue is lost. Breast reconstruction must then be accomplished by another technique at a later date. Women who smoke and those who have other risk factors such as obesity and diabetes are more likely to have this problem. However, this same group derives the most benefit from a microsurgical approach because of the superior circulation provided to the tissue by this technique. Those who have a history of back problems are also good candidates for the microsurgical option because only a small portion of one abdominal muscle is used. The loss of an entire pedicled TRAM is rare.

Complications and their prevalence are listed in Table 14-2. In general, the TRAM procedure is a larger procedure than that required for implant reconstruction, often requiring 4–10 h for completion. Unlike implant reconstruction, the mound is shaped at the initial procedure and it is possible that no further revisions of the mound would be required. Bleeding is more significant and blood transfusion may be required. If the transferred tissues have marginal or poor supply, portions of the transferred flap may not survive and instead scar or liquefy. This situation is called *fat necrosis*. Areas of fat necrosis are often removed during revisional surgery months later. Complications at the donor site may also occur, most notably bulges or hernias of the abdominal wall after harvest. Sometimes synthetic mesh is required to repair or tighten the abdomen after TRAM procedures.

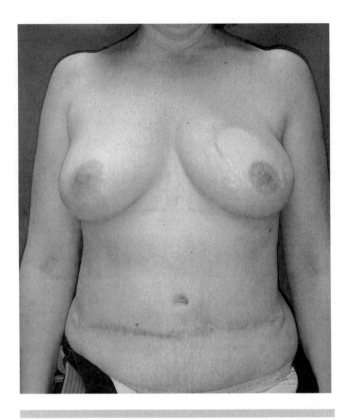

Figure 14-4 **Left breast reconstruction with free TRAM flap and nipple reconstruction to match natural breast on the right.**

Gluteal Free Flap Reconstruction

Both the upper and lower buttock are another source of skin and fat tissue for breast reconstruction.[9] These free flaps can be harvested with muscle based on the superior or inferior gluteal vessels (free superior gluteal flap or free inferior gluteal flap), or as perforator flaps leaving gluteus muscle intact (S-GAP or I-GAP flaps). There is a large scar created across the buttock with mild flattening of the buttock contour but this is imperceptible in normal clothing. The best candidates for a gluteal free flap reconstruction are healthy women who have a flat abdomen (no TRAM donor site) and a small or medium size breast with little natural sag.

Reconstruction After Radiation: A Special Situation

Some women have had radiation therapy prior to reconstruction. This is most common in those who have previously been treated by lumpectomy

Table 14-2 **Complications of TRAM Flap Reconstruction**

Flap loss
Fat necrosis
Asymmetry
Bleeding/hematoma
Infection
Seroma
Abdominal bulge/hernia
Abdominal weakness

and radiation. A mastectomy is usually recommended if a new problem develops in the same breast later. The difficulty with reconstruction is due to the detrimental effect that radiation has on skin circulation. The skin is permanently compromised and breast reconstruction performed in this setting is more prone to wound healing complications.

It is not possible to use tissue expanders to stretch radiated skin. Attempts to do so are associated with a very high failure rate. Even in those in whom expansion proves to be technically feasible, the aesthetic result is usually poor. Therefore, the best option is one that brings new skin to the reconstruction site. The latissimus flap or TRAM flap are options in this situation.

Latissimus Flap Reconstruction

The latissimus dorsi flap is named after the back muscle of the same name, based on the thoracodorsal vessels, rotated through a tunnel to supply muscle and skin for breast reconstruction. This muscle helps with upper arm motion but is not essential for normal function. Loss of latissimus muscle function is well tolerated by patients and recovery is much easier than the TRAM flap. Unlike the TRAM flap there is not enough fat volume available to form a breast mound without the addition of a breast implant. Like implant reconstruction, a tissue expander is placed at the time of the latissimus dorsi flap and the permanent implant is placed later after the new skin is expanded. Rarely, enough tissue is present in the back to build a breast to match the contralateral side with no implant.

Steps in the Process of Breast Reconstruction

Breast reconstruction can never be totally completed in a single operation, regardless of the method used. The first one or two operations create the breast mound and establish symmetry by adjustment of either the reconstructed breast, the normal breast, or both. The last step is nipple reconstruction.

The breasts are allowed to settle for several months prior to nipple reconstruction so that its position on the breast can be determined accurately.

Immediate Reconstruction Versus Delayed Reconstruction

Breast reconstruction can begin either at the time of mastectomy or several months later. The timing does not influence the quality of the result. The concept of immediate reconstruction is attractive because it saves one hospitalization, one general anesthetic, and the reconstruction is already underway while the mastectomy wound is still healing. The negative impact of mastectomy on body image is less when reconstruction is begun immediately. If radiation has been performed or is part of the plan postoperatively, breast reconstruction is delayed until adjuvant therapy is over. Recent reports have documented the negative effects of irradiating a breast reconstruction, such as progressive fibrosis and shrinkage of the irradiated mound.

Reconstruction of the Nipple and Areola

Nipple and areola reconstruction is the final step in the reconstruction process. The nipple is usually made from the skin and fat tissue of the reconstructed breast or, if the normal nipple is large enough, a portion of it can be used as a graft to make a new nipple for the reconstructed side.

The finishing touch in nipple and areola reconstruction is to establish the appropriate color. This is done using a tattoo technique. Some surgeons use skin grafts to accomplish this goal but color matching is difficult.

SUMMARY

The goal of breast reconstruction is to restore the size, shape, and appearance of the breast(s) as closely as possible after mastectomy. This aids in the restoration of body image and makes it possible for patients to wear virtually all types of clothing with confidence. As we see further refinements in microsurgery, it becomes possible to reconstruct a breast with a minimum of morbidity and a lifetime of benefit.

REFERENCES

1. Bostwick J. *Plastic and Reconstructive Breast Surgery*, 2nd ed, Vol. II. St. Louis, MO: Quality Medical Publishing, 2000.

2. Spear SL, Little JW, Lippman ME, et al. *Surgery of the Breast: Principles and Art.* Philadelphia, PA: Lippincott-Raven, Chaps. 22–48, 1998.

3. Hartrampf CR, Scheflan M, Black PW. Breast reconstruction with a transverse abdominal island flap. *Plast Reconstr Surg* 69:216–224, 1982.

4. Hartrampf CR, Bennett GK. Autogenous tissue reconstruction in the mastectomy patient. A critical review of 300 patients. *Ann Surg* 205:508–518, 1987.

5. Moon HK, Taylor GI. The vascular anatomy of the rectus abdominis musculocutaneous flaps based on the deep superior epigastric system. *Plast Reconstr Surg* 82:815–829, 1988.

6. Mathes SJ, Nahai F. *Reconstructive Surgery: Principles, Anatomy and Technique.* New York: Churchill-Livingstone, 1997.

7. Taylor GI, Corlett RJ, Caddy CM, et al. An anatomic review of the delay phenomenon. Clinical applications. *Plast Reconstr Surg* 89: 408–418, 1992.

8. Allen R, Treece P. Deep inferior epigastric perforator flap for breast reconstruction. *Ann Plast Surg* 32:32, 1994.

9. Paletta CE, Bostwick J, Nahai F. The inferior gluteal free flap in breast reconstruction. *Plast Reconstr Surg* 84:875, 1989.

ENDOCRINE SURGERY

Jennifer H. Aldrink, MD
John A. Olson, Jr., MD, PhD

EVALUATION OF THYROID DISORDERS

Clinical Manifestations

Clinical manifestations of hyperthyroidism reflect increased catabolism and excessive sympathetic activity caused by excess circulating thyroid hormones. Symptomatic manifestations of hyperthyroidism include weight loss despite normal or increased appetite, heat intolerance, anxiety, irritability, fatigue, muscle weakness, palpitations, and oligomenorrhea. Signs of hyperthyroidism include goiter, tremor, hyperreflexia, fine or thinning hair, thyroid bruit, muscle wasting, and cardiac arrhythmias such as sinus tachycardia or atrial fibrillation. The presentation of hyperthyroidism varies with age. Young patients typically present with hypermetabolism, while older patients may present primarily with tachyarrhythmias or cardiac failure. Rarely, elderly patients experience only muscle wasting, apathy, confusion, or a state of depression known as apathetic hyperthyroidism. Clinical features of hypothyroidism include cold intolerance; weight gain; constipation; edema of the hands, feet, and eyelids, dry skin; weakness; somnolence; and menorrhagia.

Biochemical Testing

Biochemical thyroid function testing confirms clinically suspected abnormalities in thyroid function. However, test results must be interpreted in the context of clinical findings. The introduction of sensitive thyrotropin assays has transformed thyroid function testing from strategies based on thyroxine (T_4) to strategies based on thyroid-stimulating hormone (TSH).[1] Currently, measurement of serum TSH level is the most accurate and efficient method for diagnosing patients with thyroid disorders. Measurement of TSH (0.3–5 mIU/L) by a second-generation sensitive TSH (sTSH) test is the single most useful biochemical test in the diagnosis of thyroid illness. In most ambulatory and hospitalized patients without pituitary disease, increased sTSH signifies *hypothyroidism*, suppressed sTSH suggests *hyperthyroidism*, and normal sTSH reflects a *euthyroid state*. Hospitalized patients who are critically ill may have transient changes in sTSH, typically an elevation, without true abnormalities in thyroid function.

Assessment of T_4 concentration corroborates identified abnormalities in TSH and provides an index of severity of thyroid dysfunction. Total T_4 measurements quantify bound and unbound hormone and do not reflect directly the small *free* or active T_4 fractions. Factors that increase the thyroxine-binding globulin (TBG) concentration, such as estrogens, pregnancy, and liver disease may elevate the total T_4 or triiodothyronine (T_3) despite a normal free hormone concentration and a euthyroid state. Androgens, severe hypoproteinemia, chronic liver disease, and acromegaly result in decreased TBG.

The resin T_3 uptake (RT_3U) test measures unoccupied thyroid hormone-binding sites on TBG by allowing radiolabeled T_3 to compete for binding between TBG and a resin. This assay provides an indirect measure of FT_4. In patients with hyperthyroidism, the resin uptake is elevated because most of the sites on TBG are occupied by T_4, so that more radioactive T_3 binds to the resin. The RT_3U is related directly to the free T_4 fraction and inversely related to the TBG-binding sites. Normal values are between 20 and 40 percent.

The FT_4 index (FT_4I) is equal to total T_4 multiplied by the RT_3U value (normal values lie between 0.85 and 3.50). It correlates more closely with the level of FT_4, eliminates ambiguity introduced by altered thyroglobulin levels, and is the preferred test to estimate FT_4. Measurement of T_3 (80–200 ng/dL) is an unreliable test in hypothyroidism. This test is useful in the occasional patient with suspected hyperthyroidism, suppressed sTSH, and normal FT_4I (T_3 thyrotoxicosis).

Antithyroid microsomal antibodies are found in the serum of patients with autoimmune thyroiditis (Hashimoto's thyroiditis). The measurement of these antibodies is helpful to diagnose this common cause of hypothyroidism. Anti-TSH receptor antibodies, which stimulate the TSH receptor, are detectable in more than 90 percent of patients with autoimmune hyperthyroidism (Graves' disease); however, their measurement is not often needed in the diagnosis of this disease.

A useful thyroid function test algorithm[2] begins with sTSH assay as the initial test. If this is normal, no further tests are performed. If sTSH is elevated, FT_4I and microsomal antibodies are measured to confirm hypothyroidism, which is often autoimmune in nature. If sTSH is suppressed, FT_4I is measured to confirm primary hyperthyroidism. If TSH is low and FT_4I is normal, T_3 is measured to diagnose T_3 thyrotoxicosis.

Thyroid Imaging

Thyroid imaging is most often accomplished with ultrasound or radionuclide scanning. Other imaging modalities, including computed tomographic (CT) scanning and magnetic resonance imaging (MRI) are useful in special circumstances.

Technetium thyroid scanning 20 min after the intravenous injection of technetium-99m (^{99m}Tc) is useful in determining the size of the thyroid and in differentiating solitary functioning nodules from multinodular goiter. Hypofunctioning areas (cyst, neoplasm, or suppressed tissue adjacent to autonomous nodules) are *cold*, whereas areas of increased synthesis are *hot*. Thyroid scans alone are not able to differentiate benign from malignant thyroid nodules. *Cold* nodules have a 15–20 percent risk of malignancy, and therefore ought to be surgically removed. *Hot* nodules are almost never malignant. ^{99m}Tc thyroid scans are most useful as adjunctive tests to assess risk of malignancy in patients with indeterminate thyroid nodule cytology or in hyperthyroid patients suspected of having a hyperfunctioning thyroid adenoma. Thyroid scanning 4–24 h after oral iodine-131 (^{131}I) is useful to identify metastatic differentiated thyroid tumors and to both confirm a diagnosis of Graves' disease and predict a response to ^{131}I radioablation. Patients with goiter and uniformly high uptake are best treated with ^{131}I radioablation.

Thyroid ultrasonography with high-frequency transducers (7.5–10.0 MHz) accurately determines gland volume as well as the number and character of thyroid nodules. Features suggestive of malignancy on ultrasound include hypoechoicity, incomplete peripheral halo, irregular margins, and microcalcifications. Ultrasound is useful to guide fine-needle aspiration (FNA) biopsy and cyst aspiration. Cysts seen on ultrasound, especially those larger than 3 cm, are malignant in one-tenth of cases.

CT scanning and MRI of the thyroid are costly and generally are reserved for assessing substernal or retrosternal masses suspected to be goiters. Iodinated contrast should not be administered to patients with known or suspected thyroid cancer since it will impair thyroid uptake of therapeutic ^{131}I for weeks after surgery.

THYROID DISORDERS

Graves' Disease

Autoimmune diffuse toxic goiter (Graves' disease) is the most common cause of hyperthyroidism and is caused by immunoglobulins directly stimulating the TSH receptor. Graves' disease may be treated with antithyroid drugs, ablation with radioactive iodine (RAI), or surgery, depending on the clinical situation.

Thionamide drugs, such as propylthiouracil (PTU) or methimazole, are the initial therapy in most cases. Ablation with RAI is the treatment of choice for most patients with Graves' disease. After treatment, the incidence of permanent hypothyroidism approaches 70 percent, which is easily managed by replacement therapy. There are virtually no other long-term side effects of RAI (i.e., no significantly increased risk of thyroid cancer, leukemia, or teratogenicity). Exceptions to radiotherapy are pregnant women, newborns, patients who refuse, or patients with low RAI uptake (less than 20 percent) in the thyroid. Treatment of children or young adults (less than 30 years) with RAI is controversial because of presumed long-term oncogenic risks.

Thyroidectomy for Graves' disease may be indicated for children or adolescents, pregnant women (late second or early third trimester), patients unresponsive to or noncompliant with medical therapy, or patients who refuse RAI. A bilateral subtotal thyroidectomy should be performed with the goal of leaving a 1- to 2-g vascularized cuff of thyroid on each side. Risks of surgery are extremely small (less than 1 percent) in experienced hands but include hypoparathyroidism and injury to the recurrent laryngeal nerve (RLN). Hypothyroidism results less frequently with surgical management than with RAI.[3] The long-term incidence of recurrent hyperthyroidism after surgery is approximately 10 percent. Patients with recurrent hyperthyroidism after thyroidectomy should be treated with RAI.

Multinodular Goiter

A large goiter or retrosternal extension can compress the trachea. Subtotal or total thyroidectomy is the treatment of choice if there are symptoms of compression or if the gland is cosmetically bothersome.

Other Causes

Toxic adenoma is an autonomously functioning thyroid nodule that produces hyperthyroidism and is treated by surgical lobectomy. Rare causes of hyperthyroidism include self-administration of excessive thyroid hormone (factitious hyperthyroidism), iodine-induced hyperthyroidism, pituitary TSH-secreting adenoma, trophoblastic tumors secreting chorionic gonadotropin, which possesses TSH-like activity, struma ovarii, and thyroiditis.

Hypothyroidism

Hypothyroidism is almost always caused by primary hypofunction of the thyroid gland. Clinically, hypothyroid patients should be separated into those without goiter (primary atrophy), those with goitrous hypothyroidism (i.e., Hashimoto's thyroiditis, drug-induced hypothyroidism, iodine deficiency, and congenital causes of dyshormonogenesis), and those with postablative hypothyroidism (after thyroidectomy or treatment with RAI). Postablative hypothyroidism and Hashimoto's thyroiditis are the most important causes of hypothyroidism encountered by the surgeon. Diagnosis rests on the characteristic clinical features and laboratory findings of an elevated TSH (usually greater than 15 U/mL) and a decreased FT_4 level. A low TSH in association with low T_4 suggests pituitary or hypothalamic failure.

Thyroiditis

Thyroiditis represents a diverse group of autoimmune and inflammatory disorders characterized by infiltration of the thyroid with inflammatory cells and subsequent fibrosis of the gland.

Hashimoto's thyroiditis is a chronic autoimmune disorder characterized by destructive lymphocytic infiltration of the thyroid. The disease is 15 times more common in women, and more than 90 percent of patients have circulating antibodies directed against thyroid microsomes and thyroglobulin. Patients are initially euthyroid, and hypothyroidism generally occurs later. A firm symmetric or asymmetric goiter is palpable and usually (but not always) nontender. Thyroidectomy is indicated for compressive symptoms or for a dominant nodule suspicious for malignancy.

Acute suppurative thyroiditis is rare and is caused by infection with *Streptococcus* or *Staphylococcus* spp. Treatment consists of appropriate antibiotic therapy and surgical drainage of abscesses.

Subacute (de Quervain's) thyroiditis is a rare condition that occurs in young women, often after a viral upper respiratory tract infection. Presenting symptoms include fatigue, weakness, and painful thyroid enlargement radiating to the patient's jaw or ear, and are treated with nonsteroidal anti-inflammatory drugs or with steroids. The condition almost always remits spontaneously within a few weeks. Thyroidectomy may be indicated in rare cases of persistent thyroiditis after months of unsuccessful steroid treatment.

Riedel's thyroiditis is a rare, progressive, inflammatory condition of the entire thyroid gland, strap muscles, and other neck structures. Its cause is unknown, and it can be associated with other fibrotic processes, including retroperitoneal fibrosis, sclerosing cholangitis, and fibrosing mediastinitis. The lymphocytic infiltrate and dense fibrous tissue reaction in the thyroid result in a firm, nontender goiter with a characteristic woody texture. Surgical excision may be required to relieve compressive symptoms or to exclude malignancy.

Solitary Thyroid Nodule

Solitary thyroid nodule occurs commonly in up to 4–7 percent of adults and is usually a benign lesion. Such nodules may be associated with a multinodular goiter or with an otherwise normal thyroid. The malignant potential of the newly discovered thyroid nodule is of justifiable concern to both physician and patient, and the goal of diagnostic testing is to separate the relatively few patients with thyroid malignancy from the larger group of patients with benign thyroid nodules. Surgical intervention is appropriate for all malignant or suspicious thyroid nodules. The frequency of cancer in surgically excised nodules is 8–17 percent.[4]

History and physical examination are invaluable in the management of the thyroid nodule. Nodules in the very young and very old (especially men) are more likely to be malignant. Exposure to ionizing radiation increases the incidence of both benign and malignant thyroid nodules and is a well-recognized risk factor for the development of thyroid carcinoma. A family history of thyroid malignancy, familial polyposis, or other endocrine disease also increases risk of cancer. Rapid nodule growth, pain, compressive symptoms, or hoarseness of voice increase the likelihood of malignancy but are nonspecific symptoms. Physical findings of a solitary nodule with firm or irregular texture or with fixation of surrounding structures suggest malignancy. Similarly, the presence of enlarged cervical lymph nodes is extremely important because this finding is highly indicative of thyroid cancer. Malignancy is uncommon in hyperfunctioning nodules, and all patients should have a serum TSH measured to exclude clinical or subclinical thyrotoxicosis.

FNA is the initial diagnostic test of choice for the euthyroid patient with a solitary thyroid nodule. This procedure is safe, inexpensive, and easy to perform, and allows the better selection of patients for operation than does any other technique.[5] Cytologic results of FNA can be benign, malignant, or indeterminate. The accuracy of these results ranges from 70 to 90 percent and is highly dependent on the skill and experience of the cytopathologist. The false-negative rate of FNA is low (less than 6 percent), and patients with negative (i.e., not cancerous or not indeterminate) cytology can be followed safely.[6] Indeterminate aspirations pose difficult management decisions because carcinoma occurs in 10–30 percent of these cases. Follicular and Hurthle cell neoplasms and the follicular variant of papillary cancer account for many indeterminate results, whereas papillary, medullary, and undifferentiated thyroid carcinomas usually have distinctive cytopathologic features.

Radionuclide thyroid scans detect areas of increased or decreased thyroid hormone synthesis but do not provide information that allows clear separation of benign and malignant nodules. Approximately 20 percent of nodules that are hypofunctioning (*cold*) on thyroid scintiscan are malignant; the majority are benign. Hyperfunctioning (*hot*) nodules carry a low risk of malignancy, but exceptions occur.

Ultrasonography is a sensitive method for determining whether a lesion is solid or cystic, but it cannot distinguish reliably between benign and malignant nodules. Although thyroid cysts have a lower likelihood of being malignant nodules, larger carcinomas can undergo cystic degeneration. Cysts may disappear after FNA, but those that persist, recur, or yield insufficient material for interpretation should be excised.

Thyroid lobectomy is indicated for (a) nodules with malignant or indeterminate aspiration cytology, (b) nodules in children, (c) nodules in patients with either a history of neck irradiation or a family history of thyroid cancer, and (d) symptomatic or cosmetically bothersome nodules.

Thyroid Neoplasms

Differentiated (papillary and follicular) thyroid cancers are among the most curable of human cancers.[7] These cancers are rare in children and increase in frequency with age. The female to male ratio is approximately 2.5:1.0. The cause of these cancers is unknown, but childhood exposure to radiation is the best known etiologic factor. Approximately 30 percent of exposed children develop thyroid nodules, and of these an estimated 30 percent are malignant. The appropriate initial procedure for a solitary thyroid nodule suspected of being malignant is lobectomy and isthmusectomy. Controversy exists about the extent of surgery that ought to be performed for patients with biopsy-proven differentiated thyroid cancer, principally because these patients have a good prognosis irrespective of the surgical treatment. Prognosis depends mostly on the patient's age as well as extent and histologic subtype of disease.

Papillary thyroid carcinoma (PTC) represents 85 percent of thyroid carcinomas and can occur in any age group, but is more common in children and women younger than 40 years. PTC is often multifocal and frequently metastasizes to cervical lymph nodes. Total thyroidectomy is appropriate for patients with gross evidence of bilateral disease, multifocal PTC, or a history of neck irradiation. Total thyroidectomy is arguably the treatment of choice for unilateral tumors larger than 1.5 cm. Advantages of total thyroidectomy include the ability to treat extrathyroidal metastases or recurrences with RAI and to use serum thyroglobulin to monitor therapy. Retrospective studies also show a decreased risk of recurrence or death with total thyroidectomy. Complications of total thyroidectomy include temporary or permanent hypoparathyroidism and RLN injury, which occur in less than 1 percent of cases. Concurrent central lymphadenectomy is useful for staging but risks hypoparathyroidism. Prophylactic lateral neck dissection is not indicated for PTC, but a modified ipsilateral neck dissection is indicated for patients with palpable metastases in cervical nodes.

Follicular thyroid carcinoma constitutes approximately 10 percent of thyroid carcinomas, is rare before 30 years of age, and has a slightly worse prognosis than does PTC. Unlike PTC, follicular thyroid cancer spreads hematogenously to bone, lung, or liver. Follicular thyroid cancer will involve regional lymph nodes, though less frequently (about 11 percent) than does PTC. Small, unilateral follicular carcinomas with limited invasion of the tumor capsule or spread along blood vessels may be treated with thyroid lobectomy, whereas multicentric tumors and tumors with more extensive invasion or distant metastases are treated with total thyroidectomy. Radioablation is indicated after total thyroidectomy, followed by lifelong thyroid hormone suppression.

Medullary thyroid carcinoma (MTC) arises from the thyroid C cells that derive from the neural crest and secrete calcitonin. MTC may occur sporadically or may be inherited either alone or as a component of multiple endocrine neoplasia (MEN) types 2A or 2B. Sporadic MTC usually is detected as a firm, palpable, unilateral nodule with or without involved cervical lymph nodes. Patients with hereditary MTC develop bilateral, multifocal tumors and often are diagnosed on the basis of family screening. MTC should be suspected if tumor calcification is noted on plain x-rays or if the patient has profuse diarrhea and episodic flushing (caused by excess calcitonin release). MTC spreads early to cervical lymph nodes and may metastasize to liver, lungs, or bone. All patients with suspected or known MTC should have a careful family history taken. In addition, they should be tested biochemically for pheochromocytoma before thyroidectomy, and be genetically tested for DNA mutations in the RET protooncogene.[8] Treatment of MTC is total thyroidectomy with removal of the lymph nodes in the central zone of the patient's neck (from the sternal notch to hyoid bone and laterally to the carotid sheaths). A modified neck dissection is indicated for clinically involved ipsilateral cervical lymph nodes.

Undifferentiated or anaplastic thyroid carcinoma (1–2 percent of thyroid carcinomas) carries an extremely poor prognosis, usually presents as a fixed, sometimes painful goiter, and usually occurs in patients older than the age of 50 years. Invasion of local structures, with resultant dysphagia, respiratory compromise, or hoarseness due to RLN involvement can preclude curative resection. External irradiation or chemotherapy may provide limited palliation.

Primary malignant lymphoma of the thyroid often is associated with Hashimoto's thyroiditis. The typical presentation is rapid enlargement of a long-standing goiter in an elderly patient. Diagnosis may be made with fine-needle or core-needle biopsy, although a surgical biopsy can be required. Radical surgical resection generally is not indicated once a diagnosis is made. Combination chemotherapy and radiotherapy is the treatment of choice for disease confined to the patient's neck, and responses usually occur rapidly.

Complications Following Thyroidectomy

Transient hypocalcemia commonly occurs 24–48 h after thyroidectomy, but infrequently requires treatment. Adult patients who are markedly symptomatic or who have serum calcium below 7 mg/dL are given one to two ampules (10–20 mL) of 10 percent calcium gluconate intravenously, followed by oral calcium carbonate. On occasion, a calcium drip may be required. To prepare this, six ampules of 10 percent calcium gluconate, each containing 90 mg elemental calcium are added to 500 cc D_5W to achieve a concentration of approximately 1 mg elemental calcium per cc. The drip is run at a cc per hour rate equivalent to the patient's weight in kilograms to achieve replacement of 1 mg/kg/h.

Permanent hypoparathyroidism is uncommon after total thyroidectomy. Normal parathyroid tissue removed or devascularized at the time of total thyroidectomy may be autotransplanted into sternocleidomastoid muscle to prevent postoperative hypocalcemia.[9]

RLN injury is a devastating complication of thyroidectomy that should occur rarely (less than 1 percent). Unilateral RLN injury causes hoarseness, and bilateral injury compromises the airway, necessitating tracheostomy. Repeat neck exploration, thyroidectomy for extensive goiter or Graves' disease, and thyroidectomy for fixed, locally invasive cancers are procedures particularly prone to RLN injury. Intentional (as with locally invasive cancer) or inadvertent transaction of the RLN can be repaired primarily or with a nerve graft, although the efficacy of these repairs is not known. The external branch of the superior laryngeal nerve may be injured if not identified during ligation of the superior thyroid pole vascular bundle. This injury results in weakness of the patient's voice at high pitch. The best prevention of these injuries is a thorough understanding of the anatomy of these nerves.

Hemorrhage is a rare but serious complication of thyroidectomy that usually occurs within 6 h of surgery. Management requires control of the airway by endotracheal intubation and may mandate urgent opening of incision and evacuation of hematoma before returning to the operating room for wound irrigation and ligation of the site of bleeding.

PARATHYROID DISORDERS

Hyperparathyroidism (HPT) refers to hypercalcemia caused by inappropriate parathyroid hormone (PTH) release from the parathyroid glands. Primary HPT results from autonomous release of PTH from parathyroid adenoma or hyperplastic parathyroid glands. Secondary HPT results from a defect in mineral homeostasis (e.g., renal failure) with a compensatory increase in parathyroid function. Tertiary HPT refers to the development of autonomous, calcium-insensitive parathyroids after prolonged secondary stimulation (e.g., prolonged renal failure).

Primary HPT

INCIDENCE

Primary HPT has an incidence of 0.25–1 per 1000 in the United States and is especially common in postmenopausal women. It most often occurs sporadically, but it can be inherited alone or as a component of familial endocrinopathies, including MEN types 1 and 2A.

MANIFESTATIONS OF HPT

The more common manifestations of HPT include nephrolithiasis, osteoporosis, hypertension (HTN), and emotional disturbances. The widespread use of the multichannel autoanalyzer has led to more patients being diagnosed with *asymptomatic* hypercalcemia or with earlier symptoms, such as muscle weakness, polyuria, anorexia, and nausea. Differential diagnosis of hypercalcemia includes HPT, malignancy, granulomatous disease (e.g., sarcoidosis), immobility, hyperthyroidism, milk-alkali syndrome, and familial hypocalciuric hypercalcemia (FHH). Patients with hypercalcemia and suspected HPT should minimally have serum calcium, phosphate, creatinine, and PTH measured. The diagnosis of HPT is biochemical and requires demonstration of hypercalcemia (serum calcium greater than 10.5 mg/dL) and an elevated PTH level. Hypercalcemia without an elevated PTH can be due to a variety of causes (especially malignancy, Paget disease, sarcoidosis, and milk-alkali syndrome) that must be excluded. Radiographic features of HPT are seen in advanced cases and include decreased bone density, osteitis fibrosa cystica, and the pathognomonic sign of subperiosteal bone resorption on the radial aspect of the phalanges of the second or third digits of the hand.

Parathyroidectomy is indicated for all patients with symptomatic HPT. Nephrolithiasis, bone disease, and neuromuscular symptoms are improved more often than are renal failure, HTN, and psychiatric symptoms. Parathyroidectomy for asymptomatic HPT is somewhat controversial (Table 15-1). Accepted indications include markedly elevated serum calcium, hypercalcemic crisis, reduced creatinine clearance, asymptomatic kidney stones, markedly elevated urinary calcium excretion, and significant osteoporosis. Close observation is required for patients not treated surgically.

LOCALIZING STUDIES

The use of preoperative localization studies to guide first exploration for HPT has become increasingly popular, but is not essential. Imaging with ^{99m}Tc-sestamibi scintigraphy and/or ultrasound will localize a parathyroid adenoma in up to 85 percent of cases, allowing for directed parathyroidectomy. Preoperative localization of the hyperfunctioning parathyroid should be attempted in nearly all reoperative cases by ^{99m}Tc-sestamibi scintigraphy and ultrasound or CT scanning. These noninvasive studies are successful in localizing the missed gland in 25–75 percent of cases.[10] With combined use of CT scan, ultrasonography, and scintigraphy, at least one imaging study identifies the tumor in more than 75 percent of patients. Invasive imaging tests, including angiography, are associated with greater morbidity and measurable mortality; they should be reserved for complex cases with negative or equivocal noninvasive studies. The success of these tests in localizing the concealed tumor is highly dependent on the skill and experience of the

Table 15-1 **Guidelines for Parathyroidectomy in Asymptomatic Primary HPT**

Parameter	Recommendation
Age	<50
Serum calcium above normal value	1.0 mg/dL
24-H urinary calcium	>400 mg
Creatinine clearance	Reduced by 30%
Bone mineral density	t-score < −2.5 at any site
Any patient in whom medical surveillance is not desired or not possible	—

radiologist.[11] Localization studies should not be used as an indication for or against surgery.

Neck exploration and parathyroidectomy for HPT results in normocalcemia in more than 95 percent of patients when performed by an experienced surgeon. A thorough, orderly search and identification of all four parathyroid glands has been the traditional approach to surgical management of HPT. Recently, a focused, unilateral approach to parathyroidectomy has been popularized where removal of parathyroid tumors is guided by preoperative localization studies. In this approach, all four glands are not identified and confirmation of removal of abnormal parathyroid tissue is made by intraoperative measurement of PTH levels, which must show a 50 percent drop. Early results show equivalent outcomes to bilateral exploration, although long-term results are lacking.

Parathyroid glands are red-brown to yellow and flat or oval, with a characteristic vascular architecture; however, it may be difficult to distinguish them from fat or lymphoid tissue. Superior parathyroid glands develop from the fourth pharyngeal pouch and most commonly are located dorsally on the middle or upper thyroid lobe, near the intersection of the inferior thyroid artery and RLN. Ectopic superior glands may be found posteriorly in the tracheoesophageal groove or cranial to the superior thyroid pole. Inferior parathyroid glands develop in conjunction with the thymus from the third pharyngeal pouch, are more variable in position than are the superior glands, and usually are located at the inferior pole of the thyroid lobe within the thyrothymic ligament. Ectopic inferior glands most likely are found in the mediastinum embedded in the thymus. The normal combined weight of the parathyroid glands is 90–200 mg. Most often, a single adenomatous gland is found; the other, normal parathyroid glands should be left in place. Occasionally, multiple parathyroid adenomas are found, which should be removed, leaving at least one normal parathyroid. Management of four-gland parathyroid hyperplasia is controversial and may include total parathyroidectomy and parathyroid autotransplantation or 3.5-gland parathyroidectomy. Hypercalcemia from secondary and tertiary HPT is treated initially with dietary phosphate restriction, phosphate binders, vitamin D analogues, and occasionally calcimimetic agents. Patients with medically unresponsive symptomatic hypercalcemia (e.g., bone pain and osteopenia, ectopic calcification, or pruritus) may be surgically treated with subtotal parathyroidectomy or total parathyroidectomy and heterotopic autotransplantation.

Parathyroid Autotransplantation

Indications for total parathyroidectomy and heterotopic parathyroid autotransplantation include HPT in patients with renal failure, in patients with four-gland parathyroid hyperplasia, and in patients undergoing neck reexploration in which the adenoma is the only remaining parathyroid tissue. Parathyroid autotransplantation may be performed into either the sternocleidomastoid muscle or the brachioradialis muscle of the patient's nondominant forearm; parathyroid grafting into the patient's forearm is advantageous if recurrent HPT is possible (e.g., MEN type 1 or 2A, or secondary HPT). If HPT recurs, the hyperplastic parathyroid tissue may be partially excised from the patient's forearm under local anesthesia.

Postoperative Hypocalcemia

Transient hypocalcemia commonly occurs after total thyroidectomy or parathyroidectomy and requires treatment if severe (total serum calcium less than 7.0 mg/dL) or the patient is symptomatic. Chvostek's sign (twitching of the facial muscles when the examiner percusses over the facial nerve anterior to the patient's ear) is a sign of relative hypocalcemia but is present in up to 15 percent of the normal population. This sign is not necessarily an indication for calcium replacement. Patients with persistent hypocalcemia after total thyroidectomy or after parathyroid autotransplantation can require continued supplementation for 6–8 weeks postoperatively. Hypocalcemic tetany is a medical emergency that is treated with rapid intravenous administration of 10 percent calcium gluconate or calcium chloride until the patient recovers. Patients with severe hypocalcemia also must have correction of hypomagnesemia.

Parathyroid Carcinoma

Parathyroid carcinoma is rare and accounts for less than 1 percent of patients with HPT. Approximately 50 percent of these patients have a palpable neck mass, and serum calcium levels may exceed 15 mg/dL. Surgical treatment is radical local excision of the tumor, surrounding soft tissue, lymph nodes, and ipsilateral thyroid lobe when the disease is recognized preoperatively or intraoperatively. Patients with parathyroid carcinoma and some patients with benign HPT may develop hyperparathyroid crisis. Symptoms of this acute, sometimes fatal, illness include profound muscular weakness, nausea and vomiting, drowsiness and confusion. Hypercalcemia (16–20 mg/dL) and azotemia are usually present. Ultimate treatment of *parathyroid crisis* is parathyroidectomy; however, hypercalcemia and volume and electrolyte abnormalities should be addressed first. Treatment is warranted for symptoms or a serum calcium level greater than 12 mg/dL. First-line therapy is infusion of 0.9 percent NaCl to restore intravascular volume and to promote renal excretion of calcium. After urinary output exceeds 100 mL/h, furosemide may be given to promote further renal sodium and calcium excretion. If diuresis alone is unsuccessful in lowering the serum calcium, other calcium-lowering agents may be used. These include the bisphosphonates, pamidronate or etidronate, mithramycin, and salmon calcitonin. Orthophosphate, gallium nitrate and glucocorticoids also have calcium-lowering effects. Calcimimetic agents are also an effective, approved approach to hypercalcemia associated with parathyroid carcinoma.

ENDOCRINE PANCREAS

Pancreatic islet cell tumors are rare tumors that produce clinical syndromes related to the specific hormone secreted. Insulinomas are the most common of these tumors, followed by gastrinoma, VIPoma, glucagonoma, and somatostatinoma. Recognition of characteristic syndromes is key to the diagnosis, which must be confirmed biochemically. Islet cell tumors are often occult and their localization may be difficult, especially for small, multifocal, or extrapancreatic tumors. Islet cell tumors may occur sporadically or as a component of MEN type 1 or von Hippel-Lindau disease. Islet cell tumors may be benign or malignant, although prediction may be based on hormone produced rather than size.

Insulinoma

CLINICAL FEATURES

Patients with insulinoma develop profound hypoglycemia during fasting or after exercise. The clinical picture includes the signs and symptoms of neuroglycopenia (anxiety, tremor, confusion, and obtundation) and the sympathetic response to hypoglycemia (hunger, sweating, and tachycardia). These bizarre complaints initially may be attributed to malingering or a psychosomatic etiology unless the association with fasting is recognized. Many patients eat excessively to avoid symptoms, causing significant weight gain. Whipple triad refers to the clinical criteria for the diagnosis of insulinoma: (a) hypoglycemic symptoms during fasting, (b) blood glucose levels less than 50 mg/dL, and (c) relief of symptoms after administration of glucose. Factitious hypoglycemia (excess exogenous insulin administration) and postprandial reactive hypoglycemia must be excluded. A supervised, in-hospital 72-h fast is required to diagnose insulinoma. Patients are observed for hypoglycemic episodes and have 6-h measurement of plasma glucose, insulin, proinsulin, and C-peptide. Nearly all patients with insulinoma develop neuroglycopenic symptoms and have inappropriately elevated plasma insulin (greater than 5 pU/mL) associated with hypoglycemia (glucose less than 50 mg/dL).

LOCALIZATION

Insulinomas typically are small (less than 2 cm), solitary, benign tumors that may occur anywhere in the pancreas. Rarely, an insulinoma may develop in extrapancreatic rests of pancreatic tissue. Dynamic CT scanning at 5 mm intervals with oral and intravenous contrast is the initial localizing test for insulinoma, with success in 35–85 percent of cases. Endoscopic ultrasound is also effective but is operator dependent.[12] Indium-111 (^{111}In)-octreotide scintigraphy is less effective (approximately 50 percent) for localization of insulinoma than other islet cell tumors because insulinomas typically have few somatostatin receptors. Selective arteriography with observation of a tumor *blush* is the single best diagnostic study for the primary tumor and hepatic metastases. If a tumor is still not identified, regional localization to the head, body, or tail of the pancreas can be accomplished by portal venous sampling for insulin or by calcium angiography. Calcium angiography involves injection of calcium into selectively catheterized pancreatic arteries and measurement of plasma insulin through a catheter positioned in a hepatic vein.

TREATMENT

Treatment of insulinoma is surgical in nearly all cases. Surgical management of insulinomas consists of localization of the tumor by careful inspection and palpation of the gland after mobilization of the duodenum and the inferior border of the pancreas. Use of intraoperative ultrasonography greatly facilitates identification of small tumors, especially those located in the pancreatic head or uncinate process. Most insulinomas can be enucleated from surrounding pancreas, although those in the body or tail may require resection. In general, blind pancreatectomy should not be performed when the tumor cannot be identified. Approximately 5 percent of insulinomas are malignant, and 10 percent are multiple usually in association with MEN type 1. Medical treatment for insulinoma with diazoxide, verapamil, or octreotide has limited effectiveness but may be used in preparation for surgery or for patients unfit for surgery.

Gastrinoma

Patients with gastrinoma and the Zollinger-Ellison syndrome (ZES) have severe peptic ulcer disease (PUD) due to gastrin-mediated gastric acid hypersecretion. Most patients present with epigastric pain, and 80 percent have active duodenal ulceration at the time of diagnosis. Diarrhea and weight loss are common (40 percent of patients). ZES is uncommon (0.1–1.0 percent of PUD), and most patients present with typical duodenal ulcer. Gastrinoma and ZES should be considered in any patient with (a) PUD refractory to treatment for *Helicobacter pylori* and conventional doses of H_2-blockers or omeprazole; (b) recurrent, multiple, or atypically located (e.g., distal duodenum or jejunum) peptic ulcers; (c) complications of PUD (i.e., bleeding, perforation, or obstruction); (d) PUD with significant diarrhea; and (e) PUD with HPT, nephrolithiasis, or familial endocrinopathy. All patients considered for elective surgery for PUD should have ZES excluded preoperatively. Diagnosis of ZES requires demonstration of fasting hypergastrinemia and basal gastric acid hypersecretion. A fasting serum gastrin level of 100 pg/mL or greater with basal gastric acid output (BAO) of 15 meq/h or more (greater than 5 meq/h in patients with previous ulcer surgery) secures the diagnosis of ZES in nearly all cases. Fasting hypergastrinemia without elevated BAO is seen in atrophic gastritis, renal failure, and in patients taking H_2-receptor antagonists or omeprazole. Fasting hypergastrinemia with elevated BAO is seen in retained gastric antrum syndrome, gastric outlet obstruction, and in antral G-cell hyperplasia. A secretin stimulation test is used to distinguish ZES from these conditions. Eighty-five percent of patients with ZES have an increase in gastrin levels (greater than 200 pg/mL over baseline) in response to a secretin stimulation test, whereas patients with other conditions do not.

LOCALIZATION

Localization should be performed in all patients considered for surgery. Approximately 80 percent of gastrinomas are located within the *gastrinoma triangle* that includes the duodenum and head of the pancreas. Gastrinomas are often malignant, with spread to lymph nodes or liver occurring in up to 60 percent of cases. Approximately 20 percent of patients with ZES have familial MEN type 1; these patients often have multiple, concurrent islet cell tumors. Dynamic CT scanning, ^{111}In-octreotide scintigraphy, endoscopic ultrasound, and MRI are useful noninvasive tests to localize gastrinoma; however, preoperative localization is unsuccessful up to 50 percent of the time. Selective angiography with or without secretin injection of the gastro-duodenal, superior mesenteric, and splenic arteries and measurement of hepatic vein gastrin can localize occult gastrinoma in up to 70–90 percent of cases.

TREATMENT

Medical treatment of gastric hyperacidity with H_2-histamine receptor antagonists and omeprazole is highly effective in ZES. These medications are indicated preoperatively in patients. Surgical management of ZES is indicated in all fit patients with nonmetastatic, sporadic gastrinoma. Goals of surgery include precise localization and curative resection of the tumor. Resection of primary gastrinoma alters the malignant progression of tumor and decreases hepatic metastases in patients with ZES. Intraoperative localization of gastrinomas is facilitated by extended duodenotomy and palpation, intraoperative ultrasonography, or endoscopic duodenal transillumination. Gastrinomas within the duodenum, pancreatic head, or uncinate process are treated by enucleation, whereas tumors in the body or tail of the pancreas can be removed by distal or subtotal pancreatectomy. Immediate cure rates are 40–90 percent in experienced hands; however, half of patients initially cured biochemically experience recurrence within 5 years.

Unusual Islet Cell Tumors

VIPomas secrete vasoactive intestinal peptide and cause profuse secretory diarrhea (fasting stool output greater than 1 L/day), hypokalemia, and either achlorhydria or hypochlorhydria (watery diarrhea, hypokalemia, and achlorhydria or Verner-Morrison syndrome). Hyperglycemia, hypercalcemia, and cutaneous flushing may be seen. Other, more common causes of diarrhea and malabsorption must be excluded. A diagnosis of VIPoma is established by the finding of elevated fasting serum vasoactive intestinal peptide levels and secretory diarrhea in association with an islet cell tumor. Octreotide is highly effective to control the diarrhea and correct electrolyte abnormalities before resection. Most VIPomas occur in the distal pancreas and are amenable to distal pancreatectomy. Metastatic disease is commonly encountered (50 percent); nevertheless, surgical debulking is indicated to alleviate symptoms.

Glucagonomas secrete excess glucagon and result in type 2 diabetes, hypoaminoacidemia, anemia, weight loss, and a characteristic skin rash, necrolytic migratory erythema. Diagnosis is suggested by symptoms and biopsy of the skin rash but is confirmed by elevated plasma glucagon levels (usually greater than 1000 pg/mL). Tumors are large and are readily seen on CT scan. Resection is indicated in fit patients after nutritional support, even if metastases are present.

Somatostatinomas are the rarest of the islet cell tumors and cause a syndrome of diabetes, steatorrhea, and cholelithiasis. These tumors are frequently located in the head of the pancreas and are often metastatic at the time of presentation.

Other rare islet cell tumors include pancreatic polypeptide-, neurotensin-, and adrenocorticotropic hormone (ACTH)-secreting tumors, as well as nonfunctioning islet cell tumors. These tumors usually are large and often malignant. Treatment is surgical resection.

CARCINOID TUMORS

Carcinoid tumors are classified according to their embryologic origin: foregut (bronchial, thymic, gastroduodenal, and pancreatic), midgut (jejunal, ileal, appendiceal, and right colic), and hindgut (distal colic and rectal). Depending on the site of origin, carcinoids secrete hormones differently and have different clinical features. Carcinoid tumors most frequently occur in the gastrointestinal tract. Bronchial and thymic carcinoids occur less commonly. In general, the diagnosis of carcinoid rests on the finding of elevated circulating serotonin or urinary metabolites (5-hydroxyindoleacetic acid [5-HIAA]) and localizing studies. The single best biochemical test is an elevated urinary 5-HIAA (normal 2–8 mg/24 h). Rectal or jejunoileal tumors may be visualized by contrast studies, whereas bronchial carcinoids can be identified on chest x-rays, CT scans, or bronchoscopy. Abdominal or hepatic metastases are best identified by CT scanning, ultrasonography, or angiography. As with other neuroendocrine tumors, some carcinoids can be detected with metaiodobenzylguanidine (^{131}I-MIBG) scanning, and most are detectable by ^{111}In-octreotide scintigraphy.

Carcinoid of the appendix is by far the most common carcinoid tumor, occurring in up to 1 in 300 appendectomies. The risk of lymph node metastases and the prognosis of appendiceal carcinoids depends on the size:

tumors less than 1 cm never metastasize, tumors 1–2 cm have a 1 percent risk of metastasis, and tumors larger than 2 cm have a 30 percent risk of metastasis. Extent of surgery for appendiceal carcinoid is based on size: simple appendectomy for tumors less than 2 cm, right hemicolectomy for tumors greater than or equal to 2 cm.[13] Prognosis for completely resected appendiceal carcinoid is favorable, with 5-year survival of 90–100 percent.

Small intestinal carcinoid tumors usually present with vague abdominal symptoms that uncommonly lead to preoperative diagnosis. Most patients are operated on for intestinal obstruction, which is caused by a desmoplastic reaction in the mesentery around the tumor rather than by the tumor itself. Extended resection, including the mesentery and lymph nodes, is required, even for small tumors. Meticulous examination of the remaining bowel is mandatory because tumors are multicentric in 20–40 percent of cases, and synchronous adenocarcinomas are found up to 10 percent of the time. An almost linear relationship exists between size of tumor and risk of nodal metastases, with up to 85 percent for tumors larger than 2 cm. Prognosis depends on size and extent of disease, overall survival is 50–60 percent, which is substantially decreased if liver metastases are present. Small-bowel carcinoids have the highest propensity to metastasize to liver and produce the carcinoid syndrome.

Rectal carcinoids are typically small, submucosal nodules that are often asymptomatic or produce nonspecific symptoms of bleeding, constipation, or tenesmus. These tumors are hormonally inactive and almost never produce the carcinoid syndrome, even when spread to the liver occurs. Treatment of small (less than 1 cm) rectal carcinoids is endoscopic removal. Transmural excision of tumors 1–2 cm can be done locally. Treatment of 2-cm and larger tumors or invasive tumors is controversial but may include anterior or abdominoperineal resection for fit patients without metastases.

Foregut carcinoids include gastroduodenal, bronchial, and thymic carcinoids. These are a heterogeneous group of tumors with variable prognosis. They do not release serotonin and may produce atypical symptoms (e.g., violaceous flushing of the skin) related to release of histamine. Gastroduodenal carcinoids may produce gastrin and cause ZES. Resection is advocated for localized disease. Gastric carcinoids are grouped by whether they are associated with presence (types I and II) or absence (type III) of hypergastrinemia. Type I tumors are associated with pernicious anemia, whereas type II are associated with MEN type 1. Small (less than 1 cm) type I and II tumors are adequately treated with endoscopic resection and surveillance. There is controversy as to whether larger (1–2 cm) type I and II tumors may be treated similarly or with gastrectomy. Concurrent antrectomy may be recommended for type I gastric carcinoids to reduce the source of gastrin. Large (greater than 2 cm) type I and II as well as type III gastric carcinoids are treated with gastrectomy.

Carinoid Syndrome

Carcinoid syndrome occurs in less than 10 percent of patients with carcinoid and develops when venous drainage from the tumor gains access to the systemic circulation, as with hepatic metastases. The classic syndrome consists of flushing, diarrhea, bronchospasm, and right-sided cardiac valvular fibrosis. Symptoms are paroxysmal and may be provoked by alcohol, cheese, chocolate, or red wine. Diagnosis is made by 24-h measurement of urinary 5-HIAA or of whole blood 5-hydroxytryptamine. Surgical cure usually is not possible with extensive abdominal or hepatic metastases; however, debulking of the tumor may alleviate symptoms and improve survival, when it can be performed safely. Hepatic metastases also have been treated with chemoembolization using doxorubicin, 5-fluorouracil, and cisplatin. Carcinoid crisis with severe bronchospasm and hemodynamic collapse may occur perioperatively in patients with undiagnosed carcinoid. Prompt recognition is crucial as administration of octreotide can be lifesaving.

ADRENAL-PITUITARY AXIS

Adrenal Cortex

Cushing syndrome results from exogenous steroid administration or excess endogenous cortisol secretion. The clinical manifestations of Cushing syndrome include HTN, edema, muscle weakness, glucose intolerance, osteoporosis, easy bruising, cutaneous striae, and truncal obesity (buffalo hump, moon facies). Women may develop acne, hirsutism, and amenorrhea as a result of adrenal androgen excess.

PATHOPHYSIOLOGY

The most common of Cushing syndrome is iatrogenic, resulting from administration of exogenous glucocorticoids or ACTH. Hypersecretion of ACTH from the anterior pituitary gland (Cushing disease) is the most common pathologic cause (65–70 percent of cases) of endogenous hypercortisolism. The adrenal glands respond normally to the elevated ACTH, resulting in bilateral adrenal hyperplasia. Excessive release of corticotropin-releasing factor by the hypothalamus is a rare cause of hypercortisolism. Abnormal secretion of cortisol from a primary adrenal adenoma or carcinoma is the cause of hypercortisolism in 10–20 percent of cases. Primary adrenal neoplasms secrete corticosteroids independently of ACTH and usually result in suppressed plasma ACTH levels and atrophy of the adjacent and contralateral adrenocortical tissue. In approximately 15 percent of cases, Cushing syndrome is caused by ectopic secretion of ACTH or an ACTH-like substance from a small cell bronchogenic carcinoma, carcinoid tumor, pancreatic carcinoma, thymic carcinoma, medullary thyroid carcinoma, or other neuroendocrine neoplasm. Patients with ectopic ACTH-secreting neoplasms can present primarily with hypokalemia, glucose intolerance, and hyperpigmentation but with few other chronic signs of Cushing syndrome. Diagnosis of Cushing syndrome is biochemical. Goals are to first establish hypercortisolism and then identify the source. However, all of the available tests are complicated by a lack of specificity and an overlap in the biochemical responses of patients with the different disease states.

The best screening tests for hypercortisolism are overnight dexamethasone suppression test (1 mg dexamethasone at 11 p.m. and serum cortisol) or measurement of the urinary excretion of free cortisol. Patients with true hypercortisolism usually fail to suppress the morning plasma cortisol level to less than 5 pg/dL after receiving dexamethasone the night before. Similarly, urinary excretion of more than 100 pg/day of free cortisol in two independent collections is virtually diagnostic of Cushing syndrome. Measurement of plasma cortisol level alone is not reliable to diagnose Cushing syndrome due to overlap of the levels in normal and abnormal patients.

LOCALIZATION OF THE CAUSE

Determination of basal ACTH by immunoradiometric assay is the best test to determine the cause of hypercortisolism. Suppression of the absolute level of ACTH below 5 pg/mL is nearly diagnostic of adrenocortical neoplasms. ACTH levels in Cushing disease may range from the upper limits of normal, 15 pg/mL, to 500 pg/mL. Highest plasma levels of ACTH (greater than 1000 pg/mL) have been observed in patients with ectopic ACTH syndrome.

Standard high-dose dexamethasone suppression testing is used to discern a pituitary from an ectopic source of ACTH. Normal individuals and most patients with a pituitary ACTH-producing neoplasm respond to a high-dose dexamethasone suppression test (2 mg PO every 6 h for 48 h) with a reduction of urinary free cortisol and urinary 17-hydroxysteroids to less than 50 percent of basal values. Most patients with a primary adrenal tumor or an ectopic source of ACTH production fail to suppress to this level. However, this test does not separate clearly pituitary and ectopic ACTH hypersecretion because 25 percent of patients with the ectopic ACTH syndrome also have suppressible tumors.

Additional tests that may be useful include the metyrapone test (an inhibitor of the final step of cortisol synthesis) and the corticotrophin-releasing factor infusion test. Patients with pituitary hypersecretion of ACTH respond to these tests with a compensatory rise in ACTH and urinary 17-hydroxsteroids, whereas patients with a suppressed hypothalamic-pituitary axis (primary adrenal tumor, ectopic ACTH syndrome) usually do not have a compensatory rise.

IMAGING

Imaging tests are useful to identify lesions suspected on the basis of biochemical testing. Reliance on radiologic studies to diagnose the cause of Cushing syndrome should be discouraged. Gadolinium-enhanced MRI of the sella turcica is the best imaging test for pituitary adenomas suspected of causing ACTH-dependent hypercortisolism. Patients with ACTH-independent hypercortisolism require thin-section CT scan or MRI of the adrenal gland, both of which identify adrenal abnormalities with more than 95 percent sensitivity. Patients with ACTH-dependent hypercortisolism and either markedly elevated ACTH or a negative pituitary MRI should have CT scan of the chest to identify a tumor-producing ectopic ACTH.

Bilateral inferior petrosal sinus sampling can delineate unclear cases of Cushing disease from other causes of hypercortisolism. Simultaneous bilateral petrosal sinus and peripheral blood samples are obtained before and after peripheral intravenous injection of 1 µg/kg corticotropin-releasing hormone. A ratio of inferior petrosal sinus to peripheral plasma ACTH of 2.0 at basal or of 3.0 after corticotropin-releasing hormone administration is 100 percent sensitive and specific for pituitary adenoma.

SURGICAL TREATMENT OF CUSHING SYNDROME

Surgical treatment of Cushing syndrome involves removing the cause of cortisol excess. Transsphenoidal resection of an ACTH-producing pituitary tumor is successful in 80 percent or more of cases of Cushing disease. Treatment of ectopic ACTH syndrome involves resection of the primary lesion. Primary adrenal causes of Cushing syndrome are treated by removal of the adrenal gland containing the tumor. All patients who undergo adrenalectomy for primary adrenal causes of Cushing syndrome require perioperative and postoperative glucocorticoid replacement because the pituitary-adrenal axis is suppressed.

Primary Aldosteronism

Primary aldosteronism (Conn syndrome) is a syndrome of HTN and hypokalemia caused by hypersecretion of the mineralocorticoid aldosterone. This uncommon syndrome previously accounted for less than 1 percent of unselected patients with HTN. However, recent data examining routine screening suggest that aldosteronism may be the cause of up to 15 percent of cases of HTN. An aldosterone-producing adrenal adenoma (APA) is the cause of primary aldosteronism in two-thirds of cases and is one of the few surgically correctable causes of HTN. Idiopathic bilateral adrenal hyperplasia (IHA) causes 30–40 percent of cases of primary aldosteronism. Adrenocortical carcinoma and autosomal dominant glucocorticoid-suppressible aldosteronism are rare causes of primary aldosteronism. Secondary aldosteronism is a physiologic response of the renin-angiotensin system to renal artery stenosis, cirrhosis, congestive heart failure, and normal pregnancy. In these conditions, the adrenal gland functions normally.

DIAGNOSIS

Aldosterone-mediated retention of sodium and excretion of potassium and hydrogen ion by the kidney causes hypokalemia and moderate diastolic

HTN. Edema is characteristically absent. Laboratory diagnosis of primary aldosteronism requires demonstration of hypokalemia, inappropriate kaliuresis, and elevated aldosterone with normal cortisol. The ratio of the plasma aldosterone concentration (PAC) to plasma rennin activity (PRA) is now considered the best test to diagnose aldosteronism. A PAC to PRA ratio greater than 20–25 further suggests primary hyperaldosteronism. Upright plasma renin activity (PRA) less than 3 ng/mL/h corroborates the diagnosis. Confirmation of primary aldosteronism involves determination of serum potassium, PRA, and a 24-h urine collection for sodium, cortisol, and aldosterone after 5 days of a high-sodium diet. Patients with primary hyperaldosteronism do not demonstrate aldosterone suppressibility after salt loading. Alternatively plasma aldosterone and PRA can be measured before and 2 h after oral administration of 25 mg of captopril. Failure to suppress plasma aldosterone to less than 15 ng/dL is a positive test. Differentiation between adrenal adenoma and IHA is important because unilateral adenomas are treated by surgical excision, whereas bilateral hyperplasia is treated medically. Because suppression of the renin-angiotensin system is more complete in APA than in IHA, an imperfect separation (approximately 85 percent accuracy) of these two disorders is provided by measuring plasma aldosterone and PRA after overnight recumbency and then after 4 h of upright posture. Patients with IHA usually have an increase in PRA and aldosterone in response to upright posture, whereas in patients with adenoma, PRA usually remains suppressed, and aldosterone does not change or falls paradoxically. In practice, this test usually is not necessary because, after a biochemical diagnosis of primary hyperaldosteronism, sensitive imaging tests are used to localize the lesion or lesions.

LOCALIZATION

High-resolution adrenal CT scan should be the initial step in localization of an adrenal tumor. CT scanning localizes an adrenal adenoma in 90 percent of cases overall, and the presence of a unilateral adenoma larger than 1 cm on CT scan and supportive biochemical evidence of an aldosteronoma are generally all that is needed to make the diagnosis of Conn syndrome. Uncertainty regarding APA versus IHA after biochemical testing and noninvasive localization may be definitively settled by bilateral adrenal venous sampling for aldosterone and cortisol during ACTH infusion. Simultaneous adrenal vein blood samples for aldosterone and cortisol are taken: A unilateral adenoma is suggested by a fourfold elevation of aldosterone (corrected for cortisol) in blood obtained from one adrenal vein versus the other.

TREATMENT

Surgical removal of an aldosterone-secreting adenoma approach results in immediate cure or substantial improvement of HTN and hyperkalemia in more than 90 percent of patients with Conn syndrome. Laparoscopic adrenalectomy is a preferred surgical approach for aldosteronoma. The patient should be treated with spironolactone (200–400 mg/day) or eplerenone preoperatively for 2–3 weeks to control blood pressure and to correct hypokalemia. Patients with IHA should be treated medically with spironolactone (200–400 mg/day). A potassium-sparing diuretic, such as amiloride (5–20 mg/day), and calcium channel blockers have also been used. Surgical excision rarely cures bilateral hyperplasia.

Acute Adrenal Insufficiency

Acute adrenal insufficiency is an emergency and should be suspected in stressed patients with a history of either adrenal insufficiency or exogenous steroid use. Adrenocortical insufficiency is most often caused by acute withdrawal of chronic corticosteroid therapy but can result from autoimmune destruction of the adrenal cortex, adrenal hemorrhage (Waterhouse-Friderichsen syndrome), or rarely from infiltration with metastatic carcinoma.

SIGNS AND SYMPTOMS

Signs and symptoms include fever, nausea, vomiting, severe hypotension, and lethargy. Characteristic laboratory findings of adrenal insufficiency include hyponatremia, hyperkalemia, azotemia, and fasting or reactive hypoglycemia.

TREATMENT

Treatment of adrenal crisis must be immediate, based on clinical suspicion, before laboratory confirmation is available. Intravenous volume replacement with normal or hypertonic saline and dextrose is essential, as is immediate intravenous steroid replacement therapy with 4 mg dexamethasone. Then, a rapid ACTH stimulation test is used to test for adrenal insufficiency. Synthetic ACTH (250 (g) is administered intravenously and plasma cortisol levels are measured at 0, 30, and 60 min later. Normal peak cortisol response should exceed 20 g/dL. Thereafter, 100 mg hydrocortisone is administered intravenously every 6–8 h and is tapered to standard replacement doses as the patient's condition stabilizes. Subsequent recognition and treatment of the underlying cause, particularly if it is infectious, usually resolves the crisis. Mineralocorticoid replacement is not required until intravenous fluids are discontinued and oral intake resumes.

PREVENTION

Patients who have known adrenal insufficiency or have received supraphysiologic doses of steroid for at least 1 week in the year preceding surgery should receive 100 mg hydrocortisone the evening before and the morning of major surgery followed by 100 mg hydrocortisone every 8 h during the perioperative 24 h.

Adrenal Medulla: Pheochromocytoma

PATHOPHYSIOLOGY

Pheochromocytomas are neoplasms derived from the chromaffin cells of the sympathoadrenal system that result in unregulated, episodic oversecretion of catecholamines. Most pheochromocytomas secrete predominantly norepinephrine and smaller amounts of epinephrine.

CLINICAL FEATURES

Approximately 80–85 percent of pheochromocytomas in adults arise in the adrenal medulla, whereas 10–15 percent arise in the extra-adrenal chromaffin tissue, including the paravertebral ganglia, posterior mediastinum, organ of Zuckerkandl, or urinary bladder. Symptoms of pheochromocytoma are related to excess sympathetic stimulation from catecholamines and include paroxysms of pounding frontal headache, diaphoresis, palpitations, flushing, or anxiety. The most common sign is episodic or sustained HTN, but pheochromocytoma accounts for only 0.1–0.2 percent of patients with sustained diastolic HTN. Uncommonly, patients present with complications of prolonged uncontrolled HTN (e.g., myocardial infarction, cerebrovascular accident, or renal disease). Pheochromocytomas can occur in association with several hereditary syndromes that include MEN types 2A and 2B and von Hippel-Lindau syndrome. Tumors that arise in familial settings frequently are bilateral.

BIOCHEMICAL DIAGNOSIS

The biochemical diagnosis of pheochromocytoma is made by demonstrating elevated plasma fractionated metanephrines or by measuring 24-h urinary excretion of catecholamines and their metabolites (metanephrines, vanillylmandelic acid). Plasma catecholamines also are elevated during the paroxysms of HTN, but they are more difficult to measure and interpret and therefore have limited clinical application.

IMAGING

CT scanning is the imaging test of choice and identifies 90–95 percent of pheochromocytomas larger than 1 cm. MRI scanning can also be useful because T_2-weighted images have a characteristic high intensity in patients with pheochromocytoma and metastatic tumor compared to adenomas. Scintigraphic scanning after the administration of ^{131}I-MIBG provides a functional and anatomic test of hyperfunctioning chromaffin tissue. MIBG scanning is very specific for both intra- and extra-adrenal pheochromocytomas.

SURGICAL TREATMENT

The treatment of benign and malignant pheochromocytomas is surgical excision. Preoperative management includes administration of an α-adrenergic blocker to control HTN and to permit reexpansion of intravascular volume. Phenoxybenzamine, 10 mg PO bid, is initiated and increased to 20–40 mg PO bid until orthostasis is encountered. Postural HTN is expected and is the desired endpoint. β-Adrenergic blockade (e.g., propranolol) may be added if tachycardia or arrhythmias develop but only after complete α-adrenergic blockade.

The classic operative approach for familial pheochromocytomas is exploration of both adrenal glands, the preaortic and paravertebral areas, and the organ of Zuckerkandl through a midline or unilateral subcostal incision. In patients with MEN type 2A or 2B and a unilateral pheochromocytoma, it is acceptable policy to remove only the involved gland.[14] In patients with sporadic, unilateral pheochromocytoma localized by preoperative imaging studies, adrenalectomy is best performed laparoscopically although an anterior or posterior open approach may be used.

Adrenocortical Carcinoma

Adrenocortical carcinoma is a rare but aggressive malignancy; most patients with this cancer present with locally advanced disease. Syndromes of adrenal hormone overproduction may include rapidly progressive hypercortisolism, hyperaldosteronism, or virilization. Large (greater than 6 cm) adrenal masses that extend to nearby structures on CT scanning likely represent carcinoma. Complete surgical resection of locally confined tumor is the only chance for cure of adrenocortical carcinoma. Definitive diagnosis of adrenocortical carcinoma requires operative and pathologic demonstration of nodal or distant metastases. Often, patients with adrenocortical carcinoma present with metastatic disease, most often involving the lung, lymph nodes, liver, or bone. Palliative surgical debulking of locally advanced or metastatic adrenocortical carcinoma may provide these patients with symptomatic relief from some slow-growing, hormone-producing cancers. Chemotherapy with mitotane may be somewhat effective. Overall, the prognosis for patients with adrenocortical carcinoma is poor.

Incidental Adrenal Masses

Incidental adrenal masses are detected in 0.6–1.5 percent of abdominal CT scans obtained for other reasons. Most incidentally discovered adrenal masses are benign, nonfunctioning cortical adenomas of no clinical significance. Because of the high morbidity and relative frequency of pheochromocytoma and hypercortisolism, biochemical testing in asymptomatic, normotensive patients should be limited to screening for these disorders. Hypertensive patients should also be screened for aldosteronoma. Lesions that are solid, homogeneous, and nonfunctioning on endocrine testing and are smaller than 5 cm may be followed conservatively with a repeat CT scan in 3–6 months.[15] Functioning lesions or nonfunctional tumors larger than 5 cm should be resected. Some authors advocate removal of any adrenal mass, functional or nonfunctional, that is larger than 3.5 cm, to avoid late diagnosis of adrenocortical carcinoma.[16]

REFERENCES

1. Klee GG, Hay ID. Biochemical thyroid function testing. *Mayo Clin Proc* 69:469, 1994.
2. Klee GG, Hay ID. Role of thyrotropin measurements in the diagnosis and management of thyroid disease. *Clin Lab Med* 13:673, 1993.
3. Sridama V, McCormick M, Kaplan EL, et al. Long-term follow-up study of compensated low-dose ^{131}I therapy for Graves' disease. *N Engl J Med* 311:426, 1984.
4. Mazzaferri EL. Management of a solitary thyroid nodule. *N Engl J Med* 328:553, 1993.
5. Gharib H, Goellner JR. Fine-needle aspiration biopsy of the thyroid: an appraisal. *Ann Intern Med* 118:282–289, 1993.
6. Grant CS, Hay ID, Gough IR, et al. Long-term follow-up of patients with benign thyroid fine-needle aspiration cytologic diagnoses. *Surgery* 106:985, 1989.
7. Schlumberger MJ. Papillary and follicular thyroid carcinoma. *N Engl J Med* 38:297, 1998.
8. Donis-Keller H, Dou S, Chi D, et al. Mutations associated in the RET proto-oncogene are associated with MEN 2A and FMTC. *Hum Mol Genet* 2:851, 1993.
9. Olson JA Jr, DeBenditti MK, Baumann DS, et al. Parathyroid autotransplantation during thyroidectomy. Results of long-term follow-up. *Ann Surg* 223:478, 1996.
10. Miller DL, Doppman JL, Shawker TH, et al. Localization of parathyroid adenomas in patients who have undergone surgery. Part I. Noninvasive imaging methods. *Radiology* 162:133, 1987.
11. Miller DL, Doppman JL, Shawler TH, et al. Localization of parathyroid adenomas in patients who have undergone surgery. Part II. Invasive procedures. *Radiology* 163:138, 1987.
12. Rosch T, Lightdale CJ, Botet JF, et al. Localization of pancreatic endocrine tumors by endoscopic ultrasonography. *N Engl J Med* 326:1721, 1992.
13. Moertel CG, Weiland LH, Nagorney DM, et al. Carcinoid tumor of the appendix: treatment and prognosis. *N Engl J Med* 317:1699, 1987.
14. Lairmore TC, Ball DW, Baylin SB, et al. Management of pheochromocytomas in patients with multiple endocrine neoplasia type 2 syndromes. *Ann Surg* 217:595, 1993.
15. Copeland PM. The incidentally discovered adrenal mass. *Ann Intern Med* 98:940, 1983.
16. Belldegrun A, Hussain S, Seltzer SE, et al. Incidentally discovered mass of the adrenal gland. *Surg Gynecol Obstet* 163:203, 1986.

HERNIAS

Keshava Rajagopal, MD, PhD

INTRODUCTION

A hernia may be operationally defined as the abnormal protrusion of a structure through a defect in the tissues that normally contain that structure. Hernias become clinically significant by virtue of chronic sequelae—stable symptoms, and progressive enlargement with or without symptoms, or due to acute complications—*incarceration* and *strangulation* of the herniated structures. Broadly, these sequelae comprise the indications for operative repair of hernias. The most common hernias encountered clinically are those of abdominal contents. Sir Astley Cooper's description of abdominal hernias in 1804 is apt: "A protrusion of any viscus from its proper cavity is called a hernia. The protruded parts are generally contained in a bag, formed by the membrane with which the cavity is naturally lined."[1] Groin or *inguinal* hernias represent the most common type of abdominal hernia, and inguinal hernia repair is the most commonly performed surgical procedure in the United States. This chapter discusses the anatomy, natural history, diagnosis, and treatment of abdominal hernias, with a particular focus on inguinal hernias. Additionally, the results of various types of hernia repairs are reviewed, and modern *evidence-based* approaches to hernia management are discussed.

HISTORICAL OVERVIEW

Hernias are among the earliest pathologies identified in medical history, and among the first surgically treated. The history of hernia surgery is truly a history of surgery, associated with many of the most illustrious names in surgery. The Edwin Smith papyrus, dating to the sixteenth century B.C., demonstrated the ancient Egyptians' knowledge of inguinal hernia, and the usage of local application of heat to facilitate manual reduction.[2] There is also evidence to suggest that the Egyptians operatively repaired inguinal hernias, based on the mummy of the pharaoh Memeptah. Later, in ancient Greece, Hippocrates of

Kos identified *etru rhexis*, or rupture of the abdominal wall, and is thought to have first used the term hernia.[3] Subsequently, Susruta, a physician and surgeon of the Gupta era civilization of ancient India, in the first medical treatise devoted to surgery (Susruta samhita), also discussed approaches to surgical repair of hernias.

The Renaissance ushered in detailed human anatomic investigation and the forerunners of modern surgical techniques. The famed sixteenth century French battlefield surgeon Ambroise Pare, who pioneered the field of trauma surgery (specifically by introducing concepts of sterile technique and wound care)[4], repaired an inguinal hernia using a gold wire cerclage, and repaired an incarcerated inguinal hernia. Over the next three centuries, inguinal anatomy was elucidated, with individual structures acquiring some of the most recognizable eponyms in surgery. Scarpa and Camper lent their names to superficial fascial layers, while each of the major ligaments acquired the following names: (1) inguinal—Poupart's, (2) lacunar—Gimbernat's, and (3) iliopectineal—Cooper's. Finally, the triangle through which direct inguinal hernias classically occur (see section Direct Inguinal Hernia) acquired Hesselbach's name.

ANATOMY

For an understanding of hernias, it is essential to be conversant with the anatomy of the abdominal wall. In this section, the anatomy of the anterior/lateral abdominal wall and groin are reviewed and diagrammed, and the abnormalities present in direct and indirect inguinal hernias are reviewed and diagrammed afterward.

Anatomy of the Anterior/Lateral Abdominal Wall

The layers of the anterolateral abdominal wall are displayed in Fig. 16-1. It is useful to organize the structures from superficial to deep, as one would encounter them operatively. Anteriorly, above the arcuate line (*linea semicircularis*), the termination of the posterior sheath of the rectus abdominis muscles, the layers (excluding interspersed fat) are as follows: skin, Camper's fascia, Scarpa's fascia, anterior rectus sheath, rectus abdominis muscle, posterior rectus sheath, transversalis fascia, and parietal peritoneum. The rectus sheaths fuse in the midline, forming the *linea alba*. Below the arcuate line, the posterior rectus sheath is absent. Lateral to the rectus abdominis, the lateral border is termed the *linea semilunaris*, the layers are: skin, Camper's fascia, Scarpa's fascia, external oblique muscle, internal oblique muscle, transversus abdominis muscle, transversalis fascia, and parietal peritoneum. Finally, the transversus abdominis and internal oblique muscles fuse inferomedially to form the conjoint tendon, also known as the *falx inguinalis*.

Anterior abdominal wall: Superficial dissection

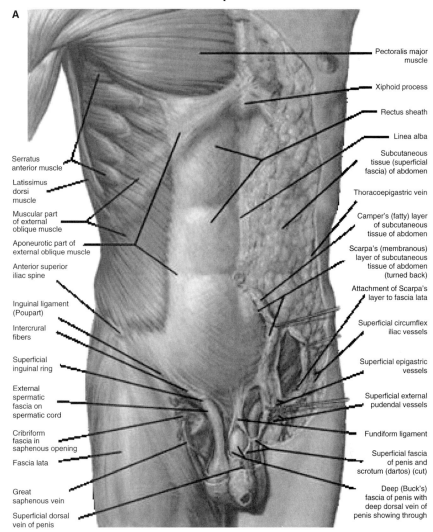

A

Pectoralis major muscle

Xiphoid process

Rectus sheath

Linea alba

Subcutaneous tissue (superficial fascia) of abdomen

Thoracoepigastric vein

Camper's (fatty) layer of subcutaneous tissue of abdomen

Scarpa's (membranous) layer of subcutaneous tissue of abdomen (turned back)

Attachment of Scarpa's layer to fascia lata

Superficial circumflex iliac vessels

Superficial epigastric vessels

Superficial external pudendal vessels

Fundiform ligament

Superficial fascia of penis and scrotum (dartos) (cut)

Deep (Buck's) fascia of penis with deep dorsal vein of penis showing through

Serratus anterior muscle

Latissimus dorsi muscle

Muscular part of external oblique muscle

Aponeurotic part of external oblique muscle

Anterior superior iliac spine

Inguinal ligament (Poupart)

Intercrural fibers

Superficial inguinal ring

External spermatic fascia on spermatic cord

Cribriform fascia in saphenous opening

Fascia lata

Great saphenous vein

Superficial dorsal vein of penis

Figure 16-1 **Anatomy of the anterior abdominal wall. (A) Anterior view of superficial dissection of the anterior abdominal wall. (B) Intermediate dissection. (C) Transverse section through the abdominal wall above the arcuate line, demonstrating the layers of the anterior abdominal wall. Below the arcuate line, the posterior rectus sheath is absent.** (*Source:* The Netter Collection. Icon Learning Systems.)

Anterior abdominal wall
Intermediate dissection

B

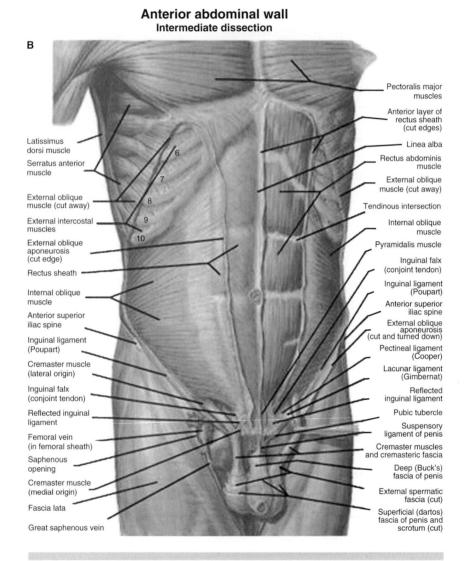

Pectoralis major
muscles

Anterior layer of
rectus sheath
(cut edges)

Linea alba

Rectus abdominis
muscle

External oblique
muscle (cut away)

Tendinous intersection

Internal oblique
muscle

Pyramidalis muscle

Inguinal falx
(conjoint tendon)

Inguinal ligament
(Poupart)

Anterior superior
iliac spine

External oblique
aponeurosis
(cut and turned down)

Pectineal ligament
(Cooper)

Lacunar ligament
(Gimbernat)

Reflected
inguinal ligament

Pubic tubercle

Suspensory
ligament of penis

Cremaster muscles
and cremasteric fascia

Deep (Buck's)
fascia of penis

External spermatic
fascia (cut)

Superficial (dartos)
fascia of penis and
scrotum (cut)

Latissimus
dorsi muscle

Serratus anterior
muscle

External oblique
muscle (cut away)

External intercostal
muscles

External oblique
aponeurosis
(cut edge)

Rectus sheath

Internal oblique
muscle

Anterior superior
iliac spine

Inguinal ligament
(Poupart)

Cremaster muscle
(lateral origin)

Inguinal falx
(conjoint tendon)

Reflected inguinal
ligament

Femoral vein
(in femoral sheath)

Saphenous
opening

Cremaster muscle
(medial origin)

Fascia lata

Great saphenous vein

Figure 16-1 **(Continued)**

Normal Inguinal Anatomy

Figure 16-2 depicts normal anatomy of the inguinal region. The surgically relevant structures will be reviewed in the following order: (1) fascial structures, (2) vasculature, (3) spermatic cord structures, and (4) nerves.

The inguinal ligament is formed from the aponeurosis of the external oblique muscle, and extends from the anterior superior iliac spine to the

Rectus sheath
Cross section above arcuate line

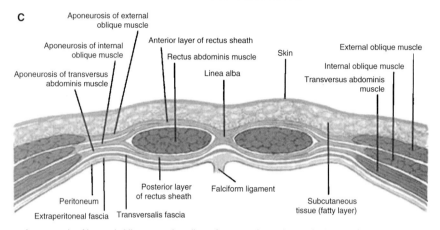

Aponeurosis of internal oblique muscle splits to form anterior and posterior layers of rectus sheath. Aponeurosis of external oblique muscle joins anterior layer of sheath; aponeurosis of transversus abdominis muscle joins posterior layer. Anterior and posterior layers of rectus sheath unite medially to form linea alba

Figure 16-1 (***Continued***)

pubic tubercle. Posteromedially, the inguinal ligament forms the lacunar ligament, which extends from the pubic tubercle to the iliopectineal line. Further posteriorly, the lacunar ligament connects with the iliopectineal ligament, which runs along mediolaterally along the superior pubic ramus.

The inguinal ligament and the iliopectineal ligament form two sides of a triangle, with the lacunar ligament at one vertex. The third side of the triangle is formed by the iliopsoas muscle. The external iliac artery (lateral) and vein (medial) lie on the anterior surface of the iliopsoas, and course through this fascial triangle (termed the femoral sheath), deep to the inguinal ligament. Once the vessels pass posterior to the inguinal ligament, they are renamed the common femoral artery and vein, respectively. Medial to the external iliac/ common femoral vein is the femoral canal. Femoral hernias occur through this space. Finally, the inferior epigastric vessels are the last branches of the external iliac vessels, prior to their passage under the inguinal ligament.

The spermatic cord in the male and round ligament in the female pass from posterior to anterior through the deep inguinal ring laterally, and then through the superficial inguinal ring medially. The deep inguinal ring is a foramen in the transversalis fascia lateral to the inferior epigastric vessels, while the superficial ring is a foramen in the external oblique fascia. Finally, the nerves of concern in inguinal hernia are the genitofemoral and ilioinguinal.

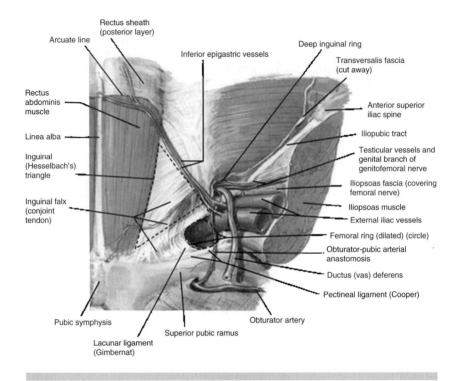

Figure 16-2 **Normal inguinal anatomy. The right inguinal region is viewed from posterior to anterior.** (*Source:* The Netter Collection. Icon Learning Systems.)

The genitofemoral nerve is derived from roots L1-2, and runs on the anterior surface of the iliopsoas muscle, and divides into genital and femoral branches. The genital branch passes through the deep inguinal ring, and supplies the cremaster muscle. The femoral branch passes through the femoral sheath and supplies skin overlying the femoral triangle. The ilioinguinal nerve is derived from roots T12-L1, and is formed with the iliohypogastric nerve. It runs along the iliacus muscle, and then passes the anterior iliac crest *en route* to lying between the internal and external oblique muscles. The nerve then passes through the superficial inguinal ring, and supplies the superomedial thigh and superior portion of the scrotum.

Direct Inguinal Hernia

A direct inguinal hernia occurs within the boundaries of Hesselbach's triangle. Consequently, it is a *medial* hernia, that is, it is medial to the inferior epigastric vessels. As a result, it classically occurs through the superficial inguinal ring with or without a defect in the conjoint tendon, in contrast to indirect inguinal hernia. Direct inguinal hernias are generally oriented in a posteroanterior fashion, unlike indirect hernias.

Indirect Inguinal Hernia

An indirect inguinal hernia occurs outside Hesselbach's triangle; thus, it occurs lateral to the inferior epigastric vessels. Furthermore, an indirect inguinal hernia is through the deep inguinal ring, in contrast to a direct inguinal hernia. The indirect hernia is generally oriented in a lateral-to-medial fashion, in contrast to direct hernia.

Classification Systems

There is not an all-encompassing classification system that stratifies etiology and/or treatment for hernias. However, two classification systems predominate for categorizing inguinal hernias, the Aachen[5,6] and Nyhus[7] systems. These are displayed in Tables 16-1 and 16-2, respectively. In the Aachen system, four types of hernias are recognized: *lateral* (L), *medial* (M), *combined* (Mc), and *femoral* (F). Each type of hernia is subcategorized based on hernia size: I denotes an orifice less than 1.5 cm in diameter, II denotes an orifice from 1.5 to 3 cm, and III corresponds to orifices greater than 3 cm. In the Nyhus system also, four types of hernias are recognized. Type 1 is an indirect hernia without dilation of the internal ring, while type 2 is an indirect hernia with dilation of the internal ring. Three subtypes of type 3 hernias are present: (a) direct hernia with a backwall defect, (b) indirect hernia with a backwall defect, and (c) femoral hernia. All recurrent hernias are classified as type 4.

The purpose of disease classification systems is to distinguish different disease states based on anatomic and/or physiologic features that in turn usually (but not always) correlate with or dictate therapeutic options. The Aachen and Nyhus systems are of value in this context. However, it is important to note that data are continuing to emerge regarding inguinal hernia repair, and that furthermore, anatomic heterogeneity exists within the

Table 16-1 **The Aachen Hernia Classification System**[a]

L	Lateral
M	Medial
Mc	Combined
F	Femoral
I	Hernia orifice <1.5 cm
II	Hernia orifice 1.5–3.0 cm
III	Hernia orifice >3.0 cm

[a]See text for details.

Table 16-2 **The Nyhus Hernia Classification System**[a]

Class	
1	Indirect—intact internal inguinal ring
2	Indirect—dilated internal inguinal ring
3a	Posterior—direct
3b	Posterior—indirect
3c	Posterior—femoral
4a	Recurrent inguinal hernia—direct
4b	Recurrent inguinal hernia—indirect
4c	Recurrent femoral hernia
4d	Recurrent combined

[a]See text for details.

classes of hernias. Thus, decisions regarding operative management of hernias are often made on a case-by-case basis.

ETIOLOGY AND PATHOGENESIS

Direct Inguinal Hernia

Direct inguinal hernias are generally acquired in origin, arising as a result of an imbalance between intra-abdominal stresses and the strength of the abdominal wall. The stresses alone cause weakening of the wall, and when the strength of the abdominal wall is exceeded, herniation occurs. The etiologic factors in direct hernia thus relate to conditions with high intra-abdominal pressure (and thus, wall stresses), and loss of structural integrity of the abdominal wall.

High intra-abdominal pressure may arise due to extra-abdominal or intra-abdominal pathology. Extra-abdominal pathology that results in elevated intra-abdominal pressure generally is comprised of mechanical diseases of the lungs and/or pleura.[8] Obstructive lung diseases, either due to excessively high lung compliance (emphysema) or elevated airways resistance (chronic bronchitis), necessitate the development of high pleural pressures during expiration in an attempt to maintain adequate expiratory airflow rates. Since the thorax and abdomen are effectively a single cavity separated by the diaphragm, contraction of the abdominal wall muscles can aid in the development of positive intrathoracic pressure. This can result in concentration of stresses at points of pre-existing structural weakness in the abdominal wall. In those patients with emphysematous characteristics, elevated lung volumes and the inferior steady-state displacement of the diaphragm confine minimally compressible abdominal contents in a small space, increasing basal intra-abdominal pressure. Furthermore, emphysematous disease may be a marker for loss of systemic tissue integrity due to imbalances in proteolytic systems and their regulation in favor of proteolysis.[9] Restrictive and obstructive lung diseases with profoundly increased airways resistance necessitate the development of highly negative pleural pressures during inspiration in an attempt to maintain adequate inspiratory airflow rates. For this same reason described for expiration, stresses can concentrate in weaknesses in the abdominal wall. That is, high-amplitude fluctuations in pleural pressure during inspiration and/or expiration can load the abdominal fascia such that hernias may occur. Obesity and ascites may also increase intra-abdominal pressure, by increasing the volume of abdominal contents.

Poor abdominal wall structural integrity may be genetic or acquired in origin. Heritable connective tissue disorders include Ehlers-Danlos syndrome[10,11] and similar disorders of collagen synthesis and processing.[12] Acquired etiologies include malnutrition,[13] usage of steroids,[8] and other medications that impair healing. However, the most common mechanisms underlying abdominal wall weakness are traumatic,[14] either acute or due to chronic wear.

Indirect Inguinal Hernia

Unlike direct inguinal hernia, indirect inguinal hernia is congenital in origin, arising from a developmental defect, namely, patency of the *processus vaginalis*.[14] Additionally, it is predominantly found in males, occurring in a male: female ratio of 4:1. This was first reported by the renowned British surgeon John Hunter in 1756. The processus vaginalis is an outpouching of peritoneum that in the male passes through the deep and superficial inguinal rings and into the scrotum. During the eighth month of *in utero* life, the testicle descends from an abdominal position; the processus vaginalis precedes it into the scrotum and clears a path for testicular descent. Once the testicle has reached a scrotal position, the processus vaginalis is obliterated normally. Persistence of the processus vaginalis results in an ability of the peritoneum-lined abdominal structures to enter the scrotum, by definition a hernia. For this reason, indirect inguinal hernia is also referred to as a *communicating hydrocele*. In some cases, the processus vaginalis may obliterate with a fluid collection present in the scrotal remnant; this is termed as *noncommunicating hydrocele*.

In the female, the round ligament is analogous to the spermatic cord, and passes through the deep and superficial inguinal rings to terminate in the labium majus. The labium majus is the Müllerian analogue of the scrotum. The patent processus vaginalis in this setting is termed the *canal of Nuck*.

In summary, direct and indirect inguinal hernias have distinct etiologies. Direct hernias are acquired, and are a consequence of an imbalance between intra-abdominal stresses and abdominal wall strength. Indirect inguinal hernias, which are more common and preferentially occur in males, occur due to patency of the processus vaginalis. These etiologic distinctions may translate to differences in clinical presentation.

CLINICAL PRESENTATION AND DIAGNOSIS

As the understanding of molecular mechanisms underlying disease increases, the utility of and dependence on sophisticated diagnostic assays has increased in parallel. This is particularly true in diseases with complex underlying pathophysiologic mechanisms. Nevertheless, thorough histories and physical examinations continue to form the basic framework of diagnosis, and are invaluable. The diagnosis of a hernia is one that is still most often made by history and physical examination, in the absence of imaging studies. Consequently, the pertinent aspects of history taking and physical examination in the context of a suspected hernia (with focus on inguinal hernia) are reviewed in this section. Diagnostic studies are discussed afterward.

History

The evaluation of any patient in the non-emergent setting begins with the history. The history is essential in the formulation and stratification of a differential diagnosis, and this is also the case in various general surgical disorders. Specifically, it is directed toward answering whether the patient likely has a condition that requires or will benefit from surgery, and if so, with what urgency operative intervention needs to be undertaken. Thus, it is important to know how hernias present, and particularly, how they present differently in the chronic setting versus the acute setting. It is also requisite to obtain a complete previous medical and surgical history with review of systems, family history, medication regimen, and adverse drug reactions. This allows for evaluating operative/postoperative risk, and furthermore, is crucial in guiding the pre- and postoperative care of the patient.

Risk factors for hernia are important to investigate in the prospective general surgical patient, in whom other information may suggest the presence of a surgical disease. The principal clinical risk factors for hernia are thought to be: (1) any disorder associated with increased intra-abdominal pressure; (2) disorders associated with impaired structural tissue integrity, (3) male sex[15,16], (4) age[15,17,18], (5) known history of previous hernia, (6) family history of hernias[19,20], and (7) smoking.[18]

The majority of presentations of hernias are in the outpatient setting, with chronic symptoms. Patients with inguinal hernias most commonly complain of groin pain or discomfort, and often report groin swelling or the presence of a new or enlarging mass. Both of these symptoms may be exacerbated by standing or actively increasing intra-abdominal pressure (e.g., lifting weight, coughing, or Valsalva maneuver)[16]. Patients commonly report that the mass is reducible, that is, it can be returned to an intra-abdominal position. However, some patients report so-called *intermittent incarceration*, when the mass appears fixed for a period of time, only to be reduced later.

In evaluating a patient presenting with pain and an inguinal mass consistent with a possible inguinal hernia, it is important to better characterize these two cardinal symptoms. First, the following attributes of groin pain must be identified: (1) character, (2) location, (3) timing and onset, (4) improving/exacerbating stimuli, and (5) radiation. Next, the mass must be characterized based on appearance and tactile findings (see section Physical Examination).

Acutely, the presentation of hernias is due to specific complications, namely those of *incarceration* and *strangulation*. Incarceration refers to immobility and irreducibility of the hernia, while strangulation constitutes a subset of incarceration in which ischemia of the herniated contents occurs as a consequence of incarceration. It is essential to understand that left untreated, the natural history of an incarcerated hernia is to often progress to strangulation. For this reason, all suspected incarcerated hernias mandate intervention—either nonoperative reduction (which if successful, the hernia was not truly incarcerated) or operative repair. Those incarcerated hernias in which strangulation is suspected require urgent operative exploration.

Patients with incarceration classically present with a history of acute-onset groin pain, usually worse than previous episodes not associated with incarceration. The pain is typically described as sharp and constant. Unlike previous episodes that the patient may have experienced, which are relieved by manual reduction of the hernia, pain in the setting of incarceration is often unrelenting. Constitutional symptoms, specifically fevers, should raise the suspicion of strangulation. Gastrointestinal symptoms, in particular those associated with bowel obstruction, make up the remainder of significant symptoms. Incarcerated hernias are the second to fourth most common cause of small bowel obstruction,[21,22] with inguinal hernias accounting for the majority of these. Symptoms associated with bowel obstruction include nausea, emesis, abdominal pain, obstipation (failure to pass flatus), and constipation. Of note, incarcerated Richter hernias, discussed later, do not present with bowel obstruction.

Physical Examination

The findings of physical examination in the hernia patient, like the history, are different in the chronic setting versus the acute setting. It is important to conduct a thorough physical examination with vital signs, including a cardiovascular and pulmonary assessment. However, the present discussion will focus on the abdominal/inguinal examinations.

The approach to the abdominal and inguinal examinations consists in inspection, palpation, and auscultation. In the chronic setting, an isolated inguinal hernia is seen as a unilateral groin enlargement. Direct hernias are often observed medially and superiorly, in contrast to indirect hernias, which are seen to extend laterally and inferiorly. On palpation, hernias in the chronic (i.e., not incarcerated) setting are generally soft, mobile masses that can be either partially or fully reduced; they are rarely tender. Auscultation may reveal bowel sounds present over the hernia. The remainder of the abdominal examination should be performed in a similar fashion. Particular attention should be paid to evaluation for other abdominal hernias (see section Other Abdominal Hernias), and inspection for surgical incisions.

In the acute setting, the important features of examination are those that argue for or against incarceration, with or without strangulation. Inspection may reveal erythematous skin changes overlying the hernia, which should raise concern for possible strangulation. The position of the hernia is typically similar to that seen in the chronic setting. Palpation is essential, with its purpose being evaluation for incarceration and possible strangulation. Incarcerated hernias are often tender to palpation, particularly when strangulation has occurred. However, the diagnosis of incarceration centers on the palpatory findings of irreducibility and to a lesser extent, immobility. Auscultation over the hernia may reveal obstructive or even absent bowel sounds when incarceration of bowel has occurred. Finally, the remainder of the abdominal and groin examinations should be performed to evaluate for other processes that may present similarly, and equally importantly, to evaluate for peritonitis, which suggests incarceration and mandates immediate surgical intervention. Other etiologies of bowel obstruction and their severity must be evaluated on physical examination. Thus, examination for abdominal distension, masses that may or may not be tender to palpation, abdominal surgical incisions, auscultation of the abdomen with characterization of bowel sounds (as either present, absent, or obstructive), and palpation of the abdomen to evaluate for peritoneal signs is essential.

Differential Diagnosis

The differential diagnosis of an inguinal mass is listed in Table 16-3. Of note, vascular pathologies manifesting with inguinal masses are rare, but are potentially of high morbidity and associated mortality. These include external iliac or femoral arterial aneurysms and pseudoaneurysms (and even rarer, venous aneurysms and pseudoaneurysms), and fascially contained hemorrhage. Also uncommon and of equally high morbidity and mortality are hematologic malignancies manifesting as groin masses (e.g., lymphoma).

It is important to note that of the etiologies listed, hernias are by far the most common in incidence. Other common etiologies include testicular neoplasms or torsion, lipoma, and varicocele.

Nonoperative Reduction

In some cases, patients who present with an otherwise incarcerated hernia may be successfully treated by nonoperative reduction. Strictly speaking, a hernia is not incarcerated if it is reducible, but there are hernias that are temporarily incarcerated until formal nonoperative reduction is performed. The procedure for nonoperative reduction is described below.

First, the diagnosis of an incarcerated hernia must be confirmed. Second, adequate analgesia is administered. The patient is placed in Trendelenburg position, which reduces groin pressure. Ice may then be applied to reduce

Table 16-3 **Differential Diagnosis of an Inguinal Mass**

Organ System Involved	Different Diagnoses
Hernias	Inguinal
	Femoral
Urologic	Testicular neoplasm
	Testicular torsion
	Hydrocele
	Lymphocele
	Varicocele
Infectious	Psoas abscess
	Epididymitis
	Hidradenitis
	Sebaceous cyst
	Inguinal adenitis
	Femoral adenitis
Hematologic/immunologic	Lymphoma
Vascular	Aneurysm (external iliac/common femoral)
	Pseudoaneurysm (external iliac/ commonfemoral)
	Hematoma

inflammation and thus, the size of the incarcerated hernia. Then, the mass is tubularized and gently pulled outward (distracted). The mass is then slowly pushed back through the inguinal ring, in an inferomedial to superolateral direction. If this fails, operative intervention is required.

Diagnostic Studies

The majority of patients who undergo elective inguinal hernia repair do not require preoperative laboratory or imaging studies. In some cases however, due to preoperative comorbid conditions (most notably cardiovascular and pulmonary disease), preoperative assessment of cardiac and pulmonary function, as well as blood laboratory studies, are necessary. Patients with complex abdominal hernias, unlike most inguinal hernias, may need preoperative abdominal computerized tomographic (CT) scans to guide surgical planning.

Unlike elective repair, patients who undergo urgent inguinal hernia repair either require or undergo blood testing and imaging studies during the course of their preoperative workup. Useful blood tests include a white blood cell count with differential (to assess for infection/inflammation as a consequence of strangulation, particularly in febrile patients), and serum electrolytes (particularly in those patients with bowel obstruction), while urinalysis is important in febrile patients. Preoperative imaging studies include abdominal plain radiographs (to assess bowel obstruction and perforation) and for the same reasons, abdominal CT scans.

SURGICAL PRINCIPLES AND APPROACHES

Overview

Hernias are anatomic diseases, and thus the treatment of hernias centers on the restoration of normal anatomic relationships. This requires surgical intervention. In the modern era of hernia surgery, multiple surgical approaches are available, each with specific advantages and disadvantages. Broadly, hernia repairs may be classified as under tension or tension-free. Primary repairs are generally considered to be tensioned, as they rely on direct approximation of muscle/ligament layers to obliterate the defect. Mesh repairs, on the other hand, as they employ use of exogenous material to obliterate the defect, are generally considered to be tension-free. In this chapter, these various approaches will be discussed.

Primary Repairs

BASSINI REPAIR

The Bassini repair is a tensioned primary repair, first performed by the Italian surgeon Eduardo Bassini in 1884.[23] Popular modifications include the Halsted I and II repairs.[24] A Bassini repair consists of hernia reduction, and direct (sutured) approximation of the conjoint tendon to the inguinal ligament. The Halsted repairs differ from the Bassini repair in that the external oblique aponeurosis is imbricated in the Halsted operation. The Halsted I and II further differ from one another in that the spermatic cord is kept external to the external oblique fascia in the Halsted I repair, whereas the Halsted II repair maintains the normal anatomic position of the spermatic cord.

The Bassini/Halsted inguinal hernia repairs have the advantage of not requiring an indwelling foreign body. However, they are tensioned repairs, and consequently, have a higher rate of recurrence in comparison to tension-free repairs (see section Mesh-based Repairs).

MCVAY REPAIR

The McVay repair, first performed in 1948,[25] is a primary repair that may be used for both inguinal and femoral (see section Other Abdominal Hernias) hernias. It differs substantively from the Bassini/Halsted repairs in that the iliopectineal ligament is incorporated medially.[24–26] After hernia reduction, a relaxing incision is made in the rectus sheath. The conjoint tendon is suture approximated to the iliopectineal ligament medially, and a stitch transitioning the inferior margin of closure from the iliopectineal ligament to the inguinal ligament is placed at the level of the femoral canal, thereby closing it. Laterally, the remainder of the conjoint tendon/transversalis fascia is sutured to the inguinal ligament.

The McVay repair has an the advantage of being applicable to both inguinal and femoral hernias, in comparison to other tensioned repairs. Its disadvantages are identical to those for other tensioned repairs.

SHOULDICE/CANADIAN REPAIR

The Shouldice repair is essentially a modification of the Bassini operation, first performed in 1945 by Dr. E. Shouldice.[27] Unlike the Bassini and McVay repairs, which use a single-layer approximation of the conjoint tendon and transversalis fascia to the inguinal ligament, the Shouldice repair involves a layered closure.[24,27] The abdominal wall is dissected into its distinct layers and incised, yielding medial and lateral edges. Then, closure is performed by overlapping separate layers of external oblique, internal oblique, transversalis fascia, and transversus abdominis. In this imbricated layer approach, the spermatic cord is still maintained under a layer of external oblique fascia.

The Shouldice repair has, by design, the lowest tension of the tensioned repairs. This results in a lower recurrence rate than other primary repair techniques (see section Mesh-based Repairs). However, this is yet higher than the tension associated with a mesh-based repair. Like all primary repairs, the Shouldice repair has the advantage of the absence of an indwelling foreign body.

NYHUS/ILIOPUBIC TRACT REPAIR

Unlike the previously discussed primary repairs, all of which are anterior approaches, the Nyhus or iliopubic tract repair is a posterior-based repair.[24,28] Reported in 1959, it is related to operations for inguinal hernia first performed by Cheatle in 1920. Posterior approaches such as the Nyhus repair may also be performed using mesh. In the Nyhus technique, the anterior rectus sheath is incised medially, extending to the internal and external oblique aponeuroses laterally. The preperitoneal space is entered, and the hernia sac is reduced. Then, the hernia defect is repaired by directly approximating the transversalis fascia to the iliopubic tract (Bassini-like), or by directly approximating the transversalis fascia to iliopectineal ligament medially, and to the iliopubic tract laterally (McVay-like).

Posterior-based approaches have the advantage of being better suited to recurrent hernias. Primary Nyhus repairs are similar to other primary repairs in terms of benefits and risks, whereas those performed with mesh are similar to other open techniques performed with mesh.

Mesh-Based Repairs

The past two decades have been noteworthy for the development of tension-free repairs, which use a prosthesis to bridge the hernia. These are discussed below.

LICHTENSTEIN REPAIR

The most commonly performed method of inguinal hernia repair in the United States is the tension-free mesh repair introduced in the 1980s by Irving Lichtenstein.[24,29,30] It involves placing a piece of mesh, typically polypropylene, to fill the space between the conjoint tendon/transversalis fascia superiorly, and the inguinal ligament inferiorly. The mesh scars in place, and the scar acts to prevent recurrence. The conjoint tendon/transversalis fascia are sutured to the mesh patch superiorly, and the inguinal ligament is sutured to the mesh patch inferiorly; inferomedially, the patch may be anchored to the pubic tubercle and/or the iliopectineal ligament. A neoinguinal ring is fashioned by making two *legs* laterally in the patch, which wrap around the spermatic cord.

MESH PLUG TECHNIQUES

Other techniques for mesh repair include so-called *mesh plugs* in which the hernia is reduced and a plug of mesh occupies the defect and is affixed to the adjacent tissues; this has been championed by Rutkow,[31,32] among others. This may be performed with or without overlay or small under- or overlay mesh patches.

Laparoscopic Repairs

The advent of laparoscopic surgery has resulted in the development of laparoscopic techniques for hernia repair. The primary disadvantage of these approaches is the requirement of general anesthesia, and a possibly higher risk of major vascular injury and recurrent in less experienced hands.[33,34]; this is in contrast to the previously discussed approaches, which employ local and/or regional anesthesia. Advantages include smaller incisions, decreased postoperative pain, and decreased length of postoperative stay.[33–35]

TRANSABDOMINAL PREPERITONEAL REPAIR

A transabdominal preperitoneal (TAPP) repair, as its name implies, involves accessing the preperitoneal space.[36,37] This is accomplished by incising the peritoneum laterally from the medial umbilical ligament, and anterior to the hernia. The hernia sac(s) is(are) then reduced, and then a fashioned mesh patch is laparoscopically stapled in place. Importantly, the mesh is stapled superiorly, medially, and inferomedially, but no lateral (particularly inferolateral) stapling of the mesh to the iliopubic tract is performed due to the risk of injury to the external iliac/femoral vessels.

TOTAL EXTRAPERITONEAL REPAIR

In contrast to a TAPP repair, a total extraperitoneal (TEP) repair does not violate the peritoneum, and has the argued advantage of lower risk of visceral injury. The laparoscopic trocars do not enter the peritoneal cavity, but are dissected through the preperitoneal space.[37,38] The hernia is identified laparoscopically and then reduced. A mesh repair is then undertaken as would be performed via an open approach.

RESULTS OF SURGICAL TREATMENT

Multiple studies have been published regarding the various strategies for achieving inguinal hernia repair, and their advantages and disadvantages. The best evidence, however, is that derived from randomized controlled trials (RCTs) and relevant meta-analyses. These are briefly reviewed in this section. Some of the information in this section is from a recent editorial by Jacobs.[39]

Results of Clinical Trials

First, comparisons between tensioned and tension-free repairs will be discussed. Within tensioned repairs, two RCTs have shown superior outcomes after the Shouldice operation in comparison with the Bassini operation,[40,41] with substantially lower recurrence rates. Three RCTs from 1998 to 2002 comparing the Shouldice repair with the Lichtenstein repair have shown that generally, the Lichtenstein repair is easier to learn and has a shorter operative time.[42–44] Also, although both repairs have a low (approximately 5 percent or less) rate of recurrence, the Lichtenstein repair has a lower rate of recurrence. Comparisons between open and laparoscopic approaches have yielded mixed results. An RCT from 1997 comparing all open repairs with laparoscopic repairs demonstrated superior outcomes after laparoscopic repair[45]; however, the majority of patients who underwent open repair in this study underwent tensioned repairs. A more recent RCT from 2004 demonstrated an increase in morbid outcomes and mortality following laparoscopic inguinal hernia repair, consistent with the requirement for general anesthesia.[46] Furthermore, most of the patients who underwent open repair had mesh repairs performed, and no improvement in recurrence was documented.

Complications

Hernia surgery is generally low risk and performed on an outpatient basis. However, there is a known incidence of postoperative complications. These are reviewed in detail by Eubanks.[16] In brief, complications may either be local or systemic. The most common operative/perioperative (local) complications are low-grade bleeding with hematoma formation and nerve injury. The most deleterious consequences are vascular injury (to the external iliac/femoral vessels) and visceral injury, both of which are rare and may be more common in laparoscopic repairs. Systemic complications are uncommon, and of these, the most frequent complications are postoperative atelectasis and superficial thrombophlebitis.

OTHER ABDOMINAL HERNIAS

While inguinal hernias account for the majority of abdominal hernias, other hernias are often seen as well. These are briefly summarized below.

Femoral Hernia

Femoral hernias are second in incidence and prevalence to inguinal hernias. They occur through the femoral canal, which is formed by the convergence of the three major ligaments of the groin, and is laterally bounded by the common femoral vein. The *anterior border* is the inguinal ligament, the *posterior border* is the iliopectineal ligament, and the *medial border* is the lacunar ligament. Unlike inguinal hernias, femoral hernias occur primarily in females. Furthermore, they are more likely to incarcerate than inguinal hernias. Repair is typically accomplished by the McVay technique, which closes the femoral canal after reduction of the hernia.

Epigastric Hernia

Epigastric hernias are generally thought to be a type of congenital hernia that arise due to incomplete development of the abdominal wall in the midline (i.e., the linea alba), between the xiphoid process and the umbilicus. Repair may be accomplished with or without mesh.[47]

Umbilical Hernia

Umbilical hernias are also congenital in etiology, and are defects in the abdominal wall at the umbilicus. The natural history of these hernias, when identified in infancy, is to close within 5 years. Symptomatic umbilical hernias in patients over 5 years of age may be repaired. Primary repair is commonly performed, but mesh may be used if necessary.[47,48]

Littre Hernia

A Littre hernia, first reported in 1700, is the eponym given to any abdominal hernia in which the sac contains a Meckel diverticulum. Repair is accomplished by any appropriate repair of the anatomic hernia observed.

Obturator Hernia

Obturator hernias, first described by Roland Arnaud de Ronsil in 1772, occur through the obturator foramen, and are bounded by the obturator vessels and nerve. They are acquired in origin, and occur predominantly in women. Like femoral hernias, a high incidence of incarceration is observed, and mortality is as high as 25 percent.[49] Physical examination is noteworthy for presence of the Howship-Romberg sign, which is inner thigh pain that is relieved by thigh flexion.[50] Repair is achieved by either a pre- or transperitoneal approach, with defect closure either primarily or with mesh.[49]

Lumbar Hernia

Two types of lumbar hernias can occur, through either the superior (Grynfeltt, described in 1866) or inferior (Petit, described in 1774) lumbar triangle. Blunt trauma to the abdomen is a common etiologic factor.[51] Lumbar hernias through the superior triangle are more common. Common approaches to repair include layered primary closure or mesh repair.[52]

Richter Hernia

A Richter hernia is defined as an abdominal hernia in which the contents of the sac include a portion of bowel, but not its full circumference. The important functional consequence is that an incarcerated Richter hernia does not present with obstruction.[53] In other words, a patient with an incarcerated hernia with bowel involvement may not necessarily have bowel obstruction. Furthermore, strangulation of the herniated portion of bowel may occur in the absence of obstruction. Richter hernias may thus pose diagnostic challenges. Repair is achieved by the previous approaches discussed depending on the location of the hernia.

Spigelian Hernia

A Spigelian hernia occurs at the junction of the lateral border of the rectus abdominis (linea semilunaris) and the arcuate line (linea semicircularis). This is a site of anatomic weakness in the normal abdominal wall. These hernias are acquired in origin. Spigelian hernias are often difficult to diagnose as hernias, and patients frequently undergo preoperative abdominal CT scanning. Repair is generally accomplished with mesh.

Incisional Hernia

Incisional hernias represent a common etiology of hernia, and are an iatrogenic complication of laparotomy (and to a much lesser extent, laparoscopy). As these hernias are often complex in anatomy, preoperative imaging studies are often useful. Repair is most commonly achieved with mesh prostheses. Recently, however, the technique of *component separation* has been developed, in which relaxing incisions are placed to separate the different layers of the abdominal wall from one another, and then these layers are stretched to achieve primary closure, and the layers are reapproximated in the new position.[54] Incisional hernias have a significantly higher rate of recurrence than other hernias.[8]

Internal Hernia

An internal hernia does not involve the abdominal wall, but rather, is herniation of intra-abdominal structures through a mesenteric defect, which often occurs as an iatrogenic complication of abdominal surgery. This commonly manifests as a small bowel obstruction (abdominal pain, nausea, vomiting, obstipation, constipation) in the absence of a palpable external hernia on examination. These hernias obviously cannot be nonoperatively reduced. Repair centers on reduction of the hernia and primary closure of the mesenteric defect.[55]

REFERENCES

1. Cooper A. *Treatise on Hernia*, 1804.

2. Atta H. Edwin Smith surgical papyrus: the oldest known surgical treatise. *Am Surg* 65:1190–1192, 1999.

3. Dorairajan N. Inguinal hernia—yesterday, today and tomorrow. *Indian J Surg* 66:137–139, 2004.

4. Eustace D. Premier Chirugien du Roi: the life of Ambroise Pare. *J R Soc Med* 85:585, 1992.

5. Schumpelick V, Tons C, Kupczyk-Joeris D. Operation of inguinal hernia. Classification, choice of procedure, techniques and results. *Chirurg* 62:641–648, 1991.

6. Schumpelick V, Treutner K, Arlt G. Inguinal hernia repair in adults. *Lancet* 344:375–379, 1994.

7. Nyhus L. Classification of groin hernias: milestones. *Hernia* 8:87–88, 2004.

8. Dunne J, Malone D, Tracy J, et al. Abdominal wall hernias: risk factors for infection and resource utilization. *J Surg Res* 111:78–84, 2003.

9. Cannon D, Read R. Metastatic emphysema: a mechanism for acquiring inguinal herniation. *Ann Surg* 194:270–278, 1981.

10. McEntyre R, Raffensperger J. Surgical complications of Ehlers-Danlos syndrome in children. *J Pediatr Surg* 12:531–535, 1977.

11. Liem M, van der Graaf Y, Beemer F, et al. Increased risk for inguinal hernia in patients with Ehlers-Danlos syndrome. *Surgery* 122:114–115, 1997.

12. Pans A, Albert A, Lapiere C, et al. Biochemical study of collagen in adult groin hernias. *J Surg Res* 95:107–113, 2001.

13. Lee B, Thurmon T. Nutritional disorders in a concentration camp. *J Am Coll Nutr* 16:366–375, 1997.

14. Skandalakis J, Colborn G, Androulakis J, et al. Embryologic and anatomic basis of inguinal herniorrhaphy. *Surg Clin North Am* 73:799–836, 1993.

15. Primatesta P, Goldacre M. Inguinal hernia repair: incidence of elective and emergency surgery, readmission, and mortality. *Int J Epidemiol* 25:835–839, 1996.

16. Eubanks W. Hernias. In Townsend C, ed., *Sabiston Textbook of Surgery*, Vol. 1. Philadelphia, PA: W.B. Saunders, 2000:783–801.

17. Rutkow I. Epidemiologic, economic, and sociologic aspects of hernia surgery in the United States in the 1990s. *Surg Clin North Am* 78:941–951, 1998.

18. Sorensen L, Hemmingsen U, Kirkeby L, et al. Smoking is a risk factor for incisional hernia. *Arch Surg* 140:119–123, 2005.

19. Liem M, van der Graaf Y, Zwart R, et al. Risk factors for inguinal hernia in women: a case-control study. The Coala Trial Group. *Am J Epidemiol* 146:721–726, 1997.

20. Ikeda H, Suzuki N, Takahashi A, et al. Risk of contralateral manifestation in children with unilateral inguinal hernia: should hernia in children be treated contralaterally? *J Pediatr Surg* 35:1746–1748, 2000.

21. Mucha Jr P. Small intestinal obstruction. *Surg Clin North Am* 67:597–620, 1987.

22. Miller G, Boman J, Shrier I, et al. Etiology of small bowel obstruction. *Am J Surg* 180:33–36, 2000.

23. Cervantes J. Inguinal hernia in the new millennium. *World J Surg* 28:343–347, 2004.

24. Nathan J, Pappas T. Inguinal hernia: an old condition with new solutions. *Ann Surg* 238:S148–S157, 2004.

25. McVay C, Chapp J. Inguinal and femoral hernioplasty: the evaluation of a basic concept. *Ann Surg* 148:499–510, 1958.

26. McVay C. Inguinal and femoral hernioplasty. *Surgery* 57:615–625, 1965.

27. Shouldice E. The Shouldice repair for groin hernias. *Surg Clin North Am* 83:1163–1187, 2003.

28. Nyhus L. Iliopubic tract repair of inguinal and femoral hernia. The posterior (preperitoneal) approach. *Surg Clin North Am* 73:487–499, 1993.

29. Lichtenstein I. Herniorrhaphy. A personal experience with 6321 cases. *Am J Surg* 153:553–559, 1987.

30. Lichtenstein I, Schulman A, Amid P, et al. The tension-free hernioplasty. *Am J Surg* 157:188–193, 1989.

31. Rutkow I, Robbins A. Tension-free inguinal herniorrhaphy: a preliminary report on the mesh plug technique. *Surgery* 114:3–8, 1993.

32. Rutkow I, Robbins A. The mesh plug technique for recurrent groin herniorrhaphy: a nine-year experience of 407 repairs. *Surgery* 124:844–847, 1998.

33. McCormack K, Scott N, Go P, et al. Laparoscopic techniques versus open techniques for inguinal hernia repair. *Cochrane Database Syst Rev* 1:CD001785, 2003.

34. The MRC Laparoscopic Groin Hernia Trial Group. Laparoscopic versus open repair of groin hernia: a randomised comparison. The MRC Laparoscopic Groin Hernia Trial Group. *Lancet* 354:185–190, 1999.

35. Memon M, Cooper N, Memon B, et al. Meta-analysis of randomized clinical trials comparing open and laparoscopic inguinal hernia repair. *Br J Surg* 90:1479–1492, 2003.

36. Birth M, Friedman R, Mellulis M, et al. Laparoscopic transabdominal preperitoneal hernioplasty: results of 1000 consecutive cases. *J Laparoendosc Surg* 6:293–300, 1996.

37. Crawford D, Phillips E. Laparoscopic repair and groin hernia surgery. *Surg Clin North Am* 78:1047–1062, 1998.

38. Bringman S, Ramel S, Heikkinen T, et al. Tension-free inguinal hernia repair: TEP versus mesh-plug versus Lichtenstein: a prospective randomized controlled trial. *Ann Surg* 237:142–147, 2003.

39. Jacobs D. Mesh repair of inguinal hernias—redux. *N Engl J Med* 350:1895–1897, 2004.

40. Paul A, Troidl H, Williams J, et al. Randomized trial of modified Bassini versus Shouldice inguinal hernia repair. The Cologne Hernia Study Group. *Br J Surg* 81:1531–1534, 1994.

41. Beets G, Oosterhuis K, Go P, et al. Longterm followup (12-15 years) of a randomized controlled trial comparing Bassini-Stetten, Shouldice, and high ligation with narrowing of the internal ring for primary inguinal hernia repair. *J Am Coll Surg* 185:352–357, 1997.

42. Barth Jr R, Burchard K, Tosteson A, et al. Short-term outcome after mesh or shouldice herniorrhaphy: a randomized, prospective study. *Surgery* 123:121–126, 1998.

43. McGillicuddy J. Prospective randomized comparison of the Shouldice and Lichtenstein hernia repair procedures. *Arch Surg* 133:974–978, 1998.

44. Nordin P, Bartelmess P, Jansson C, et al. Randomized trial of Lichtenstein versus Shouldice hernia repair in general surgical practice. *Br J Surg* 89:45–49, 2002.

45. Liem M, van der Graaf Y, van Steensel C, et al. Comparison of conventional anterior surgery and laparoscopic surgery for inguinal-hernia repair. *N Engl J Med* 336:1541–1547, 1997.

46. Neumayer L, Giobbie-Hurder A, Jonasson O, et al. Open mesh versus laparoscopic mesh repair of inguinal hernia. *N Engl J Med* 350:1819–1827, 2004.

47. Muschaweck U. Umbilical and epigastric hernia repair. *Surg Clin North Am* 83:1207–1221, 2003.

48. Kurzer M, Belsham P, Kark A. Tension-free mesh repair of umbilical hernia as a day case using local anesthesia. *Hernia* 8:104–107, 2004.

49. Bergstein J, Condon R. Obturator hernia: current diagnosis and treatment. *Surgery* 119:133–136, 1996.

50. Yip A, AhChong A, Lam K. Obturator hernia: a continuing diagnostic challenge. *Surgery* 113:266–269, 1993.

51. Esposito T, Fedorak I. Traumatic lumbar hernia: case report and literature review. *J Trauma* 37:123–126, 1994.

52. Heniford B, Iannitti D, Gagner M. Laparoscopic inferior and superior lumbar hernia repair. *Arch Surg* 132:1141–1144, 1997.

53. Steinke W, Zellweger R. Richter's hernia and Sir Frederick Treves: an original clinical experience, review, and historical overview. *Ann Surg* 232:710–718, 2000.

54. Shestak K, Edington H, Johnson R. The separation of anatomic components technique for the reconstruction of massive midline abdominal wall defects: anatomy, surgical technique, applications, and limitations revisited. *Plast Reconstr Surg* 105:731–738, 2000.

55. Garignon C, Paparel P, Liloku R, et al. Mesenteric hernia: a rare cause of intestinal obstruction in children. *J Pediatr Surg* 37:1493–1494, 2002.

HEAD AND NECK

SURGERY

RECONSTRUCTION

Steffen Baumeister, MD
L. Scott Levin, MD, FACS

INTRODUCTION

Surgery of the head and neck comprises various topics such as

- Congenital anomalies and defects
- Reconstruction of the head and neck in the setting of
  - Trauma
  - Tumor
  - Burns
  - Infection
- Aesthetic surgery

RECONSTRUCTION OF THE HEAD AND NECK

The following chapter outlines reconstruction of the head and neck. Principles of plastic surgery are emphasized.

Reconstruction of the head and neck is a major challenge to the reconstructive surgeon because it represents anatomically and functionally the most complex area of the body.

Defect Etiology

A defect or destruction in the head and neck is caused by one of the following conditions:

1. Tumor or osteoradionecrosis
2. Trauma
3. Burn
4. Infection
5. Congenital deformity

The first requirement for any reconstruction is to define the size and shape of the defect. Debridement of untidy wounds is required to convert irregular contours to a geometrically smoother contour as well as to eliminate nonviable tissue or tumor from the wound.

Principles of Debridement

Debridement usually requires making larger defects out of a smaller one. Without tools for reconstruction the surgeon might be reluctant to increase a wound's size or depth. However, experience shows that a well-debrided and well-perfused wound has the best chance of healing without complications. Debridement before wound closure or reconstruction is essential.

TUMORS

Radical extirpation is important in tumor surgery. Surgery is performed as a two-team approach. The extirpative team performs resection of the cancer with the only goal of obtaining tumor-free margins. The resecting team is thereby not inhibited from performing a wide excision. The reconstructive team performs the reconstruction after extirpation.

Histopathologically, tumors in the head and neck can derive from any tissue in this area, so they can be epithelial, mesenchymal, lymphoid, or hematologic in origin. It is beyond the scope of this chapter to discuss the histologic types of malignancies in detail. The vast majority (90–95 percent) of malignancies occurring in the oral cavity are squamous cell carcinomas (SCC). The remaining tumors are predominantly of salivary gland origin. Many malignant tumors are not specific for the head and neck region. Skin tumors, however, are common in the sun-exposed face or scalp. Relevant and common tumors of the skin are basal cell carcinoma, melanoma, and SCC. Malignant lymphoma (Hodgkin and non-Hodgkin lymphoma) commonly presents in cervical lymph nodes. Soft tissue and bone tumors are overall not common in the head and neck. Rhabdomyosarcomas in the head and neck occur most commonly in childhood (80 percent). Furthermore, malignancies can always be metastatic from primary tumors elsewhere in the body.

Classification is currently based on a *TNM* system. *T* describes the two-dimensional tumor size, *N* describes the nodal status in the cervical region, and *M* describes the metastatic disease beyond the cervical lymph nodes. On the basis of the TNM classification, all tumors can be assigned to a clinical stage (0–IV). The TNM and staging classifications depend on the type of tumor. Clinical staging is used for planning the treatment regimen, for assessing the prognosis for tumor control, recurrence and patient survival as well as for comparing outcome of different treatment regimens and institutions.

The basic goals of cancer treatment are to control the cancer, minimize the likelihood of secondary recurrence, and achieve an acceptable quality of life. Treatment consists of an individualized combination of surgery, chemo- and radiotherapy. Surgical therapy consists of precise removal of tumor and a margin of normal-appearing tissue around the tumor. Immediate reconstruction following radical tumor resection is preferable to secondary reconstruction. Adjuvant radiotherapy and potential chemotherapy are useful adjuncts in the patients with advanced disease.

TRAUMA

In trauma patients, visible soft tissue destruction is often an indicator of further underlying pathology such as facial or cervical fractures, intracranial bleeding, destruction of dentition or ocular damage. These associated injuries maybe life threatening and cause blindness or tetraplegia when undetected. Thorough diagnosis for exclusion of such comorbidities is essential.

Once concomitant injuries are excluded, soft tissue defects are closed primarily. Meticulous debridement is important to prevent infection and ensure the best cosmetic result.

BURNS

The surgical treatment of burns requires the acute treatment of the injury, such as debridement of burned tissue and subsequent coverage of the defects, as well as the secondary reconstructive issues such as contracture release, treatment of scar ectropion, or microstomia.

In the acute setting, the decision to operate and debride a burn depends on the depth of a burn, which can be classified into four degrees: 1-, 2a-, 2b-, and 3-degree burn.

If a burn involves only the upper dermis (2a) spontaneous reepithelialization occurs from the epithelial appendages such as hair bulbs which are located in the deeper dermis. The healing requires no surgery and is completed within 2–3 weeks without scar formation. If a burn involves the deep dermis (2b) no spontaneous reepithelialization will occur. Healing involves scar formation.

The differentiation between 2a and 2b burns is thus essential for the decision to wait for spontaneous healing or to operate, debride (= necrectomy), and skin graft the wound.

Therefore, if there is any doubt about the depth of a burn, one should wait for 7–10 days after the trauma to decide whether a necrectomy is necessary or not. Although this applies to burns anywhere in the body, it is common to wait longer in the face than anywhere else due to two reasons: (1) In the face and particularly in the cheek, perioral and chin area, the skin is thicker than in most other parts of the body with deeply located hair bulbs. Spontaneous healing of these areas is common and differentiation between 2a and 2b burns requires significant experience. (2) Operative treatment and skin transplantation to the face has a huge effect on esthetic appearance and social reintegration of the patient and therefore it should be avoided if there is any chance for spontaneous healing.

When operative debridement is performed, skin transplantation is the method of choice for coverage provided there is a well-perfused wound.

RECONSTRUCTION

Historical Review

Early reports about reconstruction of the head and neck date back as far as 1597, when Tagliacozzi replaced skin in the face by suturing the upper arm in an elevated position to the face. Another early reconstructive report is the so-called *Indian method* for reconstruction of the nose. A pedicled flap from the forehead was transferred to the nose. These pedicled flaps were divided after a few weeks.

At the beginning of the twentieth century, advances in tumor surgery with the establishment of radical neck dissection and the experiences during and after World War I boosted head and neck surgery. The modern father of plastic surgery Sir Harold Gilles outlined a series of principles for reconstruction, such as the replacement of *like with like*. During the 30s and 40s he relied on tubed flaps transferred sequentially from one part of the body to another.

For a long time, pedicled flaps remained the mainstay of surgical reconstruction. In 1965, Bakamjian introduced the deltopectoral flap,[1] in 1979, Ariyan described the pectoralis major musculocutaneous flap.[2] Quillen described the pedicled latissimus dorsi flap[3] and Conley (nachschauen1 in article) described the superior trapezius musculocutaneous flap for head and neck reconstruction.[4]

In the late 1970s, microsurgery was popularized, facilitated by small vessel anastomosis using the operating microscope. The first free flaps to the head and neck was described in 1973.[5] Composite microsurgical transplantation evolved in the 1980s. Since then, microsurgical reconstruction has become the standard of reconstruction. Although it is most complex and difficult surgical option, the success rates are about 94–97 percent.[6,7]

Goals

The principles of reconstructive surgery in the head and neck region are identical to those elsewhere in the body. The goals of any reconstruction are *restoration of form* and *function*. However, these goals are particularly challenging in the head and neck. The interaction among form, function, and appearance is greater in this anatomic site than anywhere else. In the head and particularly the face, appearance and cosmesis is obviously of utmost importance as the face is exposed and conveys the first contact with others.

The importance of the face in social interactions cannot be overestimated. Likewise, the ability to speak and swallow are central to quality of life.

The functional aspects of reconstruction are more prevalent in the head and neck than in most other parts of the body. These are the abilities of communication by speech formation, articulation, as well as facial expression. It involves hearing, seeing, eating, maintaining oral continence, chewing, swallowing, and breathing with a fine-tuned coordination of these various functions.

The goal of reconstructive surgery is to restore these complex functions. The techniques for head and neck reconstruction relies on a team approach that includes head and neck extirpative surgery, oral surgery and dentistry, craniofacial surgery and reconstructive plastic surgery, ophthalmologists, speech therapists, and social workers.

In addition to the complexity of function and appearance, complex regional anatomy in the head and neck pose further challenges. In tumor surgery, oncologic issues take precedence over the concept of saving normal tissue. Therefore, the defects after tumor removal can be very large, not respecting any anatomic border. Pre- and postoperative radiation can cause fibrosis and scarring of surrounding tissues, friability of blood vessels, ankylosis of the temporomandibular joint, and adversely affect healing. Maintenance of oral competence is often difficult, with resultant fistulae formation.

Reconstructive Principles

After debridement it is obvious which layers of tissue and what structures are missing. Optimally, each layer of absent tissue should be repaired with like tissue, for example, the cutaneous defects should be closed with skin of similar thickness, color, and texture, cartilaginous defects should be repaired with a cartilaginous graft of similar characteristics.

The plastic surgeons armamentarium to cover defects is extensive: Defects can be closed by primary suture, partial- or full-thickness skin grafts, local flaps, regional flaps, or free flaps. Typically, the reconstruction begins with simple methods such as primary closure or skin grafts and progresses to local tissue, regional tissue reconstructions, and finally free tissue transfer. This reconstructive concept is described by the term *reconstructive ladder* which refers to an escalation from the simple to the most complex surgical option to achieve a successful reconstruction which is measured by an improvement in the patient's function, structure, and appearance. If a simple procedure serves this adequately it should be chosen, if not, the next step on the ladder should be evaluated.

However, in many patients the ideal approach requires skipping steps of the ladder and starting with the most complex option. A free flap may sometimes be the easiest technique to perform. Experience has confirmed that the complication rate of local flaps is similar to that of free flaps. Figure 17-1 gives an overview of the reconstructive ladder with examples.

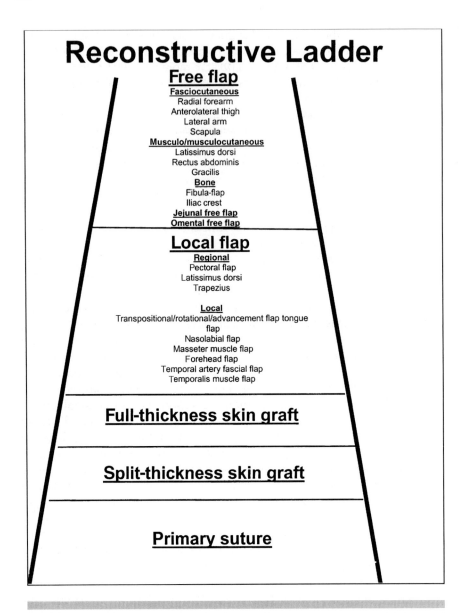

Reconstructive Ladder

Free flap

Fasciocutaneous
Radial forearm
Anterolateral thigh
Lateral arm
Scapula
Musculo/musculocutaneous
Latissimus dorsi
Rectus abdominis
Gracilis
Bone
Fibula-flap
Iliac crest
Jejunal free flap
Omental free flap

Local flap

Regional
Pectoral flap
Latissimus dorsi
Trapezius

Local
Transpositional/rotational/advancement flap tongue
flap
Nasolabial flap
Masseter muscle flap
Forehead flap
Temporal artery fascial flap
Temporalis muscle flap

Full-thickness skin graft

Split-thickness skin graft

Primary suture

*Figure 17-1 **Reconstructive ladder showing reconstructive principles and options for head and neck reconstruction.***

Reconstructive Ladder

DIRECT, PRIMARY CLOSURE

Direct suture of a wound is the easiest and best way to close a defect. The limiting aspect is the size of the defect after debridement. The mobility of the surrounding tissue must allow for direct closure without tension or distortion of surrounding anatomic units. The lower eyelid is particularly susceptible to deformity and if too much tension in the cheek or nasal area is applied there is the risk of an ectropion (outward scarring of the lower lid).

If direct closure is possible it is important to remove the stitches earlier than in other parts of the body, generally on the fifth postoperative day in the face, to avoid epithelialization of the stitch canals. Direct closure of deeper defects requires meticulous reconstruction of any involved tissue layer, for example, three-layer closure in perforating wounds of the cheek (mucosa, muscle, and skin).

Skin Transplantation

Skin grafts are transplanted without their intrinsic vascular supply. Nutritional supply is initially by perfusion from the wound bed. It therefore requires a well-perfused wound to allow for a skin transplantation. Exposed vessel, nerves, tendons, cartilage, bone, or foreign material are contraindications for a skin graft.

Skin grafts can either be full-thickness or partial-/split-thickness skin grafts. Full-thickness skin grafts contain the entire thickness of skin excluding the subcutis. Advantages are stable coverage, less contraction, and better cosmesis than with a split-thickness graft. However, the donor site requires direct closure and availability is therefore restricted. Therefore, only small defects can be covered. The thinnest skin can be obtained from the eyelid, followed by postauricular, preauricular, supraclavicular, antecubital, lateral upper arm, and groin skin. Groin skin may contain hair bulbs which are undesirable for transplantation into the face. For cosmetic reasons, there are few indications for skin grafts in facial reconstruction, but more in scalp and neck reconstruction. Indications for full-thickness grafts can be the release of contractures in the cervical, oral, or eyelid area (e.g., ectropion) or defects in elderly patients where skin grafting is the quickest and easiest option, and cosmesis is not a major issue.

A split-thickness skin graft contains the epidermis and part of the dermis (0.2–0.4 mm). The donor site reepithelializes spontaneously from the remaining epithelial appendages in the lower dermis such as hair bulbs. The supply of split-thickness skin grafts is almost unlimited. Split-thickness grafts contract more than full-thickness skin grafts, and esthetics are poorer. Although a scar does not remain on the donor site, the patient should be aware of hyper- or hypopigmentation. In children, the scalp is an excellent donor site which will be invisible with subsequent hair growth.

Flaps

Flaps are indicated when bone, vessels, nerves, tendons, or any foreign material or osteosynthesis material is exposed. Flaps are further indicated when thick, pliable, and well-vascularized tissue is needed. Flaps have their own vascular network and they may help to cover defects resulting from radiation or scarring.

Flaps can be classified in various ways according to their

1. Blood supply (pedicled flap [randomized or axial vascular supply] vs. free flap)
2. Location (local, regional, distant)
3. Tissue components (cutaneous, adipocutaneous, muscular, musculocutaneous, fascial, fasciocutaneous, bony)

ANATOMIC BLOOD SUPPLY

Pedicled Flap

If a flap is transposed to another part of the body with the supplying vessels remaining intact it is a pedicled flap.

Pedicled flaps can be subdivided as random pattern flaps or axial pattern flaps. *Random pattern flaps* derive their blood supply through the cutaneous dermal-subdermal plexus. There is no defined vessel in the pedicle, but the vessels are random. The surviving length of such a flap is related to the vessels perfusion pressure and the vascular supply of the particular part of the body. The normal ratio of length to width is 1:1. However, a flap designed in the head and neck region where vascularity is optimal, length to width ratio increases up to 2.5 or 3:1 (Fig. 17-2). However, the surgeons always need to be cautious and consider risk factors for poor vascularity such as age of the patient, atherosclerosis, previous radiation, or smoking. Examples for random pattern flaps are rotational, transpositional, or advancement flaps.

Axial pattern flaps contain a direct axial vessel running in the pedicle. The length of these flaps can be as long as the supplying vessel runs in the flap. Therefore, it can be much longer. Examples of axial pattern flaps in the face are the temporal fascia flap containing the superficial temporal vessels, the forehead flap containing the supraorbital vessels, or the glabella flap containing the supratrochlear vessels.

In the head and neck, with respect to the distance between defect and donor site these pedicled flaps can be local, when the flap is designed immediately adjacent to or near the location of the defect (e.g., nasolabial flap [Fig. 17-3] and temporal muscle flap). They can be regional (trapezius, latissimus dorsi, pectoralis major) or distant (upper arm). In the regional or distant flaps, the pedicle is usually cosmetically or functionally disturbing and needs to be divided. This is done about 3 weeks after transposition of the flap.

In small defects local flaps are the method of choice. Transposition is usually safe with regard to the vascular supply and the tissue lying adjacent to the defect matches best in texture, hair, color, and thickness. However, regional flaps from the patient's chest or back have largely been replaced by free flaps as the latter offer more flexibility with no higher complication rate.

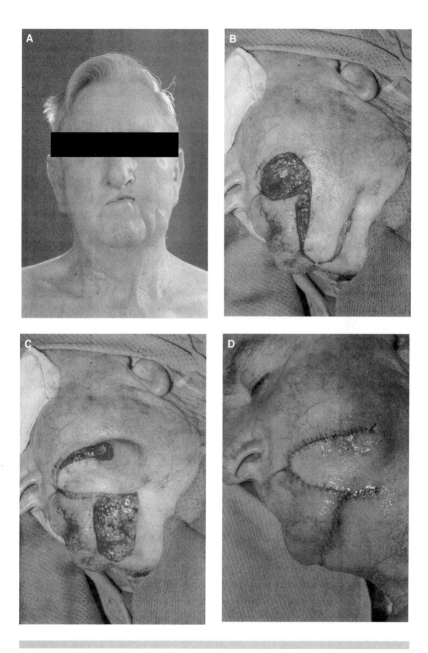

Figure 17-2 **(A) Postoperative result after excision of a SCC at the modiolus with resultant scarring and microstomia; (B and C) defect coverage with a randomized rotational flap; (D) flap in place; (E) result after 9 months.**

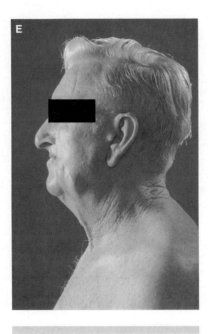

Figure 17-2 **(Continued)**

Free Flap

If a flap is transplanted from another part of the body with microvascular anastomosis it is free flap. These can de classified according to the consisting tissue (cutaneous, fascial, muscular, bone) (Fig. 17-1). Free flaps have become a standard in reconstruction of the head and neck. Their variability in size, character, consistency, thickness, tissue components, and function make them the first reconstructive option in many cases particularly since a high success rate is achievable. Free tissue transfer enables selection of the most appropriate type of tissue in the required amount.

Complications of free flap reconstruction are either flap related or general medical complications.[6–9] Flap-related complications can be subdivided into *flap* and *donor site* complications.

The most severe complication of a microvascular flap surgery is vascular thrombosis and flap loss. Viability of a free tissue transfer is based primarily on clinical observation, with normal capillary refill confirming vascular patency. Other methods of monitoring such as the laser Doppler and the implantable Doppler flow probes that are coupled around the vessels assist in assuring high degrees of patency. Confirmation of flap viability should be performed hourly in the postoperative period. As soon as vascular compromise is recognized,

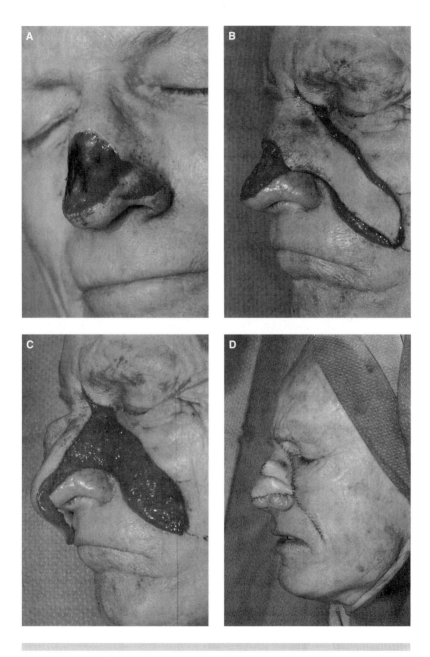

Figure 17-3 *(A) Soft tissue defect on the nose in a male patient following excision of a SCC treated with a nasolabial flap; (B) harvest of nasolabial flap; (C) rotation into the defect; (D and E) flap in place.*

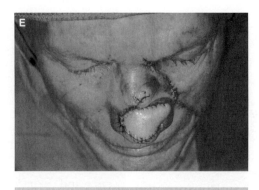

Figure 17-3 **(Continued)**

the patient should be taken back to the operating room (OR), the anastomoses explored, and vessels thrombectomized.

To avoid vascular problems, large recipient vessels in the head and neck
are selected. Recipient vessels include the superficial, temporal, facial, superior thyroid, lingual, or external carotid arteries. For venous drainage, the
superficial temporal, facial, and jugular veins are options.

General medical complications such as respiratory problems with pneumonia, prolonged intubation requiring tracheostomy, cardiac or thrombotic
problems are not infrequent in this patient population.

Decision-Making Process

The reconstructive surgeon has to consider these general reconstructive principles as well as to make a detailed assessment of the individual patient and
defect to outline his or her reconstructive plan. Various reconstructive methods
exist for every site that needs restoration. It is not the aim of this chapter to
name all of them, but give an impression of the reconstructive variability,
options, and considerations.

For the therapeutic decision, analysis of the defect and the individual
patient profile help to choose the appropriate reconstructive option out of
the vast reconstructive armamentarium: What is destroyed, what structures
need to be replaced for an anatomic and functional reconstruction?

- Defect
  - Depth
  - Size
  - Location/functional impairment
    - Oral cavity
    - Pharynx

- Mandibular
  - Craniofacial
    - Base of the skull
    - Scalp and cranium
    - Midface

DEFECT

Depth

The depth of the defect is an important factor determining which category of the reconstructive ladder (skin graft vs. flap) can be used. If there is adequate subcutaneous tissue or a perfused wound, skin grafts either split thickness or full thickness are possible. They can be used for oral or nasal mucosal defects to provide inner lining. However, even if a skin graft is technically possible for external defects such as in the face, flaps achieve a better cosmetic outcome and are therefore preferred.

Size

The size of a defect is an important factor determining within one category of the reconstructive ladder which skin transplant (split thickness vs. full thickness) or which flap (local vs. single free flap vs. combined free flap) can be used.

Full-thickness skin grafts can only be used in smaller defects, as the availability is limited as outlined above. There is no size limitation for the use of split-thickness skin grafts.

Small defects in the face, on the skull, or neck as well as mucosal defects can be reconstructed by local or regional flaps. Larger defects require a free flap. Again the size of the defects determines whether a required cutaneous free flap can be a radial flap or needs to be bigger such as an anterolateral thigh flap or even a combined scapular/parascapular flap. For muscular requirements, a small defect might be closed by a gracilis flap, a larger defect may require a rectus abdominis or even a latissimus dorsi muscular or musculocutaneous free flap.

Location/functional Impairment

The site of reconstruction in the head and neck largely influences the associated functional impairment and thus reconstructive requirements.

ORAL CAVITY

Defects of the oral cavity affect eating, chewing, food movement, maintaining oral continence, and the initiation of swallowing and speech formation. It requires reconstruction of an inner (mucosa) and outer lining (skin).

Reconstruction of the oral cavity is a matter of flap reconstruction,[10] the role of skin grafts is only supplementary, for example, to reconstruct an inner lining on a transplanted free flap.

The Radial Forearm Flap

In 1981, Yang described the radial forearm flap and it is therefore referred to as the *Chinese flap*.[11,12] It is the most commonly used free flap to the head and neck. The flap is harvested on the radial artery and its venae comitantes. The cephalic vein can be additionally taken to augment venous drainage. The radial forearm flap provides a large, thin, pliable, and predominantly hairless flap for intraoral and oropharyngeal lining (Figs. 17-4 and 17-5). The skin has the capacity to become sensate with microanastomosis of the antebrachial cutaneous nerve. Bone or tendons can be included to provide oral support such as in lower lip reconstruction. Furthermore, its pliable skin allows for the folding and contouring that are necessary to recreate the nasopharyngeal sphincter and the conduit to the hypopharynx. Before harvesting the radial artery, adequate collateral ulnar artery circulation has to be confirmed either preoperatively by an Allen test (manual occlusion and sequential release of radial and ulnar vessels at the wrist) or intraoperatively by clamping the radial artery before dissection. However, donor site problems are well recognized particularly an unsightly donor site defect which is usually skin transplanted.

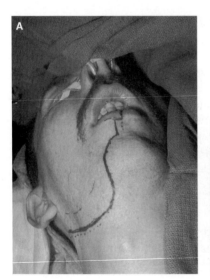
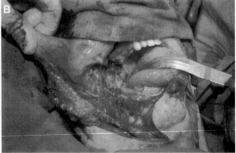

Figure 17-4 **A 43-year-old male patient with an intraoral SCC. (A) Preoperative; (B) after tumor extirpation; (C) donor site at the forearm showing a radial forearm flap; (D) intraoperative view after inset of the flap; (E) postoperative intraoral view after 1 year.**

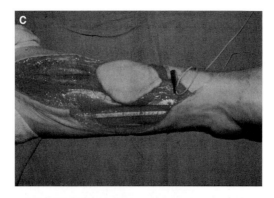

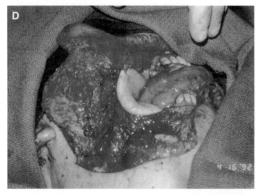

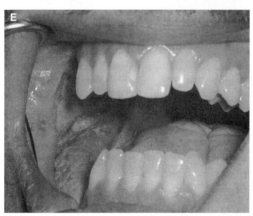

Figure 17-4 **(Continued)**

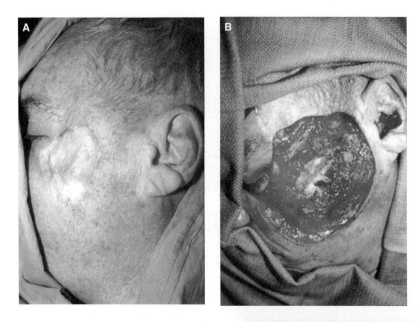

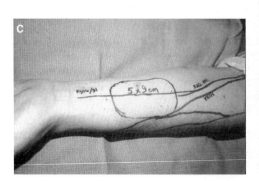

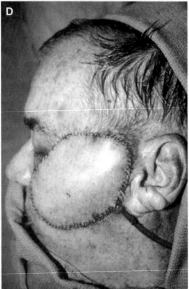

Figure 17-5 *(A) A 73-year-old patient with a recurrent malignant melanoma and a history of split-thickness skin graft and radiation; (B) midfacial defect after tumor resection; (C) outline of the radial forearm flap; (D) flap in place; (E) result after 1 year without any revision surgery of the flap.*

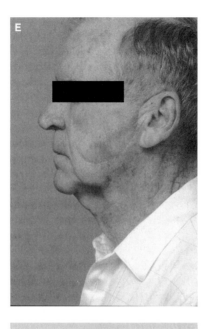

Figure 17-5 **(Continued)**

The Scapular Flap/parascapular

An alternative adipocutaneous flap is the scapula flap which is located over or at the lateral border of the scapula. It is supplied by the arterial system of the subscapular artery, which branches in the circumflex scapular (supplying scapula/parascapular flap) and the thoracodorsal artery (supplying the latissimus dorsi flap). The flap can be larger than the radial artery flap. The donor site can be hidden. A disadvantage is that the patient may need to be turned intraoperatively.

The lateral arm flap[13] is a further alternative providing a thin adipocutaneous flap from the lateral aspect of the upper arm. It is smaller than the radial artery flap but the donor site is usually more acceptable.

The anterolateral thigh flap[14] provides a large and thin cutaneous flap based on the descending branch of the lateral circumflex femoral artery. The dissection is more difficult than with the radial forearm flap, but it is increasingly becoming popular.

Second-line options are pedicled flaps, such as the pectoralis major, pedicled latissimus, or deltopectoral flap. The deltopectoral flap is located on the upper chest ranging from the sternal border up to the deltoid muscle. The first four perforating branches of the internal mammary artery supply the flap. It is an adipocutaneous flap that can reach up the oral cavity for reconstruction.

Glossal Defect

It has been shown that speech is a primary factor determining quality of life. Quality and intelligibility of speech largely depends on tongue mobility. Furthermore, the tongue serves swallowing and airway protection. To restore these functions it requires a bulky, voluntary mobile and possibly sensate flap. The goals are almost impossible to achieve.

Regional flaps such as the pectoralis major musculocutaneous flap have been described for tongue reconstruction. However, free flaps have become the method of choice. Various flaps have been described such as the radial forearm flap, the free groin flap, or anterolateral thigh flap. As outlined above, a bulky flap is favorable for tongue reconstruction, so with all of these flaps, muscle has been incorporated such as the brachioradialis muscle in the forearm flap, the sartorius in the groin flap, or the vastus lateralis in the anterolateral thigh flap to give the bulkiness for restoring the tongue.

Alternatives are predominant muscular flaps with a cutaneous component such as musculocutaneous rectus abdominis or the latissimus dorsi flap.

PHARYNX

Defects of the pharynx affect swallowing, prevention of aspiration, and coordination of breathing and eating.

In the oropharyngeal area it requires a flexible reconstruction to allow narrowing for adequate velopharyngeal function, which means a separation of oronasopharynx during swallowing. This can be served by a folded radial forearm flap which is further sutured to the back of the pharynx.

In the lower pharynx or cervical oesophagus a tubed, mobile but stable reconstruction allowing for transportation of food is required. The first choice is the free jejunal flap containing a segment of the jejunum. With a jejunal free flap the swallowing function is better compared to other reconstructive options. Additionally, it provides the secretion of mucous. It has been shown, in view of its good blood supply, to tolerate postoperative radiotherapy well.[15]

MANDIBLE

Defects of the mandible affect dental and oral closure as well as eating. It requires a bony reconstruction with adequate strength to allow—if necessary—for subsequent dental reconstruction with osseointegrated implants. Furthermore, an associated mucosal or skin defect needs to be covered. Vascularized bone grafts are the method of choice.

Fibula Flap

The vascularized fibula based on the peroneal artery was described by Taylor in 1975,[16] and the reliability of skin further characterized by Yoshimira, Beppu, and Wei. The osteocutaneious fibula flap has become the mainstay of the mandibular reconstruction providing both oral lining as well as bony structure to the resected mandible (Figs. 17-6 and 17-7). Large segments of up to

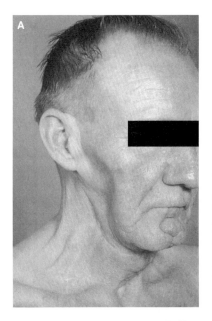

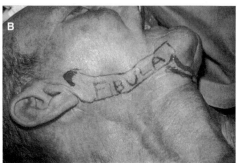

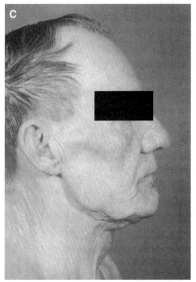

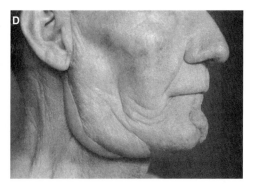

Figure 17-6 *(A) A 70-year-old male patient status posthemimandibulectomy and radiation for cancer; (B) secondary reconstruction with osteoseptocutaneous fibula for contour cosmesis and restoration of mandibular balance; (C and D) postoperative results.*

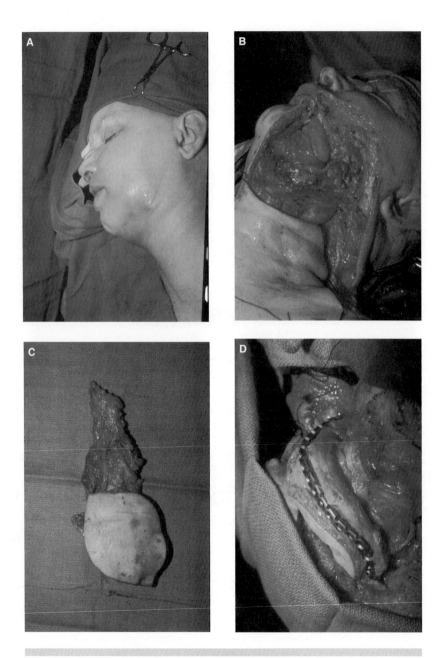

Figure 17-7 **(A) Patient with SCC; (B) excision of tumor with hemi-mandibulectomy; (C) harvest of osteoseptocutaneous fibula free flap; (D) inset of free flap. A skin paddle was required for the extraoral soft tissue defect; (E) postoperative result.**

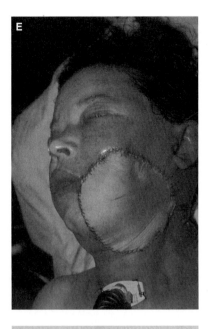

Figure 17-7 **(Continued)**

25 cm can be obtained. One of the major disadvantages is the limited availability of the skin and soft tissue necessary for reconstructing mucosal defects. In the elderly, one has to be aware of associated vascular and atherosclerotic disease.

The free circumflex iliac osteocutaneious flap is an alternative bone flap based on the deep circumflex iliac vessels (Fig. 17-8). Associated soft tissue can be bulky. Furthermore, the radial forearm flap can be harvested with radial bone, the scapula flap can include scapular bone if needed, and the free serratus anterior flap can be harvested with ribs.

A pedicled alternative is the pectoralis major flap which can include a rib segment.

CRANIOFACIAL DEFECTS

Craniofacial reconstruction includes restoration of

1. The base of the skull
2. The scalp and cranial area
3. The midface

Defects affecting the base of the skull need adequate coverage to protect and seal off the neurocranium. Muscular flaps provide better vascularization in infected, radiated, or scarred tissue.

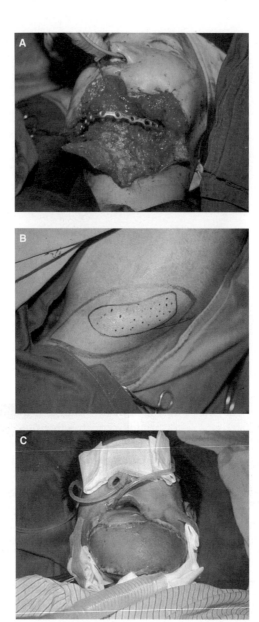

Figure 17-8 **A 45-year-old male patient with mandibulectomy and bilateral radical neck dissection for SCC. (A) Reconstruction with plate to recreate the mandibular contour; (B) donor site showing the hip region. An osteocutaneious deep circumflex iliac artery (DCIA) flap is marked containing part of the iliac crest; (C) flap in place.**

The latissimus dorsi muscular or musculocutaneous flap is the largest muscular free flap. It is supplied by the large calibered thoracodorsal artery, a branch of the subscapular vessels. The harvest is uncomplicated and the donor site can be closed primarily. However, as with a scapula flap, turning the patient is necessary prolonging operative time.

Defects of the scalp and osseocranium cranium affect stability and protection of the neurocranium. It requires adequate and stable coverage either with soft tissue alone or combined with vascularized bone. For soft tissue defects, muscular flaps such as the latissimus, rectus abdominis, or gracilis are favorable options. Large defects can be covered with the free omental flap. The free omentum provides a pliable and well-vascularized tissue which needs an additional split-thickness skin graft (Figs. 17-9 and 17-10).

For a combined osteocutaneious coverage, the serratus anterior muscle flap with the anterior half of several ribs provides an elegant way to reconstruct calvarium.

Defects affecting the midface may impair sight, nasal breathing or respiration, eating, oral continence, and—importantly—esthetics. Cutaneous flaps and in particular local flaps provide best cosmesis, because skin characteristics are similar. If the defect is larger, the radial forearm flap again is the method

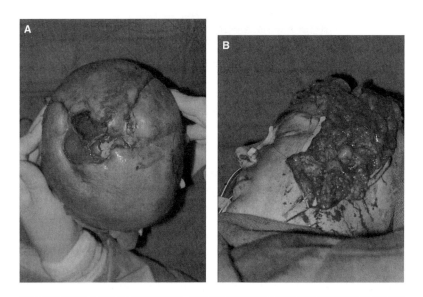

Figure 17-9 (A) Osteomyelitis of the skull following radiation for brain tumor; (B) insetting of an omental free flap; (C) result after 1 year. Patient wears a wig.

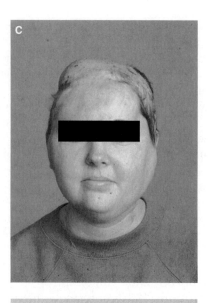

Figure 17-9 **(Continued)**

of choice (Figs. 17-4 and 17-5). It is beyond the scope of this chapter to outline the nasal or orbital reconstructive options.

Complex Injuries

Complex injuries imply multifocal or multistructural defects. The latter can involve the simultaneous injury of soft tissue, nasal destruction with cartilaginous injury, mucosal defects, joint (e.g., temporomandibular) or bone injury (e.g., maxilla, mandible, and skull), or muscular destruction (e.g., facial muscles and tongue). Complex defects occasionally require more than a single free flap due to the size or a compound, multicomponent flap for a successful reconstruction.[17] This might be the combination of a local flap with a free flap, the usage of different tissue components within a single flap (e.g., bone), or the combination of several free flaps on a single or more than one pedicles. Some examples have been given above such as the radial forearm flap containing tendon, muscle or bone or the circumflex iliac free flap containing iliac crest, or sartorius muscle. The largest tissue reservoir is provided by the subscapular vascular axis. The scapular, parascapular, latissimus dorsi, serratus muscle, or fascia flap can be combined with additional scapular or rib bone.

Patient Profile

All reconstructive options have to be discussed with the patient, either before debridement in a one-stage reconstruction or after radical debridement in a two-stage procedure. Sometimes the patient has wishes as far as donor site

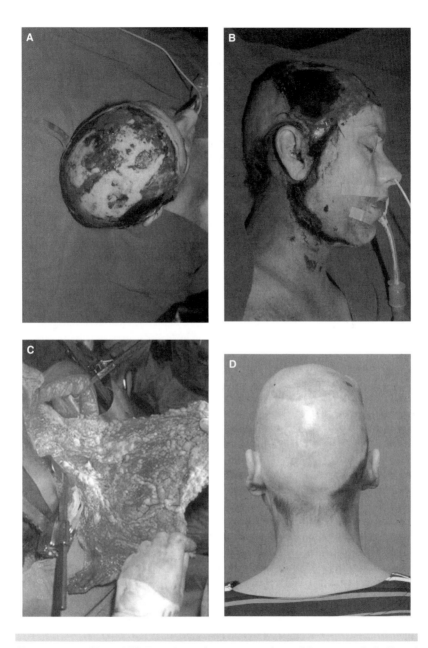

Figure 17-10 **(A and B) Female patient presenting with exposed skull and unstable scars and necrosis after a scalp avulsion injury; (C) defect coverage with a free omental flap; (D) postoperative result; (E) the patient wears a wig.**

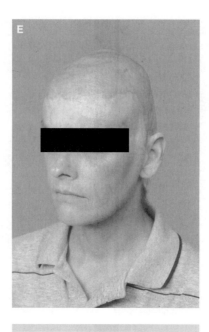

Figure 17-10 (**Continued**)

morbidity or perioperative risk is concerned, preclude the use of local flaps
even if adequate or vice versa. The functional and nutritional status of the
patient, the level of disease burden, as well as the patient's social support system all need to be considered. The specific risk factors for the possible coverage options have to be evaluated on an individual basis. If the patient is older
and comorbid, a long operative procedure may not be possible without a substantial risk to the patient. Two operating teams may be necessary to save
operating time, one team to debride the defect and the other team to simultaneously harvest the flap. The choice of flap may also be influenced when
changing positions during the operation such as from a lateral to a supine
position costing too much time. If the patient is an alcoholic or noncompliant
patient, one may need to find a compromise and perform a pedicled flap
rather than a free flap.

REHABILITATION

A successful reconstruction with restoration of function can only be achieved
with adequate rehabilitation. Treatment does not stop with successful operation. Examples are speech therapy after oropharyngeal surgery, or compression therapy and prevention of contractures after burn injuries.

REFERENCES

1. Bakamjian VY. A two-stage method for pharyngooesophageal reconstruction with a primary pectoral skin flap. *Plast Reconstr Surg* 36:173–184, 1965.

2. Ariyan S. The pectoralis major myocutaneous flap. A versatile flap for reconstruction in the head and neck. *Plast Reconstr Surg* 63:73–81, 1979.

3. Quillen CG, Shearin JC Jr, Georgiade NG. Use of the latissimus dorsi myocutaneous island flap for reconstruction in the head and neck area: case report. *Plast Reconstr Surg* 62:113–117, 1978.

4. Conley J. Use of composite flaps containing bone for major repairs in the head and neck. *Plast Reconstr Surg* 49:522–526, 1972.

5. Kaplan EN, Buncke HJ, Murray DE. Distant transfer of cutaneous island flaps in humans by microvascular anastomoses. *Plast Reconstr Surg* 52:301–305, 1973.

6. Eckardt A, Fokas K. Microsurgical reconstruction in the head and neck region: an 18-year experience with 500 consecutive cases. *J Craniomaxillofac Surg* 31:197–201, 2003.

7. Nakatsuka T, Harii K, Asato H, et al. Analytic review of 2372 free flap transfers for head and neck reconstruction following cancer resection. *J Reconstr Microsurg* 19:363–368, 2003.

8. Genden EM, Rinaldo A, Suarez C, et al. Complications of free flap transfers for head and neck reconstruction following cancer resection. *Oral Oncol* 40:979–984, 2004.

9. Haughey BH, Wilson E, Kluwe L, et al. Free flap reconstruction of the head and neck: analysis of 241 cases. *Otolaryngol Head Neck Surg* 125:10–17, 2001.

10. Harashina T, Fujino T, Aoyagi F. Reconstruction of the oral cavity with a free flap. *Plast Reconstr Surg* 58:412–414, 1976.

11. Shpitzer T, Goldberg I, Stern Y et al. Radial forearm free flap in head and neck reconstruction. *Isr J Med Sci* 29:735–738, 1993.

12. Yang G, Chen B, Gao Y. Forearm free skin transplantation. *Natl Med J China* 61:139–141, 1981.

13. Sullivan MJ, Carroll WR, Kuriloff DB. Lateral arm free flap in head and neck reconstruction. *Arch Otolaryngol Head Neck Surg* 118:1095–1101, 1992.

14. Miller MJ, Reece GP, Marchi M, et al. Lateral thigh free flap in head and neck reconstruction. *Plast Reconstr Surg* 96:334–340, 1995.

15. Wei WI, Lam LK, Yuen PW, et al. Mucosal changes of the free jejunal graft in response to radiotherapy. *Am J Surg* 175:44–46, 1998.

16. Taylor GI, Miller GD, Ham FJ. The free vascularized bone graft. A clinical extension of microvascular techniques. *Plast Reconstr Surg* 55:533–544, 1975.

17. Conley J. Use of composite flaps containing bone for major repairs in the head and neck. *Plast Reconstr Surg* 49:522–526, 1972.

FUNDAMENTAL
PROCEDURES

FUNDAMENTAL

PROCEDURES

STERILE TECHNIQUE/UNIVERSAL
PRECAUTIONS

Jose L. Trani, Jr., MD

A discussion of sterile technique and universal precautions for invasive or operative procedures is a discussion of the use of a barrier for two different but related purposes. In the application of sterile technique, the primary goal is in protecting the patient from nosocomial infection during a procedure that both penetrates a major body defense against disease, the skin, and simultaneously diminishes the immune defense system. The importance of preventing surgical site infections (SSIs) is illustrated by the fact that they are the third most frequently reported source of nosocomial infection. SSIs account for approximately 15 percent of all nosocomial infections among hospital patients.[1] Between 1986 and 1996, hospitals participating in the Centers for Disease Control (CDC) National Nosocomial Infection Surveillance system reported 15,523 SSIs after 593,344 procedures.[2] Besides the morbidity and mortality associated with these infections, patient stays and costs associated with the lengthened stay increased with this added treatment. In promoting and following universal precautions, the barrier serves to protect both the medical team and the patient from infectious spread from inadvertent contact with bloodborne, or body fluids/tissues that have potential to transmit disease. The importance of protecting both parties is highlighted by the fact that transmission to a naive host may lead to the development of a chronic carrier state and its associated morbidity and mortality.

Sterile Technique

HISTORY

The first physician to establish an effective antisepsis technique was Joseph Lister, an English surgeon, who successfully translated Pasteur's principle of germ theory into a viable format by substituting chemical antiseptic for heat sterilization. By 1865, Lister was routinely applying his most famous antiseptic agent, pure carbolic acid, directly onto wounds and dressings and using an aerosolized form to reduce bacterial load in the operative theatre. A second contribution of Lister's involved the use of sterile absorbable sutures during operative procedures. He correctly predicted that a major source of infection among his contemporaries resulted from the use of contaminated suture material. The use of antiseptic and eventually aseptic technique would prove to be of a greater advancement in surgery than that of another advancement developed around the same time, that of anesthesia. While anesthesia reduced a patient's discomfort, permitting an increase in technical expertise and more advanced exploration, the reduction in local infection more significantly impacted both morbidity and mortality. Germans advanced Lister's pioneering work in this field further by applying heat sterilization to operating room instruments and attire. By 1890, these principles had gained widespread acceptance in both European and American operating rooms, and these techniques helped to establish the position of surgeons and surgery within the medical community.

PATIENT PREPARATION

Patient preparation begins with proper selection and workup of anyone who is a candidate for surgery. With few exceptions, patients harboring an infection or infectious process should not undergo elective procedures. After this, the next step in reducing postoperative infection is the administration of preoperative antibiotics. Studies have determined that administration of appropriately selected antibiotics leads to a decrease in SSIs when the antibiotic is administered 1 h prior to the initial incision.[3] Following these guidelines, adequate drug levels are achieved in the bloodstream to reduce the microbial burden to a manageable level for host defense in light of surgical manipulation. Although this precaution is fairly easy to accomplish, recent evidence shows that only 55.7 percent of patients receive a preoperative antibiotic at the appropriate time.[4]

Two main aspects of patient body site preparation for surgery include the removal of body hair at the proposed surgical site and the preparation of the skin with the use of an antiseptic agent. Clippers are preferred over a razor or depilatory agent for the removal of hair at the operative site. Shaving hair results in microscopic cuts that can serve to break down skin barrier protection and result in foci of bacterial multiplication.[5] Although depilatory agents produce lower rates of surgical infection than shaving or clipping,[6,7] their use is discouraged due to hypersensitivity reactions in some patients.[6] As with the administration of preoperative antibiotics, the timing of the hair removal procedure plays an important role in decreasing SSI. Hair should be clipped immediately before the operation rather than 24 h in advance. This practice has been shown to reduce SSI rates from 4.0 to 1.8 percent.[8,9]

There are a number of antiseptic agents available for skin preparation at the surgical site. All are designed to decrease the bacterial load of naturally occurring flora on the skin surface. Traditional agents include alcohol (ethyl alcohol, 60–95 percent by volume or isopropyl alcohol, 50–91.3 percent by volume in aqueous solution),[10] chlorhexidine gluconate, and iodine/iodophor-based products. Although each of these three types of agents vary in their mechanism of action and bacterial activity, all should be applied in the same manner. The patient's skin should first be free of any gross debris or contamination. The antiseptic agent should be applied in concentric circles, moving from inside to out, beginning in the immediate area of the proposed incision.[11] The prepared area should be large enough to permit easy placement of drapes creating the sterile field, taking into account lengthening of the incision or creation of new incisions. It should also permit easy placement of drains or ostomies, if required.[10]

SURGEON PREPARATION

Surgeon preparation has evolved perhaps as long as surgery has been performed. From issues of avoiding soilage on personal articles to preventing infection of the patient, current techniques are a combination of ritual, common sense, and evidence-based practice. One traditional stereotype associated with surgery is the scrubbing of the hands. This practice, which takes place in an area adjacent to most operating rooms, decreases the number of bacteria present on a surgeon's hands and forearms just prior to donning sterile gown and gloves. Agents containing alcohol-based products combined with chlorhexidine gluconate are most effective at reducing bacterial load on the skin followed by, in order of decreasing effectiveness, chlorhexidine gluconate alone, iodophor/iodine-based products, triclosan, and plain soap.[12] This process should include a thorough cleaning under the fingernails with the first scrub of the day.[13] The hands and forearms should then be covered with the antiseptic agent of choice, as this will allow maximal time to reduce bacterial burden. Following this, the hands and forearms should be scrubbed using a sponge, not a brush, starting with the fingertips and proceeding toward the elbows. Evidence demonstrates a 2-min scrub to be as effective as a 10-min scrub in reducing bacterial load.[12] After scrubbing, the hands should be rinsed. Hands should be kept up and away from the body, permitting water to drain down the arms until a sterile towel is obtained.

Once the hands and forearms are adequately prepared and dried, a sterile gown is donned followed by sterile gloves. The area of the sterile field created by these items is from the chest to the level of the sterile field (the point where the operating room table touches the sterile gown. The arms are considered sterile from 2 in. above the elbow to the cuff. The gloves are completely sterile.[14]

Gown cuffs are not considered sterile as they are contaminated once scrubbed hands pass through them.[14] Other areas such as the neckline and axilla are areas of friction and as such are not considered sterile. The back of the gown cannot be constantly monitored and is also not considered sterile.[15] After donning sterile gloves and gown, hands should be kept above the waist and in the area of the aforementioned sterile field. The patient is now ready to be prepped using sterile drapes. Sterile drapes should be carefully placed to allow adequate exposure to the proposed incision site while covering any unprepped areas.

Universal Precautions

The guidelines set forth by the United States Department of Labor Occupational Safety and Health Administration (OSHA) are designed to protect health-care workers from infection through occupational exposure to bloodborne pathogens. An occupational exposure is defined by OSHA as, "Reasonably anticipated skin, eye, mucous membrane, or parenteral contact with blood or any other potentially infectious materials that may result from the performance of an employee's duties."[16] According to the precept of *Universal Precautions*, all human blood, blood products, and certain body fluids are to be treated as if they are contaminated materials.[17] As a result, OSHA has mandated that people in health-care occupations that place them at risk of contact with human blood or blood products, including products containing components of human blood, are required to use protective measures.[16]

OSHA policy stipulates that personal protective equipment (PPE), to be worn when an occupational exposure is anticipated, consists of gloves, masks, eye protection or face shields, and gown, apron, or other protective body clothing. OSHA also states that surgical caps and/or hoods as well as shoe covers or boots should be worn in instances where gross contamination can be anticipated.[17] It should be noted that while OSHA does not mandate the use of double gloving, they strongly recommend this practice as an additional protective measure for health-care providers participating in high-risk activities.[18] The failure rates of both single and double gloving practices during surgical procedures have been studied in a number of trials. While glove perforation rates have been reported to occur in up to half of all surgeries,[13] two more recent prospective studies place this risk between 18 and 23 percent.[19,20] While the use of double gloving did not reduce the risk of glove perforation, it reduced blood or other bodily fluid contact with the surgeon's skin from 13 percent in single glove situations to 2 percent when double gloves were used.[18] Prolonged exposure of skin surface to potentially infected source material resulting from not identifying a break in the glove barrier may increase the risk of transmission from an infected patient. Current data demonstrate that surgeons who used single gloves only were able to detect a perforation in 37–42 percent of the occurrences. Surgeons using the double gloving technique identified punctures 78–86 percent of the time, thus minimizing any effects of a breach in their barrier defense.[19,20]

The risk of infection via an occupational exposure has been well studied and varies according to the pathogen and type of exposure. Percutaneous exposures are the greatest risk of bloodborne pathogen transmission to health-care workers.[21] Of the three most concerning causes, hepatitis B virus (HBV), hepatitis C virus (HCV), and human immunodeficiency virus (HIV), only HBV has a vaccination that can prevent transmission of this virus. For unvaccinated personnel, the risk of transmission via percutaneous exposure from a HBV antigen-seropositive source is at least 30 percent.[22] For HCV and HIV, the risk of infection is far less following a percutaneous exposure, however this is more than offset by the lack of vaccination prophylaxis available at present. Recent literature places the risk of transmission after a single percutaneous exposure from a seropositive person at 0–7 percent for HCV[23–25] and at approximately 0.3 percent for HIV.[26–28] Variables that may alter the risk following exposure include titer of viral agent present in the infected blood source, the frequency of exposure, and the type of exposure.[28] Differentiating the source of contaminated sharp is important for assessing risk. Needle sticks occur with either a solid tip, such as a suturing needle, or a hollow tip, such as a phlebotomy needle. The risk of infection increases with the hollow tip exposure due to the potential for a larger volume of inoculating agent to be administered. In the event of an exposure, the CDC has recommended different approaches to postexposure prophylaxis for both HCV and HIV. While it is recommended that exposure to HIV be treated with prophylactic chemotherapy,[29] there is no evidence currently supporting the use of either antiviral agents[30] or the use of immune globulin[31] following HCV exposure.

REFERENCES

1. Emori TG, Gaynes RP. An overview of nosocomial infections, including the role of the microbiology laboratory. *Clin Microbiol Rev* 6(4):428–442, 1993.

2. Mangram AJ, Horan TC, Pearson ML, et al. Guideline for prevention of surgical site infection. *Infect Control Hosp Epidemiol* 20(4):247–278, 1999.

3. Classen DC, Evans RS, Pestotnik SL, et al. The timing of prophylactic administration of antibiotics and the risk of surgical wound infection. *N Engl J Med* 326:281–286, 1992.

4. Bratzler DW, Houck PM, Richards C, et al. Use of antimicrobial prophylaxis for major surgery. Baseline results from the national surgical infection prevention project. *Arch Surg* 140:174–182, 2005.

5. Mangram A, Horan TC, Pearson ML, et al. The Hospital Infection Control Practices Advisory Committee. Guideline for prevention of surgical site infection. *Infect Control Hosp Epidemiol* 20(4):247–278, 1999.

6. Seropian R, Reynolds BM. Wound infections after preoperative depilatory versus razor preparation. *Am J Surg* 121:251–254, 1971.

7. Hamilton HW, Hamilton KR, Lone FJ. Preoperative hair removal. *Can J Surg* 20:269–271, 274–275, 1977.

8. Alexander JW, Fischer JE, Boyajian M, et al. The influence of hair-removal methods on wound infections. *Arch Surg* 118(3):347–352, 1983.

9. Masterson TM, Rodeheaver GT, Morgan RF, et al. Bacteriologic evaluation of electric clippers for surgical hair removal. *Am J Surg* 148:301–302, 1984.

10. Food and Drug Administration. Topical antimicrobial drug products for over-the-counter human use: tentative final monograph for health-care antiseptic drug products-proposed rule (21 CRF Parts 333 and 369). *Fed Regist* 59:31441–31452, 1994.

11. Hardin WD, Nichols RL. Handwashing and patient skin preparation. In Malangoni MA, ed., *Critical Issues in Operating Room Management*. Philadelphia, PA: Lippincott-Raven, 1997: 133–149.

12. Advisory Committee and the HICPAC/SHEA/APIC/IDSA Hand Hygiene Task Force. Guideline for hand hygiene in health-care settings. Recommendations of the healthcare infection control practices. *MMWR Recomm Rep* 51(RR-16):1–56, 2002.

13. Quebbemann EJ, Telford GL, Wadsworth K, et al. Double gloving. Protecting surgeons from blood contamination in the operating room. *Arch Surg* 127:213–216, 1992.

14. Association of Perioperative Registered Nurses. Recommended practices for maintaining a sterile field. *AORN J* 73(2):477–482, 2001.

15. Pierce L. Basic principles of aseptic technique. *Plast Surg Nurs* 17:48–49, 1997.

16. U.S. Department of Labor Occupational Safety & Health Administration. Regulations (preambles to final rules), section 9–IX. Summary and Explanation of the Final Standard (Construction Industries).

17. U.S. Department of Labor Occupational Safety & Health Administration. Regulations (standards—29 CFR). Bloodborne pathogens, parts 1910, 1030.

18. Letter from Greg Watchman to Sen. Brian P. Bilbray in response to the application of glove monitoring devices to aid in the detection of glove failures, 1997.

19. Naver LPS, Gottrup F. Incidence of glove perforation in gastrointestinal surgery and the protective effects of double gloves: a prospective randomized controlled study. *Eur J Surg* 166:293–295, 2000.

20. Laine T, Aarino P. How often does glove perforation occur in surgery? Comparison between single gloves and a double gloving system. *Am J Surg* 181:564–566, 2001.

21. Cardo DM, Culver DH, Ciesielski C, et al. A case-control study of HIV seroconversion in health care workers after percutaneous exposure. *N Engl J Med* 337:1485–1490, 1997.

22. Shapiro CN. Occupational risk of infection with hepatitis B and hepatitis C virus. *Surg Clin North Am* 75:1047–1056, 1995.

23. Zuckerman J, Clewley G, Griffiths P, et al. Prevalence of hepatitis C antibodies in clinical health-care workers. *Lancet* 343:1618–1620, 1994.

24. Petrosilla N, Puro V, Ipolito G, and the Italian Study Group on bloodborne Occupational Risk in Dialysis. Prevalence of hepatitis C antibodies in health-care workers. *Lancet* 344:339–340, 1994.

25. Lanphear BP, Linneman CC, Cannon CG, et al. Hepatitis C virus infection in health care workers: risk of exposure and infection. *Infect Control Hosp Epidemiol* 15:745–750, 1994.

26. Rhodes RS, Bell DM, eds. Prevention of transmission of bloodborne pathogens. *Surg Clin North Am* 75:1047–1217, 1995.

27. Chamberland ME, Ciesielski CA, Howard RJ, et al. Occupational risk of infection with human immunodeficiency virus. *Surg Clin North Am* 75:1057–1070, 1995.

28. Marcus R, Bell DM. Occupational risk of human immunodeficiency virus. In Devita VT, Hellman S, Rosenberg SA, eds., *Aids: Etiology, Diagnosis, Treatment and Prevention*, 4th ed. Philadelphia, PA: Lippincott-Raven, 1997: 645–654.

29. Centers for Disease Control and Prevention. Update: provisional public health service recommendations for chemoprophylaxis after occupational exposure to HIV. *MMWR Morb Mortal Wkly Rep* 1998.

30. Centers for Disease Control and Prevention. Recommendations for follow-up of health-care workers after occupational exposure to hepatitis C virus. *MMWR Morb Mortal Wkly Rep* 46:603–606, 1997.

31. Krawczynski K, Alter MJ, Govindarajan S, et al. Studies on protective efficacy of hepatitis C immunoglobulins (HCIG) in experimental hepatis C virus infection [abstract]. *Hepatology* 18:110A, 1993.

SUTURE TECHNIQUE

Matthew G. Hartwig, MD

The Assyro-Babylonian civilization provides some of the earliest writings involving the practice of surgery. Although removal of the surgeon's hands following adverse outcomes, as described in the Code of Hammurabi, does not routinely occur today, the code does enlighten the reader about the thousands of years that have gone into refining current surgical technique. Irrespective of advances in knowledge and technology, the underlying principles of suturing remain consistent: apposition of wound edges until inherent healing processes provide strength and aesthetics, as well as protecting against bleeding and infection. Suture technique is a basic component of all surgical procedures and must be performed appropriately to avoid postoperative complications. Proper technique demands more than a modicum of skill and depends on practice and repetition.

Suturing typically involves a surgical needle with which to penetrate tissues and advance the suture threads. The needle consists of three major areas (Fig. 18-1). The *point* is the sharpest portion of the needle and can be *tapered* or *cut* in style. Taper points are generally used for easily penetrable tissues,

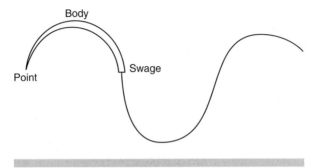

Figure 18-1 **The three major parts of a needle.**

while cutting points are used for tougher tissues, such as skin. The *body* is the middle portion of the needle, which is grasped by the needle holder. The distal section of the needle holder jaws should clutch the needle securely, approximately one-third to one-half of the distance from the swaged end to the point. The *swaged end* involves the needle and suture attachment point, and is the weakest portion of the needle.

Proper use of the needle and needle holder is a primary component of suture technique. The needle holder is held with the first and fourth digits placed through the loops in the handle, while the second digit provides stabilization by applying pressure to the fulcrum (Fig. 18-2). The needle should enter perpendicular to the surface being sutured, and subsequent force applied in the same direction as the curve of the needle. The size of the bite (the amount of wound tissue included in the closure) is determined by the size of the needle. Do not take excessively large bites of tissue. Do not grasp the point or cutting edges with the needle holders when pulling the needle through the wound. This rapidly dulls the needle for future use.

The term *suture* refers to any material used for wound closure or ligation of structures. Historically, animal sinews and certain plant fibers have been described as being used for suture material. Modern materials vary greatly in composition, but can be divided into two broad categories: *absorbable* and *nonabsorbable*. The choice of suture type is determined by the characteristics of the wound being closed. Synthetic absorbable sutures are degraded via hydrolyzation, instead of enzymatic digestion, and therefore create less tissue reaction than natural absorbable sutures. Some typical synthetic absorbable sutures in use today include polyglactin 910 (Vicryl), poliglecaprone 25 (Monocryl), and polydioxanone (PDS II). Nonabsorbable sutures are considered not to degrade within the body and can be composed of single or multiple filaments. Commonly used nonabsorbable suture materials include silk, nylon, polypropylene, and metal wire. Because of their nonabsorbable nature, these sutures are used to approximate tissues over a

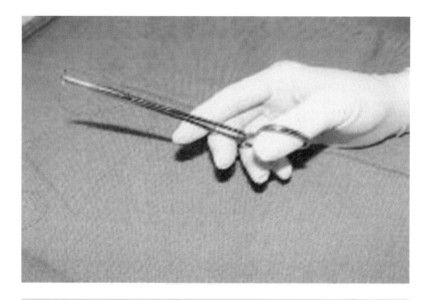

Figure 18-2 **Proper handling of the needle holder assists in stability and skillful placement of each stitch. The first and fourth digits are placed through the handle loops while the second digit rests against the fulcrum for additional support.**

long period of time. However, the lack of dissolution also serves as a possible nidus of infection, with braided nonabsorbable sutures the most likely to harbor infectious organisms.

There is an assortment of wound closure options, each with advantages and disadvantages. As with the suture material, details of the wound determine the type of closure selected by the surgeon. Wound closures can be divided into two broad categories: interrupted and continuous. With *interrupted* suturing techniques, each stitch is placed individually. In general, this allows the surgeon to make minor modifications during the closure to ensure proper alignment. Interrupted sutures also provide greater tensile strength and have a tendency to create less tissue edema. The primary disadvantage of interrupted sutures involves the longer duration of time required to close larger wounds. *Continuous*, or running, sutures involve multiple stitches being placed without interruption. Using continuous sutures can expedite the closure, but make perfect alignment more challenging and can decrease circulation to the wound. Also, dehiscence may occur if the suture were to break and unravel.

Three of the more commonly used closures include the simple, horizontal, and vertical mattress techniques. All three can be performed in an interrupted or continuous manner. The *simple* interrupted suture is the most versatile method of closing wounds (Fig. 18-3). In general, the distance between wound edges and the insertion and exit site of the needle should be equal. Also, the gap between each individual stitch should be equidistant. Typically, the base of the stitch is broader than the top. This creates a flask-shaped stitch, promotes wound eversion, and assists in avoiding excessive scarring as tissue retraction occurs during healing. The simple continuous suture provides the most rapid method of closing wounds. The first stitch is placed at one end of the wound and secured as in the simple interrupted closure. However, the suture is not cut. Instead, successive simple stitches are evenly situated along the length of the wound. The closure is finished by securing it with a knot between the tail of the suture and the loop of the last stitch placed.

Horizontal and vertical mattress sutures can both be used to support approximation of wound edges by decreasing tension. Vertical mattress stitches are a variation of the simple interrupted in which the first bite begins wide of the wound edge and travels deeply prior to exiting the wound on the opposite side (Fig. 18-4). Instead of securing the stitch at this time, the suture is brought back through the wound again, this time with entry and exit points closer and more superficial than the original bite. This technique provides superior eversion of wound edges and is able to close potential spaces deep within the

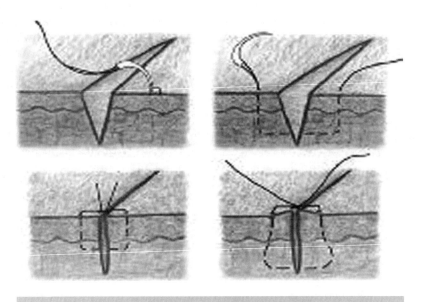

Figure 18-3 **Drawing of simple interrupted suture placement. The bottom right diagram illustrates the "flask" shape of the stitch with a wider base—optimizing wound edge eversion.** (*Source*: Adapted from Mackay-Wiggin J, Ratner D. eMedicine, 2005.)

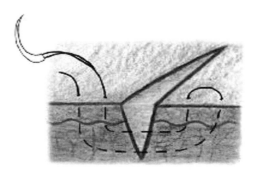

Figure 18-4 **The vertical mattress stitch includes deep and shallow bites through the wound to aid in reducing wound tension and to close any potential space at the base of the wound.** (*Source*: Adapted from Mackay-Wiggin J, Ratner D. eMedicine, 2005.)

wound. A horizontal mattress suture also can greatly reduce tension and evert wound edges when properly used (Fig. 18-5). The needle is inserted and driven through the wound as if a simple stitch was being placed. However, the needle is reinserted approximately 0.5–1.0 cm lateral to, but on the same side as the first exit site. After passing through the wound again and exiting on the side of the original needle entry location, the stitch is secured with a knot. Although useful in many situations, mattress sutures are prone to producing suture marks, tissue strangulation, and wound necrosis if not performed appropriately. In order to minimize these complications, one should tighten only enough to approximate the wound edges and then remove the sutures as early as possible based on wound strength.

In general, the continuous subcuticular suture provides the best aesthetic result for closing wounds (Fig. 18-6). It does not provide significant wound strength, and therefore should only be used in wounds under minimal tension. The technique is essentially a buried continuous horizontal mattress in which a simple stitch is placed and secured at one end of the wound. The suture is then carried the length of the wound by taking horizontal bites through the papillary dermis on alternating sides until the wound is closed. If both anchoring knots are buried, it is possible to completely conceal the suture material below the epidermis and obviate suture marks, or crosshatching.

Suture removal also requires proper technique in order to achieve the best possible outcome. Although premature removal of sutures may lead to

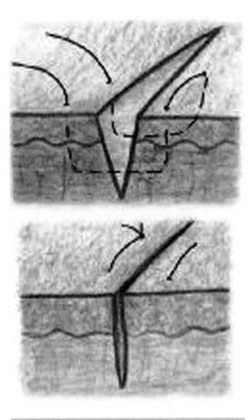

Figure 18-5 **The horizontal mattress stitch also provides additional support for wounds under tension.** (*Source*: Adapted from Mackay-Wiggin J, Ratner D. eMedicine, 2005.)

dehiscence and disappointing cosmetic results, delay in suture removal may increase tissue reaction, scar formation, crosshatching, and the risk of infection. Proper timing of suture removal depends on the amount of tension and anatomic location of the wound. Typically, sutures are removed 1–2 weeks following wound closure. Sutures on the face are usually removed within 5–7 days. On the contrary, sutures on the lower extremities or in areas of mobility may need to stay in place for 3 weeks, or more. Buried sutures with absorbable material will dissolve over time and do not require later removal. In order to remove a suture, it should be gently elevated with forceps while one side is transected with scissors. The knot can then be grasped and slowly pulled

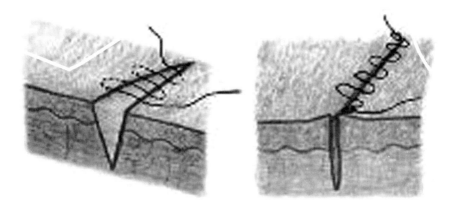

Figure 18-6 **The subcuticular stitch is a modification of the horizontal mattress in which the suture is buried beneath skin level in order to improve the aesthetic appearance of a wound.** (*Source*: Adapted from Mackay-Wiggin J, Ratner D. eMedicine, 2005.)

toward the suture line while the stitch slides free of the wound. Pulling the stitch away from the suture line may lead to wound separation. Often, sterile adhesive strips are placed on the wound following suture removal for additional support. This may help prevent spreading the wound scar.

WOUND CARE

Brian Lima, MD

A prerequisite for effective wound care is a thorough familiarity with the basic principles and mechanisms of wound healing and the clinical factors that may significantly impede this process. Briefly, the sequence of events in normal wound healing can be arbitrarily divided into four sequential phases: *inflammation, epithelialization, fibroplasia,* and *maturation.* The maximum tensile strength of a wound, which is typically reached by 8 weeks, is determined by the extent of collagen cross-linking and may approach 80 percent of the original level of strength. As will be described further below, essential components of wound healing include the maintenance of a moist environment, adequate oxygen delivery, removal of necrotic tissue, optimizing nutritional status, and immediate recognition and treatment of wound complications, such as infections and fascial dehiscence.

During the initial evaluation of a wound, certain features must be noted, such as whether the wound is *open* or *closed*, and whether the wound is *acute* versus *chronic* (greater than 3 months). These important distinctions are critical for classifying wounds and determining the most appropriate mode of therapy. Careful attention to every descriptive detail of the wound must also be documented, including the presence or absence of erythema, induration, necrotic tissue, granulation tissue, drainage (purulent, serous, feculent, or serosanguinous), severe tenderness, and overall wound dimensions (Table 18-1). Awareness of these characteristics enables timely diagnosis of wound complications as well as tracking progress, or lack thereof, for any given wound. Therefore, simply stating that a wound is *clean, dry, and intact* will not always suffice.

Closed Wounds

Perhaps the most simplistic and commonly encountered wound is a closed wound, in which the wound edges are surgically reapproximated following an operative procedure, allowing for healing to take place via *primary intention*. Usually, the skin edges are approximated using either staples, or a continuous subcuticular closure with an absorbable suture and overlying skin closure strips (Steri-Strips). Some wounds, such as traumatic lacerations or skin lesion excisions may be closed in interrupted fashion with nonabsorbable suture. Sterile dressings placed at the time of surgery are typically kept on these

Table 18-1 **Wound Assessment**

- Anatomic location
- Surgical wound classification: clean, clean-contaminated, contaminated, dirty
- Open vs. closed
- Dimensions (length, width, depth)
- Acute vs. chronic (>3 months)
- Necrotic tissue
- Granulation tissue
- Hematoma
- Erythema
- Induration
- Wound drainage: serous, sanguinous, serosanguinous, purulent, feculent
- Tenderness
- Temperature (warm compared with body temperature)

wounds for 24–48 h postoperatively to allow for completion of epithelialization and restoration of water barrier function.[1] The flexible skin closure strips are kept in place for up to 2 weeks. Staples and nonabsorbable stitches should be removed at 7–10 days postoperatively. However, staples or stitches in certain regions of the wound may need to be removed at earlier time points if there are any clinical manifestations of a wound infection or dehiscence, suggested by localized erythema, induration, drainage, heat, or tenderness. The wound can then be bluntly probed to evaluate for the presence of an abscess or fascial disruption. Management of these complications will be discussed further below.

Open Wounds

In certain scenarios, the wound edges are not approximated and thus healing occurs through *secondary intention*. A notable variation is that of *delayed primary closure*, in which a wound is intentionally left open for a defined period of time and later closed primarily. The overall process of wound healing is comparatively prolonged in open wounds partially because a well-defined bed of granulation tissue must form at the base of the wound and epithelial cells must traverse a greater distance for epithelialization of the wound to be completed.[2] Granulation tissue consists of a heterogeneous matrix of newly formed capillaries, connective tissue, and inflammatory cells. Formation of granulation tissue is dependent on adequate oxygen delivery to the region and impaired by the presence of devitalized tissue and infection. Consequently, evaluation of an open wound entails recognition and removal of necrotic tissue via local debridement. A paucity of granulation tissue is a sign of poor wound healing and may signify an underlying vascular insufficiency, inadequate nutritional status, or some other systemic factor such as potential etiologies. Another distinguishing feature of open or nonepithelialized wounds is the persistent leakage of plasma, which can serve as a rich culture medium for invading bacteria. This is an important attribute to keep in mind, particularly in the setting of deep open wounds with distant tunneled areas that are not readily accessible but must be managed with the appropriate packing and dressing.

Wound Dressing

The selection of the most suitable wound dressing or other therapeutic strategy can be undertaken only after completion of a meticulous wound assessment. Since the 1960s, empirical evidence has clearly demonstrated that epithelialization occurs more rapidly in a moist environment.[3] Moist healing prevents desiccation at the base of the wound, thereby preventing tissue necrosis and delayed epithelialization. Traditionally, wet-to-dry gauze dressings have been used for open wounds and provide an effective means of continual debridement of necrotic tissue from the wound bed. This dressing involves packing moistened gauze into the wound with overlying layers of dry gauze. The moistened gauze eventually dries out and adheres to necrotic tissue at the surface which is removed at the subsequent dressing change. Preservation of the moist healing environment requires that these dressings be changed two to three times daily.

The primary disadvantages of this approach include tape-induced irritation of adjacent skin and the need for frequent dressing changes that may be very painful for the patient. As a result, several wound care alternatives have been developed and promoted, including semipermeable films, foams, hydrogels, hydrocolloids, silicone, and dermal replacements. To date, there is no indisputable evidence favoring one method over another, as long as moist healing is achieved. One recent development that is becoming increasingly more prevalent in the management of chronic or large open wounds is a device known as the vacuum-assisted closure (VAC).[4] This promising device consists of a sponge packed into the wound with an overlying transparent film and suction tubing connected to a vacuum. Through locally applied negative pressure, the VAC promotes wound healing by preserving a moist healing environment while drawing the wound closed, stimulating granulation tissue formation, and removing interstitial fluid and necrotic tissue. In contrast to wet-to-dry gauze dressings, which must be changed two to three times daily, the VAC is changed only every 2–3 days. There are also data from prospective, randomized trials that suggest the VAC can lead to an increased rate of wound healing when compared with other conventional wound dressings.[5] The VAC clearly provides a viable option for wound care, and must be considered when contemplating management of challenging wounds.

Wound Complications

Knowledge of whether a particular wound was a clean, clean-contaminated, contaminated, or dirty wound serves as a valuable indicator for the potential risk of subsequent wound infection. Grossly contaminated wounds may have infection rates as high as 35 percent versus 4 percent in clean wounds. Clinical signs of a wound infection include fever, leukocytosis, localized erythema, induration, heat, incisional tenderness, and purulent drainage. If a wound infection is suspected, empirical antimicrobial therapy should be initiated along with Gram's stain and culture of the wound to optimize the antibiotic regimen. Infection of a closed wound necessitates opening and draining the wound. Rapidly progressive wound infections, such as necrotizing fasciitis, can be potentially lethal and may warrant immediate surgical debridement in the operating room.

Drainage of enteral contents from an abdominal wound usually represents an enterocutaneous fistula. Depending on the magnitude of output, enterocutaneous fistulas may be managed conservatively with wound dressing changes or by surgical repair. Fascial disruption results from the failure of fascial healing, leading to complete or partial wound dehiscence. There may be copious drainage of serosanguinous fluid from the wound, often exacerbated by Valsalva maneuvers. The spectrum of clinical presentation may range from minor defects with minimal drainage of peritoneal fluid to large defects with evisceration. Emergent surgical repair is usually required in cases of fascial disruption, which reemphasizes the critical nature of wound assessment and implications certain wound attributes may have on patient care.

REFERENCES

1. Lorenz HP, Longaker MT. Wounds: biology, pathology, and management. In Norton JA, Bollinger RR, Chang AE, et al., eds., *Surgery: Basic Science and Clinical Evidence*. New York, NY: Springer-Verlag, 2001:221–239.

2. Fine NA, Mustoe TA. Wound healing. In: Greenfield LJ, Mulholland MW, Oldham KT, et al., eds., *Surgery: Scientific Principles and Practice*, 3rd ed. Philadelphia, PA: Lippincott Williams & Wilkins, 2001:69–85.

3. Winter GD, Sacles JT. Effect of air drying and dressings on the surface of a wound. *Nature* 197:91–92, 1963.

4. Argenta LC, Morkywas MJ. Vacuum-assisted closure: a new method for wound control and treatment: clinical experience. *Ann Plast Surg* 38:563–576, 1997.

5. Ford CN, Reinhard ER, Yeh D, et al. Interim analysis of a prospective, randomized trial of vacuum-assisted closure versus the healthpoint system in the management of pressure ulcers. *Ann Plast Surg* 49(1):55–61, 2002.

VENOUS ACCESS

Mayur B. Patel, MD

Obtaining access to the venous vasculature is one of the most common procedures performed. Generally, catheters provide the conduit to permit the introduction or withdrawal of fluid, medications, or blood products. In order to determine catheter type, size, and placement, the intention for intravenous (IV) access must be known.

IV access can be required for many reasons, urgent and nonurgent, including delivery of fluid (crystalloid or colloid), blood products, total parental nutrition (TPN), and medications like antibiotics, chemotherapy, and pressor therapy. Catheters threaded near cardiac venous inflow, central venous catheters (CVCs), can provide right atrial pressure monitoring, blood drawing capability, as well as a passage for invasive cardiac monitoring (Swan-Ganz) or transvenous cardiac pacing.

Once the patient's IV need is determined, a peripheral versus central location can be addressed. Peripheral IV (PIV) access is the most common IV access method for short-term use. PIV catheters are short (less than 8 cm), inserted over a needle, through the skin into a peripheral vein, usually in the extremities. Uncommonly, venous cutdown is required for PIV placement. PIV catheters can be used for maintenance of IV fluid and medication delivery. Fourteen- to sixteen-gauge PIVs provide rapid volume delivery due to their relative short length and large diameter (resistance α length/radius^4), as compared to long, multilumen CVCs. PIV catheters are replaced every 72–96 h. When not in use, these catheters require a heparin lock IV (HLIV) or a low basal rate (10–30 mL/h) of maintenance fluid infusion (KVO, keep vein open). Rarely, PIVs are associated with bloodstream infections; however, phlebitis can occur with long-term use.

CVCs are long (greater than 8 cm) and percutaneously inserted over a guidewire (Seldinger technique, Fig. 18-7) into central veins, such as the subclavian, internal jugular, or femoral veins. Ultrasound and/or fluoroscopy can assist in CVC placement. Once inserted, the ideal position of the catheter tip is the junction between the right atrium and the superior vena cava (SVC). The average distance from skin to right atrium is 14.5 and 18.5 cm, for right- and left-sided cannulations, respectively. Maximal barrier precautions are mandatory during placement. Also, specialized CVC teams help decrease serious complications.

Despite best efforts and depending on location, improper CVC placement can cause pneumothorax, hemothorax, arterial or nerve injury, cardiac dysrhythmia, air embolism, catheter embolization, or thrombosis. Importantly, in patients with a prior pneumothorax or hemothorax, it is safer to attempt CVC placement on the ipsilateral injured side. This avoids harming the uninjured side and risking bilateral pneumothorax or hemothorax. It is vital that a chest x-ray be completed after any subclavian or internal jugular CVC placement or attempt (unnecessary for femoral CVC access).

Unfortunately, CVCs cause the majority of serious catheter-related infections, especially those occurring in the intensive care unit (ICU). Skin flora is the origin of most CVC infections. Early infection (3–5 days) usually results from infection of the subcutaneous tract. Later infections may have the same cause or may occur by hematogenous spread. *Staphylococcus epidermidis* and *Staphylococcus aureus* are the most common bacteria cultured. Contamination of the catheter hub contributes substantially to intraluminal colonization of CVCs. Multilumen catheters and catheter thrombosis both increase the incidence of catheter sepsis. To decrease infection risk, certain catheters are coated or impregnated with

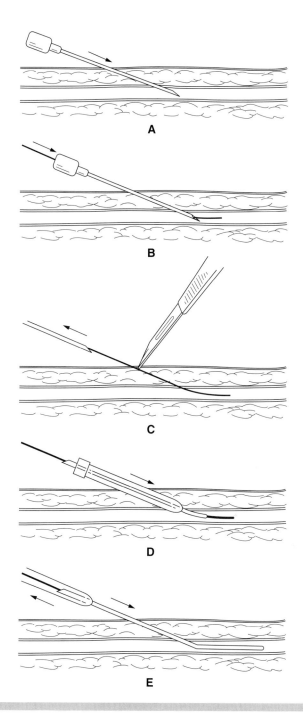

Figure 18-7 **Seldinger technique of vascular cannulation. (A) Vessel cannulation with needle. (B) Guidewire advancement. (C) Needle removal and puncture wound enlargement. (D) Subcutaneous tissue dilation. (E) Dilator removal and catheter advancement.** (*Source*: Adapted from Deitch EA. *Tools of the Trade and Rules of the Road*. Philadelphia, PA: Lippincott-Raven, 1997.)

389

antimicrobial or antiseptic agents (minocycline/ rifampin or chlorhexidine/silver-sulfadiazine), but nothing replaces sterile technique during CVC placement and subsequent dressing changes. The most common therapy for suspected catheter infection is removal of the catheter.

CVCs can deliver medications directly to the heart for immediate distribution to the body. This also avoids potential venous irritation or infiltration of substances, such as dopamine. In cases of poor PIV access or chronic IV needs, CVCs are an only option.

There are several types of CVCs, which are based on the intended lifespan, pathway from skin to vessel (tunneled versus nontunneled), and lumen number. Long-term CVCs consist of (1) Dacron cuffed, tunneled Silastic catheters (Fig. 18-8) and (2) implantable ports (Fig. 18-9). The subcutaneous tunnel isolates the venous puncture site from the skin and decreases the potential for bacterial contamination. The Dacron cuffs (one near the venous entrance site and one near the skin exit site) anchor the catheter and are also believed to inhibit colonization of the CVC by skin organisms. Hickman (single or double lumen), Broviac (small internal diameter), and Groshong (one-way valve preventing reflux) are cuffed, tunneled catheters. Cuffed, tunneled catheters can be removed at the bedside by bluntly dissecting the fibrous

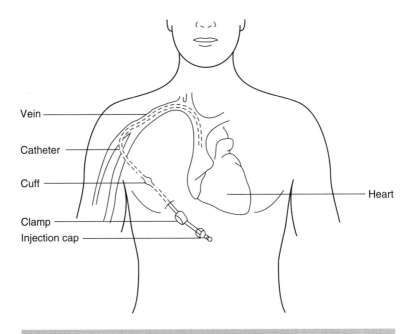

Figure 18-8 **Cuffed, tunneled catheter.** (*Source*: Adapted from The Royal Marsden NHS Foundation Trust. Central Venous Access Devices. London: Lundie Brothers Ltd., 2004.)

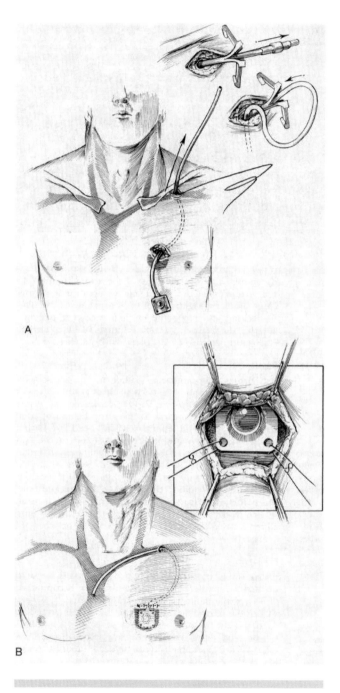

Figure 18-9 **Implantable port placement.**

ingrowth from the cuff. Other advantages of a cuffed, tunneled catheter include minimal interference with patient activity, low incidence of unintended dislodgment, and potential repair via a kit. Disadvantages include the need for regular maintenance and the fact that some patients find it cosmetically unacceptable.

Implantable ports (Port-A-Cath, Infuse-A-Port) are also tunneled, but they have a subcutaneous portal with a self-sealing septum that can be accessed by needle puncture through intact skin (Fig. 18-10). They require less manipulation and have lower complication rates than other CVCs. Ports are cosmetically superior to external tunneled catheters, require less maintenance, and afford patients greater freedom of movement. They are often used when prolonged venous access is necessary, for example, in intensive chemotherapy regimens. Disadvantages of implantable ports include the need for a specific small gauge access needle (Huber) and special training for users of the device. The Huber needle limits fluid infusion rates and increases the potential for subcutaneous extravasation.

Both cuffed CVCs and implantable ports can remain in place indefinitely until they are no longer needed, have thrombosed, become infected, or fail to function.

Peripherally inserted central catheters (PICC, Fig. 18-11) are noncuffed, nontunneled catheters and can last for months. They can be single or double lumen and can have a Groshong valve. PICC lines are generally placed in the basilic or cephalic veins proximal to the antecubital fossa. PICC line advantages include bedside placement/removal, ease of use, and simple maintenance.

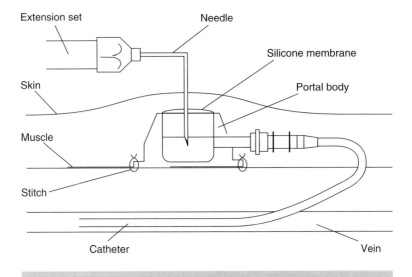

Figure 18-10 **Port schematic.** (*Source*: Adapted from The Royal Marsden NHS Foundation Trust. Central Venous Access Devices. London: Lundie Brothers Ltd., 2004.)

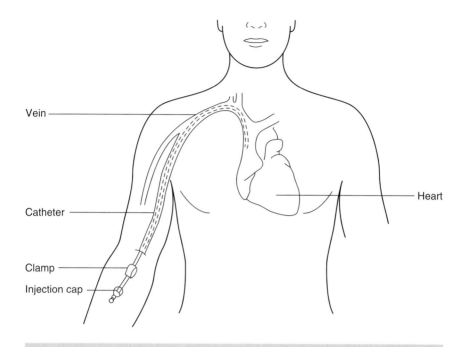

Vein

Catheter

Clamp

Injection cap

Heart

Figure 18-11 **Diagram of a PICC.** (*Source*: Adapted from The Royal Marsden NHS Foundation Trust. Central Venous Access Devices. London: Lundie Brothers Ltd., 2004.)

Short-term CVCs are frequently encountered in the operating room and ICU. These catheters are placed at the bedside and can be useful in emergencies. They are noncuffed and single (cordis introducer) or multilumen (dual or triple lumen catheters). The large diameter of cordis introducers allows large volume resuscitation and passage of smaller Swan-Ganz catheters and transvenous pacers. Multilumen CVCs are smaller in diameter and useful for multiple infusions and blood draws. Overall, short-term CVCs require constant vigilance and care to prevent infection and dislodgement.

RECOMMENDED READING

Deitch EA. *Tools of the Trade and Rules of the Road*. Philadelphia, PA: Lippincott-Raven, 1997:242–249.

Marino PL. *The ICU Book,* 2nd ed. Baltimore, MD: Lippincott Williams & Wilkins, 1997:53–93.

O'Grady NP, Alexander M, Dellinger EP, et al. Guidelines for the prevention of intravascular catheter-related infections. *MMWR Morb Mortal Wkly Rep* 51(RR10):1–26, 2002.

Roberts JR, Hedges JR. *Clinical Procedures in Emergency Medicine*, 4th ed. Philadelphia, PA: W.B. Saunders, 2004:462–466.

Townsend CM, Beauchamp RD, Evers BM, et al. *Sabiston Textbook of Surgery*, 17th ed. Philadelphia, PA: W.B. Saunders, 2004:2081–2084.

ARTERIAL PUNCTURE

Jacob N. Schroder, MD

Indications

In many situations, especially emergencies, arterial sampling is often the quickest and easiest method to obtain an adequate amount of blood for evaluation. In addition to obtaining routine laboratories, arterial blood gas (ABG) sampling aids the assessment of oxygenation, ventilation, and acid-base homeostasis. The radial artery is the most frequent site of arterial puncture and blood sampling. Its location is superficial and predictable, facilitating control of bleeding by direct compression. The radial artery has no significant paired nerve, unlike the brachial artery (with the adjacent median nerve), thus reducing the risk of neurovascular injury. Additionally, abundant collateral circulation exists at the wrist and in the digits, reducing the risk of iatrogenic ischemia. Alternative sites for arterial puncture include the brachial, femoral, and dorsalis pedis arteries. With the exception of the femoral artery in emergency code situations, these alternative sites are used less frequently and should be approached with caution.

Contraindications

The presence of cellulitis or other infection over the radial artery is a contraindication to arterial puncture. Any indication of decreased or abnormal circulation to the hand, including the absence of a palpable radial pulse, or a positive Allen's test (see Complications) is also a contraindication for the procedure. Deficiencies in clotting or coagulation, including less than 24 h postthrombolytic therapy (such as tissue plasminogen activator [TPA]), extreme thrombocytopenia, and elevated bleeding or coagulation times, are relative contraindications to arterial puncture. In these situations, the procedure can be completed, but the risks and benefits must be weighed. Extreme care must be taken when performing the procedure. The radial artery is the ideal site for puncture in these situations due to the ease of compression and ability to observe for complications.

Complications

Radial arterial puncture carries several risks including bleeding and hematoma formation, vascular thrombosis, distal embolization, vascular spasm, damage to adjacent structures, infection, distal ischemia, and infarction. In patients with normal coagulation, the risk of bleeding can be minimized by adequate manual compression and the application of a compression dressing. The risk of infection is extremely low and approaches zero when aseptic technique is used. Thrombosis and embolization are extremely rare in sites that have not been repeatedly punctured. These complications occur more frequently when arterial cannulation is performed. Frequently, the arterial pulsation transiently decreases or is lost following puncture due to vascular spasm.

To minimize the risk of ischemia and hand loss, it is necessary to check for adequate collateral circulation from the ulnar artery prior to radial puncture. More than 97 percent of patients have adequate flow through collaterals to prevent hand ischemia in the case that either the radial or ulnar flow is compromised. The *Allen's test* was first described by Dr Edgar Allen in 1929 and is used in a modified form to assess the adequacy of collateral blood flow at the wrist.[1] While the patient sits with the hand supinated and wrist slightly extended, the examiner uses both hands to gently locate the radial and ulnar pulses. The patient then squeezes the hand into a fist for 30 s. At the same time, the examiner compresses both the radial and ulnar arteries. The patient then extends the fingers while the examiner releases compression of the ulnar artery. The time it takes for color to return to the hand is then observed. A negative Allen's test (signifying normal collateral blood flow) occurs when the capillary refill is less than 6 s. The entire procedure is repeated, this time releasing, and therefore checking flow through the radial artery. Alternatively, a Doppler flow probe can be used to further enhance the detection of flow in the artery under question. If the patient has a positive Allen's test, signifying poor collateral flow, arterial puncture should be avoided on that side.

Anesthetic Use

Arterial puncture can be painful, and the use of local anesthetics to decrease this pain has been debated. Traditionally, physicians have avoided the use of local anesthetics because it was thought that the procedure itself was no more painful than injection. A few small studies have been completed to investigate the effectiveness of local anesthetics.[2,3] In one of these, 270 patients undergoing elective ABG sampling were injected with local anesthetic, saline placebo or nothing. When compared with both placebo and nothing, patients who received subcutaneous injection of 1 percent mepivicaine experienced significantly less pain (1.5 versus 3.06 and 2.8 on a pain scale, respectively, $P < 0.002$). Although this study did not include patients in emergency or critical care settings, it does indicate that infiltration of a local anesthetic may be successful in reducing the pain of arterial puncture.

Procedure

Arterial puncture, like any medical procedure, should be fully explained to the patient prior to initiation. Most hospitals have premade ABG syringe kits. If this is not available, then a 22 × 1 in. needle and a 3-cc heparinized syringe must be collected. Additionally, Betadine and alcohol prep pads, sterile gauze, and sterile gloves and tape will be needed. If local anesthetic is to be used, a 1 cc syringe with a 27-gauge needle and 0.5–1 cc of 1 percent lidocaine (all sterile) will be needed.

Assess the patient's radial pulses and perform the Allen's test on the hand with the most prominent pulse to ensure adequate collateral circulation. If the pulse is faint, extension or rotation of the wrist may help in augmenting the pulsation. Avoid puncture if there is any evidence of bruising, cellulitis, or skin lesions. Palpate the chosen radial artery at the point of maximal pulsation. Stabilize the patient's wrist in the position that presents the maximal pulse. This can be accomplished with the use of tape and an arm board or an assistant. The area should be cleaned with the Betadine prep pad, followed by an alcohol prep pad. Change to sterile gloves, repalpate the point of maximal pulsation, and create a subcutaneous wheal by infiltrating with 0.5–1 cc of lidocaine. Open the sampling kit and attach the needle to syringe. Slightly depress the plunger on the syringe (to disperses the dry heparin). Repalpate the point of maximal pulsation, and remove needle cap (palpation may be slightly more difficult after injection of the local anesthetic). At a 45° angle pierce the skin at the puncture site and slowly advance the needle in one plane. When the artery is punctured, blood will enter the syringe. Do not actively aspirate blood. If the needle is in the lumen of the artery, blood should flow smoothly. If the needle pierces through the back wall of the artery, slowly withdraw the needle until blood reappears in the syringe. If no blood appears in the syringe, withdraw the needle until the tip is just below the surface of the skin and redirect advancement in a slow smooth plane toward point of maximal pulse. Never change the direction or plane of the needle while it is fully inserted under the skin; this could result in the laceration of the artery and uncontrolled hemorrhage.

After blood has filled the syringe, withdraw the needle and immediately apply pressure directly on the site with sterile gauze and one or two fingers. Apply direct manual pressure for at least 5 min (and as long as is needed to stop bleeding) to reduce the risk of hematoma. After bleeding has stopped, apply a pressure bandage over the puncture site and assess the pulse distal to the puncture. After obtaining the ABG sample, slowly advance plunger to expel air bubbles that may be present (these may alter the values obtained) and cover it with the cap provided. The syringe should be labeled with the appropriate patient information and transported to the laboratory as directed.

REFERENCES

1. Allen EV. Thromboangiitis obliterans: methods of diagnosis of chronic occlusive arterial disease distal to the wrist with illustrative cases. *Am J Med Sci* 178:237–244, 1929.

2. Giner J, Casan P, Belda J, et al. Pain during arterial puncture. *Chest* 110:1443–1445, 1996.

3. Lightowler JV, Elliott MW. Local anaesthetic infiltration prior to arterial puncture for blood gas analysis: a survey of current practice and a randomised double blind placebo controlled trial. *J R Coll Physicians Lond* 31:645–646, 1997.

URETHRAL CATHETERIZATION

Tamarah J. Westmoreland, MD

Urethral catheterization is a useful procedure for the surgical patient. One of the more important indications for this procedure is to accurately measure urine output. Urine output is a critical parameter for the patient's hemodynamic status. Another indication is the relief of urinary retention, which could be due to medications, neurologic injury, or loss of bladder tone. Temporary treatment of urinary incontinence, collecting urine for bacterial culture, and treatment of perineal wounds are also reasons to use urethral catheterization. Urethral catheterization may also be necessary for the treatment of urinary obstruction, which may lead to hydronephrosis. Lastly, the chronically bedridden patient may require a urinary catheter for hygiene.

The judicious use of the urinary catheter is important to prevent injury to the patient.[1] Trauma to the perineal or pelvic regions can be a contraindication to the use of a urinary catheter. During the physical examination of the trauma patient, it is imperative to complete a rectal examination and closely examine the urethral meatus. If the patient has a high riding prostate or blood at the urethral meatus, a urinary catheter should not be inserted. The patient could have a posterior urethral disruption due to a pelvic fracture or an anterior urethral injury caused by straddle trauma.

To place a urinary catheter, it is imperative that you confirm that your equipment is functional. After placing the male patient in a supine position, his legs should be spread slightly. Using the nondominant hand, the penis should be grasped near the urethral meatus with mild tension. The nondominant hand is no longer sterile. Using the dominant hand, the glans, meatus, and foreskin, if present, should be prepped sterilely. The urinary catheter, which is commonly a no. 16–20 French Foley catheter, is well lubricated with K-Y jelly. The catheter should be inserted into the penis while maintaining mild tension on the penis. Insert the catheter until the sidearm for the balloon is reached. Flow of urine through the catheter confirms its placement in the bladder. If no urine is obtained after placing the catheter, suprapubic pressure should be applied and irrigation of 30 cc of fluid may be used. If the irrigation freely returns, it is highly likely that the catheter has formed a false tract in the penis and does not dwell within the urethra. If this is the case, the catheter should be removed, and a urologist should be consulted. Also, if the patient is very hemodynamically depleted, he may need hydration to produce urine. Once placement of the urinary catheter is confirmed, the balloon should be inflated with 5 cc of sterile water. If a disproportionate amount of resistance is noted when inflating the balloon, then the catheter should be removed and reinserted. Once the balloon is inflated, the catheter should be withdrawn carefully to settle the balloon at the bladder neck. The catheter should be connected to a closed drainage system. The catheter should be taped to the patient's leg to prevent dislodgement.

Female urethral catheterization uses the same sterile technique as in a male. The female patient should lie in a supine position with her legs abducted in a frog-leg position. After sterilely draping the patient, the nondominant hand should spread the labia. This hand is contaminated and should be used to maintain the labia out of the sterile field. The introitus should be prepped anterior to posterior. The lubricated catheter should be inserted to approximately 10–15 cm. Once again, return of urine confirms bladder placement. If no urine is returned, proceed with the same techniques as in the male patient. After confirming bladder placement, the balloon should be inflated with 5 cc of sterile water. The catheter should be carefully withdrawn to place the balloon at the bladder neck. The catheter should then be connected to the closed drainage system and taped to the patient's leg to prevent accidental removal.

There are many reasons urethral catheter placement may be difficult. In the awake patient, a common reason is anxiety of the patient. A urethral stricture may also be present. In the male patient, a stricture at the meatus or prostatic hypertrophy may be preventing catheterization. It is important to ensure that the catheter is well lubricated. If there is pain, a 2 percent Xylocaine jelly can be used. If the patient has continued anxiety, an anxiolytic can be used. A meatus stricture can be relieved with the use of a hemostat. A very helpful adjunct is the Coudé urinary catheter, which has a bend at the tip of the catheter. When using this catheter, it is important that the tip is pointed anteriorly. If the Coudé catheter cannot be easily passed, a urologist should be consulted. The urologist may place a catheter with cystoscopic guidance, or a suprapubic catheter may have to be used.

Careful, aseptic technique in placement of urinary catheters is critical in prevention of complications. The most common complication is the development of a urinary tract infection. This may be due to the practitioner's technique or a preexisting infection in the patient. Infection can also be caused by balloon inflation in the prostatic urethra. Quick recognition of the urinary tract infection can help prevent sepsis. Another complication is the creation of a false passage leading to urethral disruption. This can be prevented by careful technique in maintaining slight tension on the penis and by not forcing the catheter during insertion. If the vagina is inadvertently catheterized, the catheter should be removed, and a fresh, sterile catheter should be used to catheterize the urethra. If there is urine leakage around the catheter, a larger catheter may need to be placed. In addition, the balloon volume should be monitored to ensure that it has not become deflated. Hemorrhage and stricture formation are also complications that may be encountered.

Urethral catheterization is an important adjunct for the surgical patient. Proper handling of the urinary catheters and good aseptic technique can minimize the complications and maximize the benefit of this procedure.

RECOMMENDED READING

1. Bruns Jr, John J, Roussseau MB. *The Mont Reid Surgical Handbook*, 4th ed. St. Louis, MO: Mosby Year Book, 1997: 711–718.

SURGICAL AIRWAY MANAGEMENT: TRACHEOSTOMY & CRICOTHYROIDOTOMY

Rebecca P. Petersen, MD, MSc

The two procedures performed to establish a surgical airway are tracheostomy and cricothyroidotomy. *Tracheostomy* is a common elective procedure to create a surgical airway for temporary or indefinite use in patients with a secure airway. In contrast, *cricothyroidotomy* is performed emergently at the bedside when attempts to establish an airway with endotracheal intubation fail or are not possible.

Tracheostomy

INDICATIONS AND CONTRAINDICATIONS

Despite its long history and frequent use, the indications and timing for tracheostomy remain controversial. Common indications for tracheostomy include respiratory insufficiency requiring prolonged mechanical support, uncontrolled tracheobronchial secretions, relief of upper airway obstruction, and for patients undergoing a laryngectomy.[1] Requirement for prolonged mechanical support due to respiratory failure is the least clearly defined indication for tracheostomy. Although it is generally agreed that conversion of an endotracheal tube to a tracheostomy is indicated at some point during a prolonged stay in the ICU, the exact timing remains controversial. The decision to convert to a tracheostomy must be individualized and the risk-benefit ratio must be taken into account. Generally, if a patient remains intubated for 1 week and it is clear that he or she will not be extubated at anytime in the near future, a tracheostomy should be performed, assuming an acceptable surgical risk. Beyond this time period, the risk of severe laryngeal injury, need for effective pulmonary toilet, improved patient comfort, and finally, the need for a stable airway begin to shift the risk-benefit ratio toward a tracheostomy.[2-4]

ANATOMY

The trachea is a 12-cm fibrocartilaginous tube, which extends from the larynx to the roots of the lungs. There are 18–22 cartilaginous rings. The isthmus of the thyroid gland lies over the second and third tracheal rings. The inferior thyroid veins form a plexus anterior to the trachea and inferior to the isthmus. A small thyroid ima artery is present in about 10 percent of patients and ascends to the inferior border of the isthmus. The brachiocephalic trunk lies to the right of the trachea at the root of the neck. In infants and children the thymus lies anterior to the inferior part of the trachea.

PROCEDURE

A tracheostomy is performed by making a 3-cm transverse incision over the second or third tracheal ring. To identify this region the surgeon palpates the cricoid cartilage and makes an incision 1.5 cm inferior to it. The platysma is then divided and the strap muscles are separated vertically in the midline. The thyroid isthmus is then retracted superiorly. It is important to keep in mind the following important anatomic structures to avoid possible injury: the inferior thyroid veins, thyroid ima artery, left brachiocephalic vein, jugular venous arch, pleurae, and the thymus gland specifically in infants and children. After the second tracheal ring is identified, securing sutures are placed on either side of the midline between the first and second cartilages and used to retract the trachea upward. A scalpel blade is then used to make a vertical, midline incision through the second and third tracheal rings. A tracheal dilator is subsequently used to spread the divided tracheal cartilages while a lubricated tracheostomy tube is inserted through the newly created stoma. The tracheostomy tube is advanced as the endotracheal tube is carefully withdrawn. The tracheostomy tube is then confirmed to be in adequate position and subsequently sutured to the skin and tied into place with trachea around the patient's neck (Fig. 18-12).

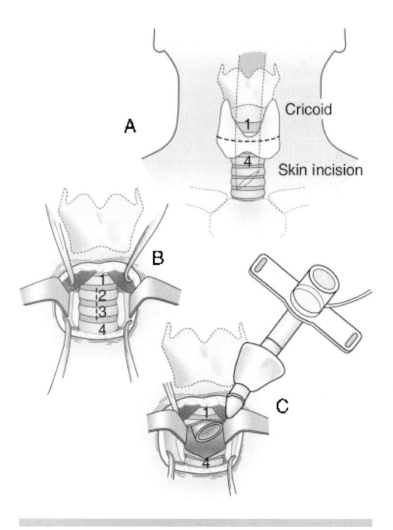

Figure 18-12 **Technique of Tracheostomy.** (*Source:* Adapted from Townsend CM, Beauchamp RD, Evers BM, et al. *Sabiston Textbook of Surgery*, 17th ed. The Netherlands: Elsevier, 2004.)

COMPLICATIONS

The complication rate following a tracheostomy is approximately 5–6 percent.[2] Acute complications of tracheostomy primarily include bleeding and infection.

Tracheoinnominate artery fistula is a rare long-term complication that occurs when a tracheostomy tube erodes into the innominate artery, resulting in life-threatening hemorrhage. An impending tracheoinnominate artery erosion may be heralded by the finding of bright-red blood during tracheal tube suctioning. The diagnosis may be confirmed with increased hemorrhage on temporary deflation of the tracheal cuff. Acutely, hemorrhage is controlled by either overinflating the tracheal cuff or by inserting a finger through the tracheostomy stoma and applying digital compression against the sternum while the patient is transferred to the operating room for repair.

Cricothyroidotomy

INDICATIONS AND CONTRAINDICATIONS

Cricothyroidotomy remains the quickest, safest, and easiest way to obtain an airway on an emergency basis when attempts at orotracheal and nasotracheal intubation have failed. It is contraindicated if any other less radical means of securing an airway is feasible. The advantages of cricothyroidotomy to secure an airway emergently are ease, safety, rapidity, and avoidance of injuring the thyroid isthmus or blood vessels that are encountered when performing a tracheostomy where the tracheal incision is made more inferiorly. Although these lifesaving benefits are specific to cricothyroidotomy in contrast to tracheostomy for establishing a surgical airway emergently, the risk of vocal cord injury and subglottic tracheal stenosis is significantly higher.

ANATOMY

The cricothyroid membrane is positioned between the thyroid cartilage superiorly and the cricoid cartilage inferiorly. It is a dense fibroelastic trapezoidal membrane bordered laterally by the cricothyroid muscles and medially by the median cricothyroid ligament. It varies in size depending on age. For adults it ranges between 22–33 mm wide and 9–10 mm high. Therefore, the endotracheal tube should not exceed 8 mm.[5] There are no major arteries, veins, or nerves in the region of the cricothyroid membrane. The cricothyroid artery arises from the superior laryngeal artery. Both the left and right cricothyroid arteries transverse the superior aspect of the membrane and usually do not pose a problem when performing a cricothyroidotomy. The vocal cords are situated 1 cm superior to the cricothyroid membrane. They are attached to the internal surface of the thyroid cartilage. The cricoid cartilage is inferior to the thyroid cartilage and is situated at level C6. It is the only complete cartilaginous ring in the larynx and trachea and serves as a stent to maintain airway patency following a cricothyroidotomy.

PROCEDURE

A cricothyroidotomy is performed with the surgeon standing to the patient's right side. The thyroid cartilage is stabilized between the thumb and middle finger of the left hand while the cricothyroid membrane is identified by palpation using the left index finger. A 2-cm vertical incision is made over the cricothyroid space. Blunt dissection is then performed using a hemostat to identify the cricothyroid membrane. Once the cricothyroid membrane is identified, a 1.5-cm transverse incision is made in the lower half of the membrane which is subsequently enlarged with a tracheal dilator. An 8-mm or less cuffed tracheostomy tube is then inserted into the trachea and adequate position is confirmed. The endotracheal tube is secured into place and suctioned. A definitive airway will be required as soon as the patient is stable. A needle cricothyroidotomy is preferred for children under the age of 12 and involves placing a 12-gauge cannula into the trachea through the cricothyroid membrane. This will allow for adequate positive-pressure ventilation for up to approximately 45 min until an expert airway can be established.

COMPLICATIONS

Complications of cricothyroidotomy can be as high as 40 percent when performed emergently.[6] However, these complications are minor compared to the devastating complication of death resulting from the inability to establish a secure airway in the acute setting. Complications include bleeding, dysphonia, and hoarseness due to injury of the vocal cords, subglottic tracheal stenosis, laryngeal damage, and thyroid cartilage fracture.

REFERENCES

1. Heffner JE, Miller S, Sahn SA. Tracheostomy in the intensive care unit. Part 1. Indications, technique, management. *Chest* 90(2):269–274, 1986.

2. Walts PA, Murthy SC, DeCamp MM. Techniques of surgical tracheostomy. *Clin Chest Med* 24:413–422, 2003.

3. Orringer MB. Endotracheal intubation and tracheostomy: indications, techniques, and complications. *Surg Clin North Am* 60(6):1447–1467, 1980.

4. Sugerman HJ, Wolfe L, Pasquale MD, et al. Multicenter, randomized, prospective trial of early tracheostomy. *J Trauma* 43:741–747, 1997.

5. Kress TD, Balasubramaniam S. Cricothyroidotomy. *Ann Emerg Med* 11:197–201, 1982.

6. McGill J, Clinton JE, Ruiz E. Cricothyroidotomy in the emergency department. *Ann Emerg Med* 11:361–364, 1982.

TUBE THORACOSTOMY

Anthony Lemaire, MD

Traumatic injury to the chest is common and the severity may range from an isolated single rib fracture to flail chest.[1] Percutaneous tube thoracostomy (PTT) is the most widely performed procedure to manage both blunt and penetrating chest trauma.[2] Although generally considered a simple procedure, placement of a chest tube is associated with numerous complications.[3] Moreover, tube thoracostomy by physicians not well experienced has been shown to lead to increased morbidity.[2] Adverse outcomes associated with PTT include thoracic empyema, undrained hemothorax or pneumothorax, improper tube positioning, posttube removal complications, and direct injuries to the lung.[4] In order to minimize risk a solid knowledge of thorax anatomy is required.

The pleural space is a potential cavity between the *visceral pleura* that envelops the lung and the *parietal pleura* that lines the chest wall. The visceral and parietal pleurae are smooth, serous membranes, continuous with each other at the lung hila and pulmonary ligaments. Under normal conditions, the parietal and visceral pleural membranes are separated by a thin layer of fluid, which functions as a lubricant and transmits the forces of breathing between lung and chest wall. Accumulations of either blood (*hemothorax*) or air (*pneumothorax*) within the pleural space are abnormalities that often require intervention by tube thoracostomy. Additional indications include clinically significant pleural effusions as well as prophylactic chest drainage in patients with severe blunt chest trauma or after elective thoracic surgery.[5]

Chest Tube Insertion Protocol

The proper application of chest tubes begins with establishing a sterile environment similar to that seen in the operating room theater. Masks, sterile gowns, and gloves must be worn at all times throughout the insertion procedure. Local anesthesia should be administered to the patient usually with 1 percent lidocaine (up to 4 mg/kg). Injection of anesthetics should be above, at, and below the planned insertion site. The pleura should be anesthetized as well. In addition, intravenous analgesia should be administered prior to tube insertion. The preferred site of insertion is at the third to fifth intercostals space, midaxillary line. The size of the chest tube varies depending on the indication for placement. In trauma, a no. 36 French (Fr) chest tube is often used to allow for proper pleural drainage and prevention from clot impediment. Prior to insertion, digital exploration should be performed to avoid lung penetration. The tube should then be directed toward the apex and posteriorly so that the last hole is 2–4 cm into the pleural cavity. The tube should then be connected to an underwater draining system and secured using 0-silk (Fig. 18-13). Petroleum gauze should then be placed around the tube at the insertion site and the tube secured with silk/adhesive tape.[5] An essential requirement after chest tube insertion is the postprocedure chest radiograph to assure correct placement.

Although standard protocols have been well established for tube thoracostomy, complications related to insertion, removal, and failures continue to occur and are reported to range from 9 to 36 percent.[6,7] The primary complications include improper placement, iatrogenic injuries to the lung, persistent air leak, and residual pneumothorax or hemothorax. The problems related to chest tube placement may require further intervention and extended hospitalization for the patient. Strategies used to limit complications should include supervised chest tube placement by senior physicians, and an establishment and observance of strict guidelines for placement.

Finally, the development of a skillful approach to chest tube placement will allow for appropriate intervention in an expeditious manner. A failure of a defined technique makes the patient susceptible to further morbidity and possible mortality.

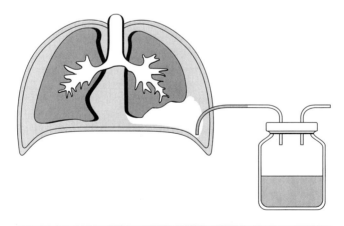

Figure 18-13 **Chest tube insertion. The tube should be directed toward the apex and posteriorly so that the last hole is 2–4 cm into the pleural cavity. The tube should then be connected to an underwater draining system and secured using 0-silk.**

REFERENCES

1. Pate JW. Chest wall injuries. *Surg Clin North Am* 69:59–70, 1989.

2. Deneuville M. Morbidity of percutaneous tube thoracostomy in trauma patients. *Eur J Cardiothorac Surg* 22:673–678, 2002.

3. Millikan JS, Moore EE, Steiner E, et al. Complications of tube thoracostomy for acute trauma. *Am J Surg* 140:738–741, 1980.

4. Etoch SW, Bar-Natan MF, Miller FB, et al. Tube thoracostomy: factors related to complications. *Arch Surg* 130:521–525, 1995; discussion 525–526.

5. Adrales G, Huynh T, Broering B, et al. Rapid atrial fibrillation following tube thoracostomy insertion. *J Trauma* 52:210–214, 2002; discussion 214–216.

6. Daly RC, Mucha P, Pairolero PC, et al. The risk of percutaneous chest tube thoracostomy for blunt thoracic trauma. *Ann Emerg Med* 14:865–870, 1985.

7. Helling TS, Gyles NR 3rd, Eisenstein CL, et al. The role of thoracoscopy in the management of retained thoracic collections after trauma. *J Trauma* 29:1367–1370, 1989.

INCISION & DRAINAGE OF CUTANEOUS ABSCESS

Jin S. Yoo, MD

Introduction

An *abscess* is defined as a local infection surrounded by inflamed tissue. The key fundamental principle of adequately treating an abscess is that a drainage procedure is essential and antibiotic therapy alone is insufficient. However, abscess smaller than 5 mm in diameter may resolve with warm soaks and compresses, which facilitates drainage of the pus material. A drainage procedure is important since the inflamed tissue around the abscess prevents the penetration of antibiotics into the site of active infection.

Incision and drainage (I&D) procedure is a common surgical technique employed by many nonsurgical physicians to primarily manage and treat cutaneous abscesses. Abscesses in other locations such as the lungs and abdomen are also managed by drainage procedures, but those topics are beyond of the scope of this chapter. The procedure described in this section is applicable to cutaneous abscesses in almost any location on the body except for extremely large abscesses, deep abscesses in very sensitive areas, abscesses involving palmar or plantar spaces, and facial abscesses involving the triangle formed by the bridge of the nose and the corners of the mouth.

Materials Needed

- No. 11 scalpel blade
- Curved hemostat
- Sterile field towels
- A container of packing material ($1/2$ in. wide)
- Sterile 4×4 gauze pads
- A bottle of povidone-iodine
- A 20–30 cc syringe
- 16-gauge needle
- 25-gauge needle
- A bottle of 1 percent lidocaine (with or without epinephrine)

Description of Procedure

First and foremost, achieving adequate local anesthesia is the most important factor which will maximize your chance of performing an adequate I&D procedure. In addition, one should always consider the use of anxiolytics in an anxious patient since anxiety can certainly exacerbate the pain.

Prepare all the instruments and materials for use prior to beginning the procedure. First, put on a sterile gown and a pair of sterile gloves. Then, set up a sterile work area on a table with all the instruments and materials laid out. Next, draw up 20–30 mL of 1 percent lidocaine in a syringe using the 16-gauge needle. Then, change the syringe to 25-gauge prior to use.

The area is prepped and draped in a sterile fashion using sterile 4×4 gauze soaked in povidone-iodine and the sterile field towels. Then, a field block is performed by injecting 1 percent lidocaine into the dome of the abscess and the syringe is held parallel to the skin and rotated to distribute the anesthetic circumferentially. The local anesthesia should be injected in the subcutaneous space above the abscess cavity and not into the cavity itself. After adequate anesthesia is obtained, a stab incision is made with the no. 11 scalpel blade and a linear incision conforming to the natural folds of the skin. Some would advocate in making the incision size the total length of the abscess; however, minimizing the incision size will decrease the time for the wound to heal secondarily and more cosmetically appealing. The incision should just be large enough to place the tip of the hemostat into the abscess to break loculations and ensure proper drainage. After all the pus is evacuated, pack the wound cavity with wet packing material to promote wound healing by performing *wet-to-dry* packing changes at least twice a day.

The patient should be instructed to follow-up in 1 week for a wound check and to continue twice-a-day wet-to-dry dressing changes with normal saline solution. The rationale for this is to frequently debride the necrotic granulation tissue in the open wound and facilitate healing by keeping the healthy granulation tissues exposed. When the *wet* packing adheres to the surface of the wound, it adheres to the underlying tissue as it dries out. Of note, a saline solution should be used to facilitate the drying process and the packing should be *just barely wet* and not *soaking wet*. If it is too wet, the wound will be too moist for the packing to adhere to necrotic tissue overlying the healthy, granulation tissue.

Wound Culture

Gram's stain and cultures of the wound are generally not performed since drainage of the pus collection will lead to resolution even without antibiotics. However, wound culture may be indicated in patients who are septic or are immunocompromised. If a wound culture and Gram's stain are needed, the sample should be collected by needle aspiration over a prepped skin area.[1,2] This allows the wound culture to be sent for anaerobic cultures as well.

Antibiotics

The use of antibiotics may have a role prior to skin incision, but it is not necessary afterward, except in patients with cellulitis and/or lymphangitis surrounding the abscess and in immunocompromised patients. These patients require at least 7 days of antibiotic treatment and possibly longer depending on their clinical response (Table 18-2).[3,4]

Special Section on Drugs

ANXIOLYTIC OF CHOICE

A common anxiolytic that is used is lorazepam (Ativan), a benzodiazepine with rapid onset and moderate duration; 0.5–2 mg IV is the recommended dose, but start with 0.5 mg at first and then give additional 0.5 mg doses every 5–10 min until the total dose is reached. Midazolam (Versed), which is commonly used for procedures such as colonoscopy, is not ideal because it is too short acting and requires frequent dosing.

LOCAL ANESTHETIC

The maximum dose of 1 percent lidocaine that one can use is 500 mg (based on 70 kg bodyweight) and 300 mg with and without epinephrine, respectively (based on 70 kg bodyweight). The duration of anesthesia is 120–360 and 30–60 min with and without epinephrine, respectively.[5] Lidocaine is available in 1 percent (5 mg/mL) or 2 percent (10 mg/mL) concentrations. Thus, you may use up to 60 mL of the 1 percent lidocaine during the procedure, but watch out for early signs of toxicity—tinnitus, dizziness, and confusion.

Table 18-2 **Antibiotic of Choice in Special Circumstances after I&D has been Performed**

	Inpatient Rx	Outpatient Rx	Most Common Organisms
Cellulitis/lymphangitis	Nafcillin or cefazolin or vancomycin + clindamycin (for serious *Streptococcus* infections)	Dicloxacillin, cefuroxime, erythromycin, clarithromycin, azithromycin	*Staphylococcus aureus Streptococcus pyogenes*
Immunocompromised	Trimethoprim/ sulfamethoxazole or piperacillin/ tazobactam ± Cipro		Above organisms + *Pseudomonas aeruginosa*

REFERENCES

1. Halvorson GD, Halvorson JE, Iserson KV. Abscess incision and drainage in the emergency department. Part I. *J Emerg Med* 3(3):227–232, 1985.

2. Meislin HW, McGehee MD, Rosen P. Management and microbiology of cutaneous abscesses. *JACEP* 7(5):186–191, 1978.

3. Llera JL, Levy RC. Treatment of cutaneous abscesses: a double-blind clinical study. *Ann Emerg Med* 14(1):15–19, 1985.

4. Cohen J, Powderly WG. et al. Cellulitis, pyoderma, abscesses and other skin and subcutaneous tissue infections. *Infect Dis* 136–141, 2004.

5. Miller RD. Local anesthetics. *Anesthesia* 575–586, 2005.

INDEX

NOTE: Page numbers followed by *f* or *t* indicate figures or tables, respectively.